EDITION 3

MEDICAL–SURGICAL NURSING CARE PLANS

nursing diagnoses & interventions

Marie S. Jaffe
Retired Nursing Faculty
University of Texas at El Paso
College of Nursing and Allied Health
El Paso, Texas

Appleton & Lange
Stamford, Connecticut

Copyright © 1996 by Appleton & Lange
A Simon & Schuster Company
Copyright © 1992 by Appleton & Lange; Copyright © 1986 by Appleton-Century-Crofts

96 97 98 99 00 / 10 9 8 7 6 5 4 3 2

Prentice Hall International (UK) Limited, *London*
Prentice Hall of Australia Pty. Limited, *Sydney*
Prentice Hall Canada, Inc., *Toronto*
Prentice Hall Hispanoamericana, S.A., *Mexico*
Prentice Hall of India Private Limited, *New Delhi*
Prentice Hall of Japan, Inc., *Tokyo*
Simon and Schuster Asia Pte. Ltd., *Singapore*
Editora Prentice Hall do Brasil Ltda., *Rio de Janeiro*
Prentice Hall, Englewood Cliffs, *New Jersey*

Library of Congress Cataloging-in-Publication Data
Jaffe, Marie S.
    Medical-surgical nursing care plans : nursing diagnoses and
interventions / Marie S. Jaffe. — 3rd ed.
        p.   cm.
    Includes bibliographical references and index.
    ISBN 0-8385-6263-9 (spiral pbk. : alk. paper)
    1. Nursing care plans—Handbooks, manuals, etc.   2. Surgical
nursing—Handbooks, manuals, etc.   I. Title.
    [DNLM: 1. Nursing—handbooks.   2. Patient Care Planning—
handbooks.   3. Surgical Nursing—handbooks.   WY 49 J23m 1996]
RT49.J34   1996
610.73—dc20
DNLM/DLC   95-4744
for Library of Congress   CIP

Acquisitions Editor: Sally J. Barhydt
Production Service: Tage Publishing Service
Production Coordinator: Elizabeth C. Ryan
Designer: Mary Skudlarek

ISBN: 0-8385-6263-9

90000

Printed in the United States of America

9 780838 562635

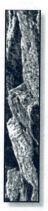

Contents

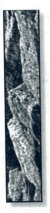

Preface

This book, as with the prior editions, was designed as a resource for nurses responsible for planning and managing the care of hospitalized adult and older adult patients. The scope is limited to care plans for common medical conditions and surgical procedures, including physical and psychological components relevant to nursing and related to both independent and dependent functions. In instances where a medical condition often leads to surgery, care for both are included. Nursing students as well as new and experienced staff nurses will benefit from the content. It is hoped that the use of this book will result in more knowledgeable, efficient, and effective practices in the application of the nursing process to the care of patients. In addition, the care plans are designed to provide the flexibility needed to individualize this care.

This third edition includes ten completely new care plans. New and existing conditions have now been combined with a number of related medical conditions and surgical procedures, bringing the total to 128 plans. The care plans are presented in twelve sections by systems (respiratory, neurologic, endocrine, etc.). The exception is the first section containing comprehensive plans applicable to conditions covered throughout the book.

Each care plan has been revised to include additional nursing problem areas and expanded to include the teaching necessary to prepare for home care as patients are now discharged earlier with ongoing and more complex care needs. Also new to this edition are system data base guides preceding each section of care plans, which provide relevant information about the specific system that can be used in care planning. These data base guides include general statements regarding past and present events, physical assessment data review, system related nursing diagnoses, diagnostic laboratory tests and procedures, medications, and geriatric considerations to serve as a guide for more specific data collection related to each area.* Data associated with a medical diagnosis or planned surgical procedure can then be selected for the identification of nursing problems and outcomes and the formulation of nursing interventions.

I wish again to express my thanks and gratitude to Appleton & Lange and staff, and Sally J. Barhydt in particular, who provided me with the opportunity to once again revise this book and present a third edition of *Medical-Surgical Nursing Care Plans: Nursing Diagnoses and Interventions.* I believe the improvements and additions will enhance the well-balanced and comprehensive content of the previous editions that have included the in-depth, problem-solving skills necessary for acute care planning.

Marie S. Jaffe

---

*Geriatric considerations included in each system data base were adapted with permission from *Geriatric Nursing Care Plans,* Skidmore-Roth Publishing, Inc., El Paso, Texas, 1991.

How to Use the Third Edition

The format for each care plan remains the same with six categories of information as follows:

TITLE
Identifies the medical condition, surgical procedure, or both by the accepted nomenclature.

DEFINITION
Briefly defines the condition and/or procedure with etiology, risk factors, effects when applicable, other pertinent information, as well as cross-references with other care plans.

NURSING DIAGNOSES
Identifies each problem area related to the title using diagnoses listed and approved by the North American Nursing Diagnosis Association (NANDA) taxonomy as of 1995. These can include related or risk factors as well as reasons for and/or results of these factors, list more than one nursing diagnosis in a given set of interventions and rationales if interrelationships exist, and provide inclusive coverage of potential problem identification in lieu of repeating similar or identical nursing interventions.

EXPECTED OUTCOMES
Provides evaluation criteria and expected evidence of outcome or goal fulfillment related to diagnoses that can be specific and/or broadly stated depending on possible repetition within the intervention section.

INTERVENTIONS
Nursing actions, both independent and dependent, divided into categories as follows:

I. Assess for:
Includes data base related to nursing diagnoses; can include nursing diagnoses defining characteristics as well as information from history, physical examination, data base guides

II. Monitor, describe, record:
Includes any ongoing collection of data or observations, usually of an objective nature

III. Administer:
Includes all medications and routes, oxygen, with the assumption that these are physician ordered, as in any dependent nursing intervention

IV. Perform/Provide:
Lists all nursing treatments and medical regimens carried out to resolve the problems identified by the related nursing diagnoses

V. Teach patient/family:
Includes all teaching aspects for hospitalizations as well as those preparing patient for discharge and home care

The designated Roman numeral for each category is used consistently in the interventions. Numerals are omitted if there is no pertinent information regarding interventions that fits a particular category.

RATIONALE
Statements of a principle or of a physiological or pathophysiological reason as to why the intervention being considered is carried out; placement is in line with and to the right of the related intervention.

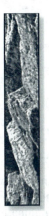

General Standards

outpatient perioperative care

DEFINITION

The physical and psychological care given prior to, during, and following a scheduled surgical procedure performed in an outpatient surgical center, hospital operating room, or physician office. With some modifications, this plan can also be used for clients scheduled for invasive diagnostic procedures both in and out of the hospital setting.

NURSING DIAGNOSIS

Anxiety related to situational crisis (impending surgery), threat to change in health status (pain, risk for complications, evidence of life-threatening condition revealed by surgery), physiological factors (presence of a chronic disease or physical impairment) resulting in inability to comply with preoperative instruction and preparation or postponement of the procedure if anxiety level is at severe or near-panic state

EXPECTED OUTCOMES

Anxiety within manageable limits (mild to moderate) evidenced by verbalizations that anxiety decreased following explanations about the procedure and what to expect, the use of relaxation techniques, statements that tension, apprehension, and fear are reduced, VS within an expected slight increase in P and BP compared to baselines

INTERVENTION	RATIONALE
I. Assess for: A. Level of anxiety, verbal expressions of fear, apprehension, uncertainty prior to surgery, and possible reasons for feelings of anxiety	A. Anxiety ranges from mild to panic levels; a moderate level is desirable as a means to mobilize internal resources helpful in coping with impending surgery

INTERVENTION	RATIONALE
B. Nonverbal expressions of anxiety prior to surgery such as shakiness, irritability, tense body and facial muscles, increased perspirations, dilated pupils, increased P and BP of >10 beats or 20 to 30 mm Hg respectively	B. May not feel comfortable or be able to communicate feelings but reveal physical/physiological responses that assist in identifying the level of and changes in anxiety
C. Perceptions of anticipated surgery as to outcome, effect on life-style, coping skills, and decision-making ability to deal effectively with perceptions	C. Identifies and clarifies ability to cope with crisis event
D. Support systems available, such as family member or friend to accompany to facility and remain with client prior to the surgery and in the home following the procedure	D. Important aspect of caring and promotes sense of well-being, assists in reducing fear and anxiety
E. Response to factual information regarding procedure and possible diagnosis and/or prognosis	E. These can increase or decrease anxiety, uneasiness about the surgery

II. Monitor, describe, record:

A. Respiratory rate, P, BP for increases as part of the preoperative assessment and return to baseline values postoperatively	A. Vital signs changes indicate the presence and degree of anxiety preoperatively and postoperative status for complications

INTERVENTION	RATIONALE
III. Administer:	
A. Prescribed sedative or anti-anxiety medications	A. Promotes sleep the night prior to or reduces anxiety the day of the procedure
IV. Perform/provide:	
A. Calm attitude of acceptance and positive response to behavior without expressing anger or impatience	A. Provides emotional support and reassurance
B. Environment that promotes trust and prevents anxiety-provoking situations	B. Decreases anxiety by avoiding additional stimuli
C. Encourage expression of feelings, fears, and concerns; listen and provide feedback to clarify behavior	C. Assists in externalizing, identifying, and acknowledging anxiety and fear
D. Allow for use of appropriate defense mechanisms	D. Helps to cope with the situation and to control environment
E. Remain with client as needed or if requested prior to surgery and postoperatively when diagnostic results or outcome are revealed	E. Promotes a feeling of safety and decreases fear, offers support if health status or role functioning is threatened
V. Teach patient/family:	
A. Relaxation techniques and their use	A. Reduces anxiety

INTERVENTION	RATIONALE
B. Information about what to expect during the procedure, the effect of the surgery, projected course of convalescence, reasons for pre- and postoperative care	B. Clarifies misconceptions about the surgical experience and allows for better acceptance of necessary treatments
C. Importance of informed consent, additional information or reinforcement of information given	C. A legal requirement prior to surgery

NURSING DIAGNOSIS

Knowledge deficit related to admission procedures and care and preoperative preparation resulting in the fear of unknown and risk for high anxiety level

EXPECTED OUTCOMES

Adequate knowledge and understanding of the preoperative experience of outpatient surgery evidenced by cooperation in routine procedures associated with admission and preparation (history, assessment, change to appropriate gown), verbalizations of expected behaviors prior to surgery, signing of necessary permits/consent forms

INTERVENTION	RATIONALE
I. Assess for: A. Mental status, ability to learn and understand information to be given	A. Provides information about level and type of communication, teaching strategies to use
B. Knowledge of proposed surgical procedure, past experiences with surgery, risks and benefits	B. Determines need for information, reinforces physician information, and clarifies misinformation

INTERVENTION	RATIONALE
III. Administer:	
A. Preoperative medications by correct route (PO, IM, eye drops, or other), correct dosage, and at the appropriate time(s) prior to surgery	A. For sedation, analgesia if ordered
IV. Perform/provide:	
A. Introduction and orientation to the facility and personnel	A. Facilitates admission to the surgical unit
B. Admission history and physical/psychosocial assessment, notify physician of any abnormalities	B. Provides information relevant to health status and risk for complications
C. Consent forms for signing after appropriate information given	C. Informed consent is a legal requirement prior to surgery
D. Privacy to change to hospital gown, place to store clothing and other articles such as jewelry, dentures, hairpins, other articles	D. Promotes comfort and ensures safe care of personal belongings to prevent loss or injury
E. Hair covering with a surgical cap and a robe over hospital gown for warmth and privacy	E. Appropriate dress for surgery
F. Accompany to surgical suite and position on the surgical table, cover with a sheet for privacy	F. Provides support and correct placement on the table

INTERVENTION	RATIONALE
V. Teach patient/family:	
A. Preparation prior to surgery such as medications, enemas, no foods or fluids for 8 to 12 hours, and bath or shower prior to surgery; provide instructions in writing	A. Provides information regarding physical preparation to ensure smooth procedures for outpatient surgery
B. Time of surgery and time to allow for the complete pre-, intra-, and postoperative care; need for transportation arrangements to and from the facility	B. Provides necessary information for the client and family
C. What to expect during and after the surgery, that postoperative care information will be available following the procedure; provide pamphlets describing the procedure and perioperative requirements.	C. Provides information and answers questions of concern
D. Reason for laboratory testing of surgical specimen and when results will be available	D. Provides diagnostic information about organ impairment or abnormality

NURSING DIAGNOSIS

Knowledge deficit related to postoperative care resulting in inappropriate treatments and procedures and risk for complications

EXPECTED OUTCOMES

Adequate knowledge and understanding of discharge plan for care following outpatient surgery evidenced by uneventful recovery postoperatively with correct performance of all procedures associated with wound care (dressings), medication administration (analgesics, antibiotics), and infection prevention, states time for expected follow-up visits (return to preoperative health status, wound healing, suture removal)

INTERVENTION	RATIONALE
I. Assess for:	
A. Readiness, willingness, and motivation, ability to listen, learn, and comply with postoperative regimen	A. Learning best takes place in the absence of anxiety or stress and is necessary to reduce risk factors that lead to complications
B. Physical status following the procedure to include VS, pain, level of consciousness, mobility, and others related to surgery performed	B. Ensures that client is in a stable condition prior to discharge home
II. Monitor, describe, record:	
A. VS q15 minutes until stable	A. Allows for early identification and intervention to prevent complications
B. Dressing for drainage, dryness, intactness prior to discharge	B. Indicates presence of risk for impaired wound healing, skin irritation, infection
III. Administer:	
A. Analgesic PO with small amount of water if ordered	A. Manages postoperative pain if present
B. Medications ordered to be given immediately following the procedure	B. Other classifications of drugs can be ordered such as diuretic, inotropic, bronchodilator, or others taken routinely that should be resumed immediately

INTERVENTION	RATIONALE
IV. Perform/provide:	
A. Place in position of rest and comfort; sitting, side-lying, or lying with head slightly elevated	A. Provides comfort and avoids tension on the wound, facilitates ventilation
B. Water, bedpan, urinal, or take to bathroom if appropriate	B. Promotes comfort and begins to replace fluids withheld prior to surgery
C. Assist to dress as needed, return personal belongings	C. Prepares client for discharge
D. Transport to car via wheelchair, remain with client until car arrives and assist into the car as needed	D. Ensures safe transportation to car for trip home
E. Support when physician reveals laboratory report if appropriate	E. Provides support while waiting for and receiving biopsy or other results
V. Teach patient/family:	
A. Fluid and dietary regimen resumption to include special inclusions and restrictions	A. Replaces fluids and maintains or adjusts dietary status
B. Medication administration to include analgesic, vitamin C, antibiotic, and others that are ordered (time, dose, frequency, side effects)	B. Resumes medication regimen and provides ordered medications for comfort and prevention of complications

INTERVENTION	RATIONALE
C. Wound care to include noting the presence of blood or drainage on the dressings and to report this, dressing change using clean technique if appropriate, protection of dressings from soiling or dampness	C. Prevents possible wound contamination and promotes early detection of wound complications
D. Refrain from strenuous exercises, lifting, or return to usual activities/occupation until advised by physician	D. Provides guidelines related to convalescence to prevent complications
E. Report persistent pain at surgical site to physician	E. Indicates need for wound inspection for possible infection
F. Make follow-up appointments; provide information and telephone numbers to access needed assistance	F. Monitors convalescence, ensures future health and well-being

preoperative care

DEFINITION
The physical and psychological care given before a scheduled surgical procedure to promote comfort and prevent complications during or following surgery

NURSING DIAGNOSES
Anxiety related to threat to self-concept (disfigurement, loss of body part), threat of death (poor risk, existing chronic condition), threat to change in health status (surgery revealing life-threatening condition, pain, complications following surgery), threat to role functioning (radical surgery, change in life-style caused by permanent disability), resulting in fear, poor response to treatments and instruction

Fear related to separation from support system in a potentially threatening situation (hospitalization and treatments) resulting in increased apprehension and tension, inability to cooperate in preoperative preparation

EXPECTED OUTCOMES
Anxiety and fear decreased and within manageable limits evidenced by ability to rest and sleep, relaxed expression and muscles, verbalization that anxiety and fear has been reduced, VS within an expected slight increase in P and BP compared to baselines

INTERVENTION	RATIONALE
I. Assess for: A. Level of anxiety, verbal expression of fear and reasons for it	A. Anxiety ranges from mild to panic state; a moderate level is desirable and helpful in coping with impending surgery

INTERVENTION	RATIONALE
B. Nonverbal expression of anxiety and fear prior to surgery such as shakiness, restlessness, irritability, pallor, tense body/facial muscles, palpitations, dilated pupils, increased P and BP of >10 beats or 20 to 30 mm Hg, respectively	B. May not be able to communicate feelings but reveal physical/psychological responses that assist to identify the level and changes in anxiety
C. Perceptions of anticipated surgery as to outcome, affect on life-style, and decision-making ability to deal effectively with perceptions	C. Identifies and clarifies ability to cope with the crisis event
D. Support systems available such as family member, spouse, friend	D. Important aspect of caring and promotes sense of well-being; assists in reducing fear and anxiety
E. Responses to preoperative preparation information and treatments	E. These can increase or decrease anxiety, uneasiness about the surgery
III. Administer: A. Sedative, anti-anxiety agent PO	A. Promotes rest and sleep the night prior to surgery
IV. Perform/provide: A. Calm attitude of acceptance and caring, positive response to behavior without expressing anger or disappointment	A. Provides emotional support and reassurance, enhances nurse–patient relationship, allows patient control of environment

INTERVENTION	RATIONALE
B. Environment that promotes trust and prevents anxiety-provoking situations	B. Decreases anxiety and fear by avoiding additional stimuli
C. Encourage expression of feeling, fears, and concerns; listen and provide feedback to clarify behavior	C. Assists to externalize, identify, and acknowledge anxiety and fear
D. Allow for use of appropriate defense mechanisms	D. Helps to cope with the situation and control environment
E. Orientation to hospital room, equipment, use of call light for assistance; information about procedures, policies, routines	E. Provides familiarity with environment and use of any equipment
F. Introduction to staff, visit from operating room personnel; visit to operating and recovery rooms if appropriate	F. Assists in becoming acquainted with staff and surgical enviroment
G. Assurance that pain medications will be administered following the surgery, care and treatments will be provided to prevent complications or prolonged recovery	G. Allays anxiety about pain and risks to health status and self-concept
V. Teach patient/family: A. Relaxation techniques and when to use them	A. Reduces anxiety by relaxing muscles and relieving feelings of fear

B. Additional information or reinforcement of information
given by the physician regarding the procedure, effects, projected course of
convalescence, reasons for
the pre- and postoperative
care

B. Clarifies misconceptions
about the surgical experience and allows for a more
receptive attitude and acceptance of necessary treatments

C. Reasons for treatments such
as enema, nasogastric tube,
catheter, intravenous, medications, lab tests, skin
preparation, and/or others

C. Allows for understanding
and better acceptance of
necessary but unpleasant
treatments and procedures

D. Importance of informed con-
sent that includes legal sig-
nature

D. A legal requirement prior to
surgery

NURSING DIAGNOSIS
Knowledge deficit related to preoperative procedures and care resulting
in risk for high anxiety level and postoperative complications

EXPECTED OUTCOMES
Adequate knowledge and understanding of expected procedures and care
evidenced by verbalizations of preoperative routines and care, demon-
strations of procedures to be performed postoperatively to prevent complications, completed and signed consent/permit forms

INTERVENTION   RATIONALE

I. Assess for:
A. Educational, developmental
level, readiness and willingness to learn

A. Provides information about
teaching strategies to use.

INTERVENTION	RATIONALE
B. Knowledge of diagnosis, proposed surgical procedure, past experiences with hospitalizations, risks and benefits of surgery	B. Prevents repetition of information and allows for clarification of misinformation
C. Knowledge if organ is to be removed or repaired, possible change in function and complications as a result of surgery	C. Allows for questions, reinforcement of physician's information
III. Administer:	
A. Preoperative analgesic, sedative, anticholinergic IM (meperidine, atropine, diazepam, or others)	A. Promotes relaxation, sleep, and as an adjunct to anesthesia and to control secretions
IV. Perform/provide:	
A. Quiet environment with adequate space and privacy	A. Conducive to learning as distractions prevent attentiveness
B. NPO status after midnight, bath or shower with antiseptic soap, scrub and cover surgical site if appropriate	B. Maintains empty stomach, prevents aspiration during induction of anesthesia, removes micro-organisms from skin at surgical site
C. Remove jewelry (except wedding ring taped to finger), hairpins, combs, dentures, glasses, contact lenses, hearing aid, other prostheses, and store in a safe place or give to a family member	C. Prevents loss of belongings or injury to patient

INTERVENTION	RATIONALE
D. Hospital gown, hair covering, anti-embolic hose	D. Provides appropriate dress in preparation for the operating room
E. Catheterization, enema, nasogastric tube	E. Cleanses bowel, empties urinary bladder and stomach prior to surgery

V. Teach patient/family:

A. Time of surgery and time to allow for the total procedure and recovery room postoperatively	A. Provides information to reduce anxiety of patient and family
B. Anesthesiologist will visit night before surgery	B. Provides information about anesthetic procedures
C. Reason for and results of preoperative routine lab tests and procedures (urine and blood tests, ECG, spirometry, chest x-ray, skin prep, N/G tube, IV, retention catheter, NPO, medications, and/or others)	C. Rules out abnormal findings or organ impairment that can postpone surgery and carries out procedures to prepare for surgery
D. Information regarding usual postanesthesia and operative care and procedures in recovery room such as vital signs monitoring, possible drains, tubes, dressings, IV and other lines in place, suction device, assessments and administration of medications for pain or nausea	D. Provides information about what to expect immediately following surgery

INTERVENTION	RATIONALE
E. Information regarding usual postoperative care and procedures such as activity limitations with gradual progression to self-care, dietary modifications with progression to general diet (beginning with liquids in 48 hours and solid foods within 48 to 72 hours), treatments (VS, breathing, wound, I&O), medications (analgesic, antibiotic, anti-emetic)	E. Provides information about what is done following surgery
F. Demonstration and return demonstration of activities to be performed postoperatively such as incentive spirometry, deep breathing and coughing exercises in supine, sitting, standing, and semi-Fowler's positions, foot and leg exercises, including calf and thigh muscles, moving in bed and changing positions using the side rails	F. Activities that prevent postoperative complications of atelectasis, thrombus formation/venous stasis
G. Progressive ambulation from sitting at side of bed, standing, and walking with assistance beginning the evening following surgery	G. Prevents hazards associated with bed rest or immobility

postoperative care

DEFINITION
The physical and psychological care given following a surgical procedure to promote safety, comfort, and return to optimal normal functioning, and the information and instruction for home care prior to discharge to ensure the return to wellness without complications

NURSING DIAGNOSES
Ineffective airway clearance related to increased tracheobronchial secretions (irritation caused by anesthetic, intubation), tracheobronchial obstruction (viscous, tenacious secretions, laryngospasm, relaxed tongue falling back and blocking the pharynx, aspiration of vomitus), decreased energy and fatigue (inability to cough, inadequate activity)

Ineffective breathing pattern related to perception or cognitive impairment (anesthesia, medications), incisional pain (positioning, distention, dressings)

Risk for aspiration related to reduced level of consciousness (medications and anesthesia), depressed cough and gag reflexes (level of consciousness, relaxed muscles resulting from anesthesia), decreased gastrointestinal motility and delayed gastric emptying (distention, vomiting)

EXPECTED OUTCOMES
Airway patency and pulmonary ventilation evidenced by rate, depth, rhythm, and ease of respirations within baseline parameters, normal clear breath sounds, secretions liquified with airway clearance maintained, progressive return to consciousness with ability to remove secretions by coughing, normal skin color, oxygen and carbon dioxide levels (ABGs)

INTERVENTION	RATIONALE

I. Assess for:

A. Respiratory status including rate (slow, rapid, tachypnea), ease (dyspnea, use of accessory muscles), depth (shallow, altered chest excursion), abnormal breath sounds (crackles, wheezes, stridor, diminished or absent), productive or nonproductive cough and sputum characteristics

A. Provides for data indicating changes from baselines resulting in airway resistance and abnormal breathing pattern, type of measures needed to improve breathing and ventilation

B. Level of pain and response to analgesia/anesthesia, level of consciousness, airway in place, return of gag reflex

B. Pain causes diminished/restricted chest expansion, airway obstruction caused by tongue falling back in throat

II. Monitor, describe, record:

A. Vital signs, respiratory quality and breath sounds auscultation q2–4h (q15–30 minutes for first 2 hours)

A. Indicates changes in respiratory status and possible complications or respiratory failure

B. Pulse oximetry for oxygen saturation or arterial blood gases (ABGs) for pO_2, skin and mucous membranes for color (cyanosis)

B. Decreased oxygen levels indicate hypoventilation, hypoxemia

III. Administer:

A. Humidified oxygen per cannula at lowest effective rate in L/min

A. Ensures oxygenation of organs and tissues

INTERVENTION	RATIONALE
B. Mucolytic agent (acetylcysteine) INH for thick, tenacious secretions by ultrasonic nebulizer or intermittent positive pressure breathing (IPPB)	B. Acts to liquify secretions for easier removal by coughing or suctioning
C. Bronchodilator (theophylline PO or nebulizer, aminophylline IV)	C. Acts by preventing bronchospasms that cause airway obstruction
D. Nasogastric tube and suction	D. Maintains compression to reduce abdominal distention that can affect breathing pattern
IV. Perform/provide: A. Continued placement of airway device until reflexes return or device is pushed out of the mouth; lift jaw upward and forward if airway obstructed by tongue	A. Ensures airway patency and prevents obstruction by relaxed tongue
B. Placement in sidelying or low semi-Fowler's positions and change q2h to allow for full chest expansion	B. Facilitates breathing, decreases the pressure of abdominal organs on the diaphragm, prevents aspiration of vomitus or secretions that can cause pneumonia
C. Coughing and deep breathing exercises q1–2h, blow bottles or incentive spirometry q2–4h; advise to splint incision during coughing to reduce pain and improve breathing effort	C. Removes secretions, prevents formation of mucus plugs that can cause atelectasis

INTERVENTION	RATIONALE
D. Humidified air, fluid intake of up to 2500 mL/day in progressive fashion if allowed	D. Liquifies secretions for easier coughing and removal, maintains moist airways and mucous membranes
E. Tracheal suctioning with frequency and duration dependent on amount of secretions and response (usually 80 to 100 mm Hg suction)	E. Removes excess secretions if unable to cough/deep-breathe, prevents aspiration (vomitus) if unable to consciously expectorate
V. Teach patient/family:	
A. Avoid smoking, environmental irritants following surgery	A. Causes airway irritation and constriction, impairs ventilation
B. Report any breathing pattern or respiratory changes immediately	B. Provides early intervention to prevent postoperative complications

NURSING DIAGNOSIS

Pain related to physical injuring agent (trauma of surgical incision, stress on incision by movement in and out of bed and breathing/coughing exercises)

EXPECTED OUTCOMES

Pain reduced and controlled evidenced by decreased requests for analgesics, verbalization that pain is decreasing or absent, ability to participate in postoperative self-care and measures to prevent complications

INTERVENTION	RATIONALE
I. Assess for:	
A. Verbal descriptors of pain including location, severity, extent, type, duration, factors that increase or decrease pain; use 1 to 10 scale to determine severity q2–3h	A. Determines type of analgesic and administer for optimal effect before pain becomes severe
B. Nonverbal descriptors of pain, including grimacing, crying, holding body part or guarding behavior, moaning, restlessness, increases in vital signs q2–3h	B. Observable clues indicating pain if patient is unable to express pain characteristics
C. Pain threshold and tolerance, situation and sociocultural factors influencing pain perception and response	C. Specific to individuals and their perception or interpretation of pain
D. Pressure from tight dressing, edema at site, bladder distention, inflammation at incisional site q4h	D. Possible postoperative causes of varied types and degrees of pain
E. Past experiences with pain and responses, measures used and their effectiveness	E. Assist in identifying and selecting relief measures known to control pain
II. Monitor, describe, record:	
A. VS q2–4h for increases	A. Indicates severity of pain

INTERVENTION	RATIONALE
III. Administer:	
A. Analgesic (meperidine, morphine) IM before pain becomes severe and withhold narcotic analgesic if respiration <12/min, PO analgesic appropriate to reduction in acute pain; self-administered analgesic (PCA) per patient-controlled device; follow gate theory in timing of analgesia administration	A. Acts by inhibiting pain pathways in CNS, alters pain perception; narcotic analgesic depresses respirations
IV. Perform/provide:	
A. Environment that controls stimuli such as optimal lighting and temperature, noise reduction, calm and positive attitude during interactions	A. Factors that can increase pain and affect response to medications, facilitates rest and sleep
B. Position for comfort and change q2h, use aids as appropriate	B. Decreases stress on incision and joints
C. Analgesic prior to planned activities and treatments, or schedule painful activities around medications	C. Allows for participation in necessary care with minimal pain
D. Comfort measures such as back rub, music, and other diversional activities, guided imagery, relaxation and breathing techniques, touch	D. Provides nonpharmacological pain-relief activities

INTERVENTION	RATIONALE
E. Positive attitude when providing analgesics and pain relief measures	E. Increases effectiveness of treatment
F. Splint, support incision, and flex knees during coughing/deep breathing, assist with position changes, ensure that any incisional drainage tubes and dressings are secure	F. Reduces tension on incision to prevent pain during activities

V. Teach patient/family:

A. Pain will be most severe for 48 hours and then subsides depending on procedure	A. Reveals what to expect and relieves fear and anxiety about pain
B. Report any pain when it begins, to request medications if not offered at regular intervals, that analgesic will be administered when needed	B. Allows for more effective relief than attempting to control severe pain, prevents anticipatory fear of pain
C. Inform of painful treatments prior to intervention and of ways to reduce known factors that increase pain	C. Reduces anxiety and associated muscle tension that cause pain

NURSING DIAGNOSIS

Altered tissue perfusion related to interruption of flow, venous (pooling/stasis of blood from inactivity and positioning), hypovolemia (blood and/or fluid loss, NPO status)

EXPECTED OUTCOMES
Adequate tissue perfusion (absence of organ impairment), peripheral evidenced by warm, normal color of extremities with palpable peripheral pulses; cardiopulmonary evidenced by vital signs within baseline levels; cerebral evidenced by mentation and consciousness within acceptable parameters for patient; renal evidenced by I&O balance within 8 hours; gastrointestinal evidenced by return of bowel sounds and absence of distention

INTERVENTION	RATIONALE
I. Assess for:	
A. Pain, swelling, redness, warmth in calf area, coolness of area distal to calf, positive Homan's sign (pain on dorsiflexion); delayed peripheral pulse, capillary refill, cold skin temperature to touch, skin color (blue or purple, mottling, pallor)	A. Signs and symptoms of deep-vein thrombosis caused by pooling/stasis associated with bed rest, anesthesia postoperatively; indicates diminished circulation to extremities
B. Restlessness, confusion or altered consciousness, headache	B. Indicates decrease in cerebral perfusion
C. Urinary output for decrease in relation to fluid intake, increase in blood pressure	C. Indicates decrease in renal perfusion
D. Nausea, vomiting, abdominal distention, absence of bowel sounds	D. Indicates decrease in gastrointestinal perfusion
E. Palpitations, dyspnea, changes in vital signs, chest pain, cardiac rhythm, cyanosis	E. Indicates decrease in cardiopulmonary perfusion

INTERVENTION	RATIONALE
F. Blood pressure decrease, pulse increase, cool, clammy skin	F. Indicates possible shock state as a result of hypovolemia (postoperative hemorrhage)

II. Monitor, describe, record:
   A. Vital signs, I&O, BUN/ creatinine, ABGs, electrolytes, enzymes, Hct/Hb, ECG; selection and frequency dependent on postoperative status

   A. Provides information about changes in circulation and tissue perfusion; reveals specific impairment as follows: heart/lung (VS, ECG, ABGs, enzymes), kidneys (I&O, electrolytes, creatinine, BUN), hemorrhage (VS, Hct/Hb)

III. Administer:
   A. Low dose anticoagulant SC (heparin) and monitor for signs of bleeding

   A. Acts to prevent clot formation following surgery by depressing synthesis of vitamin K and coagulation factors

   B. Blood or blood products IV

   B. Acts to replace blood loss resulting from hemorrhage

IV. Perform/provide:
   A. Anti-embolic hose, remove for bathing and skin assessment twice daily and reapply after elevation of legs for 10 minutes; intermittent pneumatic compression hose as an alternative if ordered

   A. Promotes blood flow and increases venous return, prevents thrombus formation

INTERVENTION	RATIONALE
B. Elevate legs and/or foot of bed, avoid using knee-gatch to raise legs	B. Promotes venous return without compromising circulation by compression
C. Movement in bed, slowly changing to upright position, and ambulate according to schedule, increase as appropriate and assist as needed	C. Promotes circulation and prevents venous stasis, syncope from postural hypotension by allowing time for regulatory mechanism to adjust to postural changes
D. Leg and feet exercises q1h; measure calves daily, and compare size with baselines and for equality	D. Increases muscle contractions and circulation; increases in measurement indicates edema associated with phlebitis
E. Increase in fluids to 2500 mL/24h if allowed, IV or PO	E. Maintains adequate fluid intake and tissue perfusion, prevents blood viscosity
F. Optimal room temperature, clothing, and bed covers for warmth	F. Prevents chilling that causes vasoconstriction
G. Measures to treat organ impairment such as elevating head, maintaining gastrointestinal decompression, avoid straining at defecation, fluid and dietary restrictions, quiet and restful environment, others dependent on organ(s) affected	G. Maximizes organ perfusion and function

V. Teach patient/family:

INTERVENTION	RATIONALE
A. Refrain from smoking	A. Smoking causes vasoconstriction and affects circulation status

INTERVENTION	RATIONALE
B. Avoid crossing legs at ankles, feet, knees when sitting	B. Places pressure on veins and constricts circulation
C. Avoid sitting or remaining in the same position for long periods	C. Encourages pooling and stasis of blood
D. Avoid trauma to extremities such as burning or bumping skin areas when bathing or ambulating	D. Precautions to prevent injury when circulation is compromised
E. Range of motion and exercises to extremities during bed rest until fully ambulatory and independent in self-care	E. Promotes circulation and improves venous return

NURSING DIAGNOSIS

Altered nutrition: Less than body requirements related to inability to ingest food (NPO status, nausea, abdominal distention, pain, lack of interest in postoperative dietary allowances), inability to digest food (vomiting, reduced bowel motility), inability to absorb nutrients (reduced tissue perfusion)

EXPECTED OUTCOMES

Adequate nutritional intake for wound healing and general health evidenced by ability to retain liquids and progress to general diet or previous special diet, and the return of appetite, strength and endurance, bowel sounds, and weight baseline for height, age, sex, and body build standards

INTERVENTION	RATIONALE
I. Assess for:	
A. Nausea, vomiting, and characteristics	A. Results from pain, distention, vagal stimulation from visceral irritation
B. Abdominal distention, gas pain, hiccoughs, presence or absence of bowel sounds, feeling of fullness in the abdomen, passage of flatus q2h	B. Gas and fluid can accumulate from decreased peristalsis resulting from manipulation of bowel, effect of medications and anesthesia; these signs and symptoms can indicate a developing paralytic ileus postoperatively
C. NPO status, nutritional intake via IV postoperatively, and subsequent oral intake over a 3-day period	C. Provides estimate of caloric intake as patient progresses to regular dietary pattern
D. Ability to chew, swallow, food likes/dislikes/ intolerances, stomatitis	D. Factors that influence intake when solid food is allowed
II. Monitor, describe, record:	
A. Weight daily to q3days, and compare to baseline standard for height, body build, sex, and age	A. Indicates weight loss or gain
B. Albumin, BUN, transferrin, iron levels if malnutrition suspected	B. Indicates nutritional deficiency if levels are low

INTERVENTION	RATIONALE
III. Administer:	
A. Anti-emetic IM or suppository (prochlorperazine) or gastrointestinal stimulant (metoclopramide)	A. Acts by blocking chemoreceptor trigger zone that affects vomiting center and reduces spasms of diaphragm if hiccoughs present; stimulates peristalsis to improve gastric emptying if nasogastric suctioning is not used to prevent paralytic ileus
B. Vitamin C	B. Acts to enhance wound healing
IV. Perform/provide:	
A. Frequent position changes and early ambulation, advise to move slowly and smoothly	A. Stimulates appetite and peristalsis, movement stimulates chemoreceptor in medulla and can cause nausea
B. Environment that is free of odors, noises, used articles or unpleasant sights, or other stimuli	B. Stimulates vomiting center or causes nausea
C. Nasogastric tube and suction if gastric distention present, vomiting continues, and bowel sounds absent; monitor for patency and maintain NPO status	C. Prevents accumulation of gas and fluid; continued vomiting causes a loss of fluid and/or ingested nutrients
D. Advise to expel flatus when need is felt, insert rectal tube or administer enema if ordered	D. Reduces accumulation of gastrointestinal gas causing distention and pain

INTERVENTION	RATIONALE
E. Advise to hold breath or breathe deeply, breathe into a paper bag	E. Provides measures to control nausea or hiccoughs
F. Clear liquids, followed by soft foods and progress to light and general diets as tolerated; include foods high in protein, calories, and vitamins	F. Begins when oral intake is allowed and bowel sounds return; protein and vitamins enhance wound healing, calories maintain weight and nourishment
G. Provide mouth care and rest before meals	G. Reduces fatigue and promotes clean mouth that enhances desire to eat
H. Offer small, frequent meals, and advise to eat slowly; supplement foods between meals	H. Prevents excessive filling that results in nausea and vomiting and provides additional caloric intake needed for the increased metabolic rate involved in wound healing
I. Offer limited amount of fluids with meals	I. Decreases amount of food intake at mealtime as fluids can fill stomach
J. Calorie count and intake analysis if nutritional status declines and weight is lost	J. Indicates adequate nutritional intake and possible need for nutritional consult
V. Teach patient/family:	
A. Avoid smoking and gum chewing, foods such as cabbage, beans, and carbonated beverages	A. Promotes air swallowing and gastric distention; gas-producing food causes gas accumulation in tract

INTERVENTION	RATIONALE
B. Avoid high-fat foods, spicy foods, beverages containing caffeine	B. Affects gastric emptying and irritates gastrointestinal mucosa
C. Avoid drinking fluids with meals, advise to eat dry foods and remain in an upright position and rest following meals	C. Assists in preventing nausea
D. Avoid drinking hot or cold fluids, advise to drink warm fluids only	D. Causes hiccoughs by irritation to phrenic nerve, warm fluids stimulate peristalsis

NURSING DIAGNOSIS

Risk for fluid deficit related to excessive losses through normal routes (vomiting), loss of fluid through abnormal routes (gastric aspirate), altered intake (NPO status, insufficient IV fluid replacement), factors influencing fluid needs (hypermetabolic state caused by wound healing), hypovolemia (hemorrhage postoperatively)

EXPECTED OUTCOMES

Fluid balance maintained at baseline level evidenced by adequate urinary output and fluid intake 24 to 48 hours postoperatively, VS within baseline levels, absence of signs and symptoms of dehydration

INTERVENTION	RATIONALE
I. Assess for:	
A. Fluid intake amount, type, and route; urinary output and determine ratio	A. Compares fluid intake and output for presence of imbalance
B. Dry mucous membranes and skin, poor skin turgor, oliguria, thirst, weakness, temperature, delay in capillary refill, concentrated urine	B. Signs and symptoms of dehydration caused by excessive fluid loss

INTERVENTION	RATIONALE
C. Decreased BP, increased P, R, cold, clammy skin	C. Signs of hypovolemia and possible approaching shock state, third spacing of fluids into extravascular space during surgery, insufficient fluid replacement during or following surgery
II. Monitor, describe, record: A. VS q5–15 min following surgery, then q30min for 4 hours, then q1h for 4 hours, then q4h for 24 to 48 hours	A. Indicates change in circulation status
B. I&O including IV fluids, drainage from wound, gastric aspirate, colostomy, vomitus, diarrhea, bleeding, urine, other sources q1–4h as appropriate	B. Determines amount of fluid loss compared to intake
C. Weight on same scale, same time, same clothing, frequency dependent on potential for fluid losses or retention	C. Determines weight loss with fluid deficit or weight gain in response to surgery caused by increase in ADH, aldosterone, cortisol levels
D. Blood for electrolytes for decreased K, Cl, albumin, Hct, Hb, total protein, urine for electrolytes, specific gravity and osmolality; guaiac of emesis, feces, drainage	D. Changes that can occur with fluid deficit, retention, hemorrhage, or electrolyte imbalance

INTERVENTION	RATIONALE
III. Administer:	
A. Blood, plasma, serum albumin, volume expanders IV	A. Replaces losses and increases volume in presence of hemorrhage
B. IV infusion of fluids at ordered amount with hourly rate checks; supplemental electrolytes in IV	B. Maintains adequate fluid replacement, lost electrolytes if needed, and prevents fluid overload
C. Anti-emetic (prochlorperazine), antidiarrheal (diphenoxylate) PO, IM	C. Controls fluid losses from vomiting or diarrhea postoperatively
IV. Perform/provide:	
A. Fluid intake of 2 to 3 L/day PO as indicated, offer a 24-hour schedule of preferred fluids and encourage to drink small amounts frequently	A. Provides fluids needed during postoperative period to maintain optimal intake and balance
B. Offer foods and fluids high in K such as citrus juices, bananas; use normal saline for irrigation purposes	B. Promotes electrolyte balance
V. Teach patient/family:	
A. Record intake of fluids on paper at the bedside	A. Assists in accurate measurement of I&O
B. Avoid flushing toilet following urination, check to be sure that bed pan has been placed under toilet seat prior to elimination (urine or diarrheal stool)	B. Assists in accurate measurement of I&O

NURSING DIAGNOSIS

Risk for infection related to inadequate primary defenses (broken skin caused by surgical incision, stasis of body fluids caused by urinary retention or pulmonary secretions), invasive procedures (IV line, urinary catheter)

EXPECTED OUTCOMES

All systems free of infectious process evidenced by temperature within baseline level, wound intact and healing, urine clear and odorless, sputum clear and easily expectorated, cultures negative for infectious agent

INTERVENTION	RATIONALE
I. Assess for:	
A. Redness, edema, warmth, fever, purulent drainage from wound; edema, pain, redness, extravasation at infusion site	A. Indicates wound infection that can result from contamination of the wound or compromised condition resulting from malnutrition, chronic disease
B. Increase in respiratory rate and pattern changes, crackles and diminished breath sounds auscultated, dullness on percussion, yellow, green or other color of sputum, fever, chills	B. Indicates pulmonary infection (pneumonia) resulting from aspirants or stasis of pulmonary secretions
C. Dysuria, frequency, urgency, foul odor and cloudiness of urine, fever	C. Indicates urinary tract infection resulting from contamination associated with indwelling catheter or urinary stasis
D. Positive sputum, urine, wound drainage culture, increased WBC, ABGs, or pulse oximetry for decreased oxygen level	D. Indicates infectious process of related organs or sites

INTERVENTION	RATIONALE
II. Monitor, describe, record:	
A. Temperature, respirations and breath sounds q4h	A. Elevation and changes occur with infection; hyperthermia can occur as a stress response to surgery, hypothermia as a result of heat loss during surgery
B. Laboratory tests, chest x ray as available (cultures, WBC)	B. Reveals abnormalities indicating a possible infection
III. Administer:	
A. Antibiotic therapy, sulfonamides (amoxicillin, sulfisoxazole) PO	A. Acts by inhibiting cell wall synthesis or interfering with biosynthesis of protein by bacteria
B. Antipyretics (acetaminophen, aspirin products) PO	B. Reduces fever by inhibiting heat-regulating center
C. Oxygen via nasal cannula at rate ordered	C. Ensures adequate oxygenation of organs and tissues
IV. Perform/provide:	
A. Handwashing with antimicrobial soap using appropriate technique prior to each contact or care activity	A. Prevents transmission of contaminants to the client
B. Wear appropriate protective wear such as mask, gloves during care	B. Prevents cross contamination to or from the patient, staff, and others

INTERVENTION	RATIONALE
C. Obtain cultures from appropriate site and send to laboratory	C. Provides for testing to identify microorganisms responsible for infection and effective antimicrobials for therapy
D. All procedures utilizing sterile technique and supplies especially for wound and catheter care	D. Prevents contamination and risk for infection
E. Postoperative respiratory physiotherapy (coughing and deep breathing, postural drainage)	E. Prevents stasis of secretions and promotes patent airways
F. Catheter and perineal care, closed drainage system and positioning of system lower than bladder level, catheter and tubing patency, catheter changes per protocol	F. Ensures sterile and functional system
G. Fluid intake of 2 to 3 L/day if allowed	G. Promotes urination and dilutes urine as a precaution against infection
H. IV site and tubing change per protocol	H. Prevents trauma and introduction of bacteria from long-term use
I. Dry dressings with changes as needed, cleanse wound with antiseptic, apply antimicrobial ointment	I. Prevents contact with microorganisms by capillary action and cleanses and protects wound from infection

INTERVENTION	RATIONALE
V. Teach patient/family:	
A. Avoid touching wound, IV site	A. Prevents contamination of sterile areas
B. Avoid contact with visitors who have upper respiratory or other infections	B. Prevents transmission of micro-organisms leading to pulmonary infection
C. Wipe genitalia and anal areas from front to back after defecation and/or urination	C. Prevents contamination leading to urinary tract infection in females
D. Wash hands following bathroom use and before meals	D. Prevents transmission of potential infectious agents
E. Report signs and symptoms of infection at any site including pain, breathing changes, burning on urination or frequency of urination, chilling, foul odor from urine or wound	E. Provides early diagnosis and therapy of postoperative infection

NURSING DIAGNOSIS

Risk for impaired skin integrity related to external factors (excretion and secretions, skin disruption caused by surgical incision, pressure from nasogastric or other tubing), internal factors (altered nutritional, metabolic, circulatory states)

EXPECTED OUTCOMES

Wound intact and healing evidenced by progressive reduction in inflammatory response associated with trauma of surgical incision (redness, swelling), approximation of wound edges, presence of granulation tissue, skin and mucous membranes free of irritation and breakdown at tube insertion sites (wound, nasogastric, oxygen cannula, IV infusion, urinary catheter, right atrial catheter)

INTERVENTION	RATIONALE
I. Assess for:	
A. Healing process of wound to include progressive resolution of redness and edema, absence of necrosis, approximation of edges, dryness of wound and around drains and tubes	A. Characterizes normal wound healing process with adequate circulation
B. Skin redness or excoriation caused by tape on skin, secretions at wound site around drainage tube	B. Indicates skin irritation and risk for breakdown
C. Separation of wound edges and protrusion of abdominal contents, statements by patient that the wound felt like it "opened up"	C. Indicates wound dehiscence and need for immediate intervention
D. Nasal mucous membranes for redness, soreness, lesions if nasogastric tube or oxygen cannula used	D. Characterizes irritation and risk for breakdown
III. Administer:	
A. Water-soluble ointment to nares	A. Lubricates mucous membranes and minimizes irritation
IV. Perform/provide:	
A. Dry bed linens free from wrinkles, change of position q2h	A. Prevents pressure on skin and promotes comfort

INTERVENTION	RATIONALE
B. Secure dressings and drainage tubes, avoid tightness; dressing changes as needed with careful removal of tape in direction of hair growth, application of skin protective barrier around tubing, use of hypoallergic tape and/or Montgomery straps for frequent dressing changes	B. Prevents injury to the wound resulting from irritation if dressing can rub against wound or if damp or soaked with drainage; tightness compromises circulation
C. Avoid positioning on tubing, ensure patency of drainage tubes, empty drainage pouch or container before they become full	C. Prevents occlusion of tubing, leakage around tubes or overflow of drainage container
D. Appropriate hydration and diet/snacks high in protein and vitamin C	D. Dry skin more prone to breakdown, nutritional inclusions promote wound healing
V. Teach patient/family:	
A. Avoid touching dressings	A. Protects wound from injury
B. Support wound during coughing and deep-breathing exercises and ambulation	B. Prevents stress on incision

NURSING DIAGNOSES

Impaired physical mobility related to pain/discomfort (surgical incision, fear of wound injury), intolerance to activity/decreased strength and endurance (bed rest status, sleep deprivation, medications/anesthesia effects)

Activity intolerance related to generalized weakness (inadequate circulatory, respiratory, nutritional status), bed rest or immobility (imposed restrictions in activities postoperatively)

Sleep pattern disturbance related to internal factor of effects of surgery (pain, difficulty in assuming comfortable/accustomed position for sleep, frequent interruptions to perform care and treatments)

EXPECTED OUTCOMES
Gradual and progressive return to physical movement and mobility within postoperative restrictions and tolerance, adequate sleep and rest necessary to sustain recuperation from the surgical procedure evidenced by increasing ambulation, participation in personal care activities without untoward effects (vital signs, fatigue, pain), verbalizations that endurance and energy are increasing, and rested feeling experienced with minimal interruption in sleep pattern

INTERVENTION	RATIONALE
I. Assess for:	
A. Energy level, fatigue, weakness, reluctance to move within environment	A. Determines endurance level and ability to move and ambulate independently
B. Response to activity (increased pulse and blood pressure, dyspnea, dizziness)	B. Indicates intolerance to activity and need to cease or reduce activity
C. Orientation, confusion, memory, sensory perceptions	C. Indicates return of mental acuity following administration of medications that can decrease mentation/movement
D. Anxiety, irritability, difficulty in falling asleep, lethargy	D. Indicates interference with or lack of sleep periods
E. Pain, swelling, warmth in extremity, Homan's sign	E. Indicates possible thrombus formation complication of surgery that can occur with reduced movement causing reduced return blood flow (stasis)

INTERVENTION	RATIONALE
II. Monitor, describe, record: A. VS prior to and following activity for increases in pulse rate of >20 and not returning to baseline within a specified time, blood pressure of >10 to 20 mm Hg	A. Indicates activity intolerance and need to decrease and monitor activity
III. Administer: A. Sedative (flurazepam) PO prior to bedtime	A. Acts to promote sleep by depressing CNS through potentiating an inhibitory neurotransmitter
B. Anticoagulant (heparin) IV or SC	B. Acts by potentiating effects of antithrombin III, prevents conversion of prothrombin to thrombin or fibrinogen to fibrin depending on dosage; administered to prevent deep-vein thrombus formation
IV. Perform/provide: A. Activity restrictions while encouraging movement in bed, ambulation, ADL	A. Promotes activity while preventing fatigue, signs, and symptoms of intolerance
B. Scheduling that alternates rest periods with activities	B. Ensures rest and prevents fatigue, rest necessary for postoperative recovery

INTERVENTION	RATIONALE
C. Activities that begin with sitting at side of bed, in chair, ambulating to bathroom and in room with assistance, then in hall with daily increases in distance, offer wheelchair, IV pole as assistive aids in ambulation	C. Slow, progressive schedule provides patient with successes and motivation to continue and increase activity
D. Schedule activities for times when analgesia or other medications are at optimal effect	D. More likely to participate in activity when free of pain and other discomforts
E. Place articles and supplies within reach and employ aids for self-care activities, assist as needed	E. Provides access to needed personal items while conserving energy
F. Uninterrupted periods of sleep at night and rest during the day, quiet, clean, odor-free, well-regulated temperature and ventilated environment	F. Establishes optimal sleep environment needed for recovery/wellness
G. Praise for all attempts at improving and increasing mobility and other activities	G. Encourages to maximize participation in all ADL, mobility in particular
H. Nonpharmacological measures such as backrub, warm beverage if allowed, relaxation music, other established bedtime rituals familiar to patient	H. Promotes relaxation and sleep

INTERVENTION	RATIONALE
V. Teach patient/family:	
A. Avoid stimuli or stimulating beverages at bedtime	A. Prevents relaxation prior to sleep
B. Utilize side rails, overhead trapeze to assist with movement in bed	B. Promotes independence in movement as needed for positions of comfort
C. Advantages of mobility and rest to all systems and rationales for early ambulation, energy conservation, and sleep/rest	C. Prevents complications associated with surgery by promoting understanding of interventions and compliance with activities
D. Avoid constricting clothing, any compression on legs (crossing legs, pillows under legs, use of knee-gatch, prolonged sitting position)	D. Compromises circulation to the extremities and predisposes to blood flow stasis and thrombus formation

NURSING DIAGNOSES

Altered urinary elimination related to mechanical trauma (retention caused by surgical procedure), neuromuscular impairment (reduced bladder muscle tone caused by anesthesia/medications)

Constipation related to less-than-adequate fluid/dietary intake (NPO status), less-than-adequate physical activity (bed rest status postoperatively), medications (narcotic analgesics for pain), emotional status (fear of incisional pain on defecation), neuromuscular impairment (reduced bowel motility caused by anesthesia and manipulation of abdominal contents during surgery)

EXPECTED OUTCOMES

Return of baseline urinary and bowel elimination patterns evidenced by voiding within 6 to 8 hours following surgery and subsequent complete emptying of the bladder; soft, brown, formed feces q1–2 days and normal bowel sounds auscultated

INTERVENTION	RATIONALE
I. Assess for:	
A. First voiding following surgery, amount, time, and subsequent frequency of voidings, ratio with fluid intake	A. Indicates normal or abnormal urinary pattern
B. Voidings of less than 50 mL, frequency with complaints of urgency, bladder fullness and discomfort, height of distended bladder palpated	B. Signs and symptoms of urinary retention
C. Bowel sounds q4h	C. Notes return of peristalsis/motility
D. First and subsequent bowel elimination and characteristics of soft/hard, dry/liquid feces, frequency, amount, color, constituents	D. Indicates normal or abnormal feces and possible constipation
E. Headache, abdominal distention, cramping, feeling of fullness or pressure in rectum, mass palpable in rectum, straining at defecation	E. Signs and symptoms of constipation
III. Administer:	
A. Stool softener, cathartic PO or suppository (docusate, bisacodyl)	A. Acts to soften feces for easier movement by stimulating peristalsis, producing fluid accumulation in the colon by altering fluid transport

INTERVENTION	RATIONALE
B. Cholinergic (bethanechol) PO	B. Acts to stimulate bladder to contract, which decreases bladder capacity in treatment of urinary retention
IV. Perform/provide: A. Privacy during urinary or bowel elimination, raise head of bed when using bedpan or urinal q2–4h (allow male to stand if possible), use bedside commode	A. Prevents embarrassment and encourages elimination
B. Increased activity and ambulation as tolerance permits	B. Increases motility and peristalsis
C. Increased fluid intake of 2 to 3 L/day if allowed, high-fiber dietary inclusion when PO intake allowed	C. Provides fluid needed to soften feces and promote urinary output, provides bulk to feces for easier elimination
D. Run water, allow to dip hands in warm water, pour warm water over genitalia	D. Actions that encourage voiding by relaxing muscles that are involved in urination
E. Single catheterization after voiding or intermittent catheterization if ordered, catheterize if voiding not established by 8 hours following surgery or sooner if severely distended	E. Determines amount of retention and empties bladder to prevent stasis that predisposes to bladder infection, catheterization reserved for inability to void or chronic retention

INTERVENTION	RATIONALE
F. Cleansing enema if ordered and suppository not effective	F. Cleases bowel of feces and prevents discomfort or impaction
V. Teach patient/family:	
A. Urinate or defecate as soon as urge is felt	A. Prevents the disappearance or delay in desire for elimination
B. Refrain from laxative use and promote elimination through other methods (fluids, foods, exercise)	B. Causes dependence on laxative for bowel elimination

NURSING DIAGNOSIS

Knowledge deficit related to lack of exposure (information regarding follow-up care on discharge to home/long-term care facility), causing increased risk for postoperative complications

EXPECTED OUTCOMES

Appropriate verbalizations and performance of care measures and treatment regimen following instruction and information about prevention of infection, life-style modifications, medications, reporting signs and symptoms of complications, follow-up appointments

INTERVENTION	RATIONALE
I. Assess for:	
A. Knowledge and understanding of surgery and rationale for treatments and preventive measures	A. Provides a basis for discharge plan and teaching techniques to utilize

INTERVENTION	RATIONALE
B. Learning readiness and abilities of patient and/or family to provide care and skills needed to perform procedures in the home	B. Provides information about need for outside assistance and referral to special professionals (social worker, physical/occupational therapist, nurse, nutritionist) and others such as nursing assistant, home aide, resources for durable equipment and other supplies, transport services
IV. Perform/provide:	
A. Written discharge plan that includes level of care, problem list, goals, interventions, and evaluation, teaching done prior to discharge	A. Provides documentation of follow-up care to ensure continuity and prevention of postoperative complications
B. Time for questions and explanations during teaching sessions	B. Provides clarification of information and demonstrations given
V. Teach patient/family:	
A. Report persistent pain in any area, temperature elevation, cough and sputum of abnormal color, loss of energy, nausea or vomiting, change in urine characteristics, difficult breathing, abnormal wound drainage, sudden weight loss or gain	A. Signs and symptoms of complications to be reported to ensure early treatment
B. Handwash technique and to use prior to meals and performing any care and following bathroom use	B. Prevents transmission of micro-organisms

INTERVENTION	RATIONALE
C. Practice coughing and deep-breathing exercises, continue with incentive spirometry if appropriate	C. Prevents pulmonary complications
D. Avoid smoking, contact with people who have upper respiratory infections	D. Smoking compromises respiratory function, avoids transmission of microorganisms that can cause infection
E. Continue physical exercises and increase as able to tolerate, stop when tired and rest	E. Promotes activity to maintain circulation status and normal function of other systems (elimination, removal of pulmonary secretions, gastrointestinal peristalsis)
F. Fluid intake of eight to ten glasses/day and dietary regimen, provide list of inclusions to fulfill specific needs such as fiber, electrolytes, vitamins, protein, nutritional supplements; include factors such as consistency of foods, frequency of meals, aids to use for self-feeding	F. Maintains fluid/nutritional status for health (wound healing, skin integrity, elimination, liquify secretions)
G. Wound care to include dressing change, cleansing, skin care, and allow to practice procedure using sterile technique; protection of wound when bathing	G. Maintains clean, dry, healing wound

INTERVENTION	RATIONALE
H. Medication administration including checking action, dose, route, frequency, side effects, food and drug interactions; to check with physician before using over-the-counter drugs, alternate liquid form that can be obtained if needed	H. Ensures compliance in administration of prescribed drugs to achieve desired effect while preventing errors in over- or underdose, continues analgesia for postoperative pain if needed
I. Modify home environment to clear pathways of rugs, furniture, provide good lighting and articles to hold onto when walking; firm and good fitting shoes	I. Safety measures to prevent falls when ambulating
J. Care and application of braces, appliances, prosthesis; care of cast	J. Ensures safe use and optimal effect of supportive aids
K. Avoid lifting, excessive exercise, check with physician for return to work	K. Precautions to prevent injury
L. Resources to obtain supplies and equipment for home care	L. Provides information and access to sterile and unsterile supplies for wound care, postoperative preventive care
M. Information and phone numbers for physician, other health care providers needed during convalescence	M. Ensures follow-up appointments and contacts for home care assistance

preventive care

....

DEFINITION
The level of care provided to control risk factors and prevent occurrence of a disease (primary), promote detection and treatment of an existing disease as well as in cases of increased risk for disease (secondary), rehabilitate to promote or restore optimal function and prevent recurrence or complications of a disease (tertiary)

NURSING DIAGNOSIS
Knowledge deficit related to risk factors associated with primary prevention and measures to take to prevent disease

EXPECTED OUTCOMES
Health status maintained evidenced by exhibiting behaviors to prevent disease/injury related to identified risk factors (screening, assessments, physical examinations, immunizations, daily health practices)

INTERVENTION

I. Assess for:
  A. Knowledge and understanding of wellness requirements and behaviors needed to prevent disease

RATIONALE

  A. Provides a basis for appraisal of health risks and need for assistance and/or referrals to modify behaviors

INTERVENTION	RATIONALE
B. General health status, personal and family history (weight problems and conditions such as diabetes, hypertension and heart disease, breast cancer and other malignancies, asthma, allergic pulmonary/skin reactions)	B. Provides information about potential genetic or biologic risk factors
C. Age, sex, race (sensory perception changes of visual and auditory acuity, mobility impairment, trauma caused by falls, malignancies, hypertension, diabetes, dental problems)	C. Provides information about risk factors associated with these areas
D. Life-style, personal habits, and environment (dietary pattern that includes fat, fiber, calcium intake, alcohol and tobacco use, rest and exercise pattern, sexual activity, exposure to noise, allergens, fumes and high-risk injury environment, drug abuse, ability to cope with stress and solve problems)	D. Provides information about risk factors associated with behaviors and ADL
V. Teach patient/family: A. Rationale for primary care measures based on personal data base	A. Promotes compliance of behaviors to prevent disease

B. Need for screening procedures such as blood pressure, weights, mammography, Pap smear, test for occult blood, blood glucose and other blood tests, skin testing, visual and hearing acuity, others and where to obtain them (health fairs, physician office, diagnostic laboratory, clinics)	B. Screening determines a potential or actual health problem based on age, sex, history, and other assessment factors
C. Avoid smoking, sun exposure, drug use, and limit alcohol use	C. Promotes behaviors that prevent health problems
D. Consume balanced diet that includes caloric, fat, cholesterol, salt, caffeine, and sugar restrictions and additional calcium, fiber/bulk foods	D. Prevents obesity, cardiovascular and other diseases while maintaining optimal nutrition
E. Engage in a regular exercise regimen that correlates with age (walking, swimming, biking, sports)	E. Promotes health status and maintains integrity of all systems
F. Practice safe sex, contraception	F. Prevents unplanned pregnancy and sexually transmitted diseases
G. Wear protective gear during work and recreational activities (goggles, helmet, radiation badge, ear plugs), use seat belts, protective clothing, and skin screen when exposed to sun	G. Protects from accidents

INTERVENTION	RATIONALE
H. Perform monthly breast, testicle examinations, obtain yearly Pap smear, annual health check-up	H. Provides for early diagnosis of health problems in age groups at risk for specific diseases
I. Dental care that includes brushing, flossing, semi-annual checks for prophylaxis and repairs	I. Promotes dental hygiene
J. Obtain immunization for pneumonia, influenza, hepatitis, and those needed prior to travel	J. Provides protection from these diseases
K. Obtain genetic counseling if appropriate	K. Provides information based on family history or personal history
L. Group support, counseling for weight control, smoking cessation, stress reduction, alcohol abstinence	L. Provides resources to prevent health problems

NURSING DIAGNOSIS

Knowledge deficit related to identification of risk factors associated with vulnerable populations and measures to take for early detection and treatment (secondary prevention)

EXPECTED OUTCOMES

Health status maintained evidenced by compliance with screenings, examinations, and counseling for early detection of a problem resulting in the absence of possible complications of an existing condition

INTERVENTION	RATIONALE
I. Assess for:	
A. General health status, risk factors associated with any existing condition or lifestyle patterns discovered in the analysis of data from the history or physical examination	A. Identifies vulnerability to disease or detects the possibility of complications
B. Potential for immobility, fluid or electrolyte imbalance, infectious process, trauma, skin breakdown, and other risk factors/complications associated with disease	B. Provides basis for secondary preventive measures
C. Genetic factors, need for screening procedures related to age, sex, race associated with disease	C. Provides additional information regarding risk factors that cannot be modified but can result in disease
V. Teach patient/family:	
A. Rationale for secondary care measures based on assessment data	A. Promotes compliance of behaviors to promote early detection of disease and prevent complications

INTERVENTION	RATIONALE
B. Need for screening procedures such as visual and auditory tests (acuity, glaucoma, cataracts), Pap smear and mammography, breast and testicular examinations, laboratory and radiographic procedures for tuberculosis, diabetes, malignancies, and others; inform of frequency of screenings based on identified risks and age	B. Determines existence of health problem based on age, sex, physical examination, and history
C. Obtain genetic counseling, information and support from groups that identify with special health problems	C. Provides information and assistance based on risk factors associated with family or personal history
D. Arrange for dental and physical check-ups with regularity based on age and vulnerability for health problems	D. Promotes early identification and treatment to prevent complications in high-risk patients

NURSING DIAGNOSIS
Knowledge deficit related to prevention of complications associated with tertiary prevention and measures to take to ensure rehabilitation

EXPECTED OUTCOMES
Optimal health status or functional state achieved evidenced by compliance with and adaptation to a prescribed rehabilitative regimen following an acute illness or surgery or as an ongoing component of a life-style behavior change in chronic disorders

INTERVENTION	RATIONALE
I. Assess for: A. Motivation, values, adaptation ability, potential for rehabilitation, sources of support and assistance	A. Provides information regarding desire and decision-making ability involved in rehabilitation practices
B. Presence of injury, surgical intervention, chronic debilitating disease, temporary debilitation caused by an acute condition	B. Provides knowledge of condition with potential for disuse and other complications and type of rehabilitation needed
III. Administer: A. Antimicrobials PO as prophylaxis prior to invasive procedures	A. Provides protection in those with immune and other system disorders such as cardiac valvular condition
V. Teach patient/family: A. Rationale for tertiary care measures based on existing conditions	A. Promotes compliance of behaviors to promote a return to wellness and to prevent recurrence or complications
B. Schedule and participate in cardiac or pulmonary rehabilitation program following myocardial infarct, cardiac bypass surgery, chronic obstructive pulmonary disease, and others as applicable	B. Promotes optimal reconstitution and maintenance of these systems

C. Participate in physical and occupational therapy following stroke, coma, limb amputation, and others as applicable; chronic conditions such as arthritis, and others

C. Promotes optimal function in ADL and general feeling of well-being; prevents disuse syndrome

D. Utilize speech pathologist, other professionals involved in the interdisciplinary team that deals with medical conditions

D. Promotes rehabilitation related to specific needs

E. Prostheses application, use, care, such as in limb prosthesis, hearing aid, eye glasses or contact lenses, eye prosthesis, dentures, and assistive aids for ADL

E. Achieves optimal movement, vision and auditory acuity to correct deficits, independence in personal care and ADL

F. Obtain necessary blood tests prior to chemotherapy, anticoagulant therapy, insulin, and intermittent testing for therapeutic drug levels, lipid panel, electrolyte panel, and others as applicable

F. Prevents untoward affects of medications administered to treat specific conditions

G. Participate in substance/ alcohol use rehabilitation programs

G. Provides support for changes in behavior needed to prevent complications and encourage adaptation to a healthy life-style

neoplasm
(chemotherapy/external and internal radiation)

DEFINITION

Neoplasm, identified in this care plan as malignancy, carcinoma, or cancer, is a tumor that invades surrounding tissue with the capability of spreading to tissues at distant site(s) in the body. This unregulated cell destruction is the result of uncontrolled and abnormal cell growth. Any system can be affected by solid tumor organ sites or blood-forming organ sites. The exact cause of cancer is unknown, however theories have been developed to explain the etiology of this pathology. Risk factors for specific cancers have been identified with preventive/detection interventions developed (see Preventive Care). Physical changes resulting from the disease process and treatments as well as psychosocial responses to the disease impact every aspect of the patient's life. These are the basis for nursing care planning strategies for all malignancies regardless of organs or systems. This care plan is an attempt to deal with the problems common to all patients with cancer and their families and/or significant others.

Surgical procedures for cancer can be preventive, curative, palliative, done for tumor staging and include cystectomy (bladder), amputation (bone), craniotomy (brain), mastectomy (breast), bowel resection (colorectal), pneumonectomy (lung), neck dissection (oral), laryngectomy (larynx), prostatectomy (prostate), gastrectomy (stomach), hysterectomy/oophorectomy (uterus, cervix, ovaries), basal cell/melanoma resection (skin), orchiectomy (testes), thyroidectomy (thyroid), enucleation (eye), hepatobiliary resection (liver, gallbladder), splenectomy (blood-forming organs). The reader is advised to refer to the chapters related to the system involved in the pathology, Preoperative Care, and Postoperative Care plans for further information regarding surgical nursing care.

Chemotherapy protocols include alkylating agents, antimetabolites, antitumor antibiotics, plant alkaloids, nitrosureas, corticosteroids, hormones, and unclassified miscellaneous and investigational drugs. These drugs can be administered by oral, intramuscular, intravenous (peripheral or central vein), intrathecal, intra-arterial, intracavity, subcutaneous, topical, intraperitoneal, or perfusion routes.

Radiation therapy can be external or internal. External therapy (teletherapy) is administered by an x-ray machine containing a radionuclide with radiation to deep tissues. Internal therapy (brachytherapy) can be sealed or unsealed permanent-type radiation. Unsealed radiation therapy is the administration of a radionuclide by the oral or intravenous route that provides a systemic treatment. Sealed temporary type radiation therapy is the surgically placed radionuclide directly into a cavity, or implantation of needles, seeds, or catheters that contain a radionuclide directly into a tumor.

NURSING DIAGNOSES

Anxiety related to threat to self-concept (changes in appearance brought about by treatments), threat of death (life-threatening disease, poor prognosis), change in health status (diagnosis of cancer, outcome or complications of treatments), threat to socioeconomic status (cost of treatments), threat to role functioning (change in life-style resulting from radical surgery or other treatment protocols)

Fear related to learned response to identified life-threatening situation and potential for premature death, separation from support system (hospitalization and treatments)

EXPECTED OUTCOMES

Anxiety and fear decreased and within manageable levels evidenced by subjective verbalizations that anxiety and fear has subsided and distress and apprehension can be controlled with progressive ability to relax and manage stress, and objective observations of reduced restlessness with improved ability to rest and sleep, relaxed muscles and facial expression

INTERVENTION	RATIONALE
I. Assess for:	
A. Level of anxiety, verbal expression such as feelings of apprehension, uncertainty, tension; fear and reasons for it (consequences of disease and/or treatments)	A. Anxiety ranges from mild to panic state with verbal expressions indicating degree and responses to expect

INTERVENTION	RATIONALE
B. Nonverbal expressions of anxiety and fear such as shakiness, restlessness, jitteriness, facial tension, poor eye contact, quivering voice, palpitations, muscle tremors	B. May not be able to communicate feelings but reveal physical/psychological responses that assist to identify the level and changes in anxiety
C. Perceptions or misconceptions of anticipated surgery or therapy protocol as to outcome, affect on life-style, self-concept, and role functioning	C. Identifies and clarifies possible reasons for anxiety and fear
D. Feelings about the body area to be irradiated or affect of chemotherapy on visible body parts	D. Identifies source of anxiety regarding body image disturbance
E. Support systems available such as family, significant other, friends	E. Important aspect of caring and promotes sense of well-being to assist in reducing fear and anxiety
F. Response to information given regarding diagnosis and treatments	F. Identifies source of anxiety and causes of uneasiness about future health status
III. Administer:	
A. Anti-anxiety agent (alprazolam) PO	A. Acts to depress the CNS to relieve anxiety
IV. Perform/provide:	
A. Calm attitude of acceptance, understanding, and caring, positive response to behavior without expressing anger or disappointment	A. Provides emotional support and reassurance, enhances nurse–patient relationship and promotes trust, allows patient control of environment

INTERVENTION	RATIONALE
B. Calm, restful, noxious-free environment, prevent anxiety provoking situations	B. Decreases anxiety and fear by avoiding additional stimuli
C. Information about the specific therapy (brachytherapy, teletherapy, chemotherapy)	C. Reduces anxiety resulting from fear of the unknown
D. Allow time and encourage to express feelings of fear or resentment, use of defense mechanisms such as disbelief, denial, and anger	D. Assists to externalize and acknowledge anxiety and fear, promotes the temporary use of defense mechanisms to control the situation and reduce fear and anxiety
E. Listen and clarify perception of diagnosis and treatment regimen, assist to sort out facts and misinformation	E. Promotes successful resolution of crisis situation, identifies the basis for fear and anxiety by providing feedback
F. Encourage questions regarding diagnosis, therapy, and expected results, prognosis	F. Promotes review and understanding of physician-provided information
G. Stress reduction and relaxation techniques (music, imagery)	G. Reduces anxiety
H. Counseling referral	H. Provides assistance in decreasing or resolving anxiety
I. Discuss possibility of visit from one who has experienced a similar or the same disease	I. Provides support from one who has had and been treated for cancer

NURSING DIAGNOSES

Anticipatory grieving related to a perceived loss of physiopsychosocial well-being and potential loss of significant other (diagnosis of cancer)

Ineffective family coping: compromised: related to temporary preoccupation by those trying to manage emotional conflicts and personal suffering and are unable to perceive or act effectively in regard to patient's needs

Ineffective individual coping related to situational crisis (diagnosis of cancer, proposed treatment and effects), and personal vulnerability (pain, fatigue, uncertainty, and threat during diagnostic tests and procedures)

EXPECTED OUTCOMES

Progressive movement through stages of grief toward resolution evidenced by expression of feelings about potential loss and the beginning adaptation to diagnosis, treatment regimen, and possible outcome; family and individual's increasing comfort and ability to cope evidenced by verbalizations of reduced anxiety, participation in treatment protocol, display of factors that assist coping (problem solving, communications, social skills and support, control, hopefulness, positiveness, need to seek information, appropriate use of defense mechanisms)

INTERVENTION	RATIONALE
I. Assess for:	
A. Anger, guilt, sorrow, denial, expression of distress, changes in eating, sleep, activity patterns	A. Presence of grief responses prior to actual loss
B. Family expressions of fear, guilt, anxiety, grief, lack of information, hopelessness, or behaviors such as disproportionate protection, withdrawal or avoidance, excessive denial, making excessive demands	B. Reactions of family members coping with the crisis of an illness of loved one

INTERVENTION	RATIONALE
C. Individual expressions of inability to cope, meet needs, or ask for help when needed, helplessness, despair, or behaviors such as inappropriate use of defense mechanisms (denial, anger), withdrawal, hostility, blaming, passive acceptance, inability to problem-solve or meet role expectations	C. Reactions of the individual coping with cancer
D. Personal and family resources to cope with stress, fear, anxiety	D. Personal strengths and support systems assist in developing coping skills and strategies
E. Factors that can help or hinder grieving and/ or coping (flexibility, pessimism/optimism, hopeless/hopeful, disengagement/open communication, self-criticism)	E. Assists in determining the course and resolution of the grieving process, behaviors that can be identified to delay or enhance coping with diagnosis and treatment
IV. Perform/provide:	
A. Calm, reassuring, noxious-free environment with acceptance and support for expressions of feelings, fear, hope, and perceptions of individual and family members	A. Allows for an atmosphere conducive to venting of feelings during stages of grieving and coping behaviors

B. Time for individual and or family members to adapt to the diagnosis, treatments, and effect on life-style, to verbalize feelings and use of defense mechanisms, work through grief in an acceptable, nonjudgmental, nondestructive manner	B. Promotes a trusting relationship and understanding of different perspectives, and allows for temporary initial coping-enhancement mechanisms
C. Listen and clarify perceptions of diagnosis and treatment protocol, assist in sorting out facts and misinformation	C. Promotes successful resolution of crisis and establishes a more positive coping pattern
D. Assist to identify and review effective coping strategies and personal strengths with honesty and sincerity	D. Promotes self-esteem and control without undermining trust
E. Encourage questions regarding diagnosis, therapy, prognosis, and the grieving process and normal responses; provide answers with honesty and sensitivity	E. Promotes understanding of physician-provided information and positive support for hope and behaviors during the grieving process
F. Include patient and family in care planning and implementation and encourage support and participation of family members	F. Provides involvement in decision making to promote and accept treatment protocol
G. Acknowledge spiritual beliefs and encourage use of clergy or other religious resources/practices	G. Provides support system

NURSING DIAGNOSES

Pain related to physical (inflammation, necrosis of tissue and organs, compression or infiltration of vessels/nerves), psychological (fear, anxiety, depression), chemical (chemotherapy, radiation therapy) injuring agents resulting from the diagnosis and/or treatment of cancer

Sleep pattern disturbance related to internal factors of illness (cancer) and side effects of therapy (pain, nausea, pruritus, diarrhea) and psychological stress (anxiety, depression resulting from effects of chemotherapy/radiation therapy)

EXPECTED OUTCOMES

Pain relieved or controlled, adequate rest/sleep achieved following pharmacological (analgesia) or nonpharmacological (relaxation techniques, diversional activity) therapy evidenced by verbalizations that pain is minimal or absent and feeling rested with uninterrupted sleep

INTERVENTION	RATIONALE
I. Assess for:	
A. Pain descriptors and cause, especially if continuous and severe, nonverbal behavior (moaning, crying, guarding, restlessness, diaphoresis)	A. Pain can be incisional at implant site, caused by effects of chemotherapy affecting gastrointestinal mucosa (stomatitis, throat, esophageal), external irradiation (skin ulceration), or effects of tumor growth (pressure, infiltration)
B. Sleep pattern and complaints of feeling tired and not well rested; nonverbal behavior (yawning, disorientation, irritability, lethargy)	B. Indicates sleep disturbance that can lead to fatigue
C. Effectiveness of pain interventions used in the past	C. Considers most effective type of pain control

INTERVENTION	RATIONALE
III. Administer:	
A. Analgesic (morphine, meperidine) IM or IV by continuous drip, (fentanyl) SC by patient-controlled device (PCA), or nonopiate analgesics PO for mild to moderate pain	A. Opiate analgesics that acts on the CNS to alter and decrease pain perception
B. Sedative (diazepam, prazepam) PO	B. Acts to depress CNS to manage anxiety and promote rest and sleep
IV. Perform/provide:	
A. Environment that controls stimuli such as optimal lighting and temperature, noise reduction, calm and stress-free	A. Pain increased by stimuli; quiet, calm and pain-free environment facilitate sleep
B. Measure pain before pain becomes severe and modify based on response	B. Follows gate theory in timing of analgesia administration
C. Positive attitude when providing analgesia and other relief measures	C. Increases effectiveness of treatment
D. Support to body parts and use comfort aids such as pillows to maintain position when needed	D. Prevents unnecessary discomfort to irradiated parts
E. Backrub, position change for comfort, guided imagery, relaxation techniques, music, touch	E. Nonpharmacological measures to reduce pain sensation and promote comfort and sleep

INTERVENTION	RATIONALE
F. Dry, clean irradiated area and place bed cradle over painful areas	F. Reduces pain associated with moist desquamation and prevents pressure on exposed nerve endings of irradiated area
G. Discourage sleep during the day, intake of stimulating beverages prior to bedtime	G. Interferes with sleep at night
H. Usual rituals prior to sleep such as bedtime, reading, TV, use of bathroom, snack	H. Promotes continuation of sleep pattern
V. Teach patient/family:	
A. Cause of pain, duration based on disease and therapy effectiveness, pain that can be expected	A. Provides information about pain and discomforts to expect
B. Report any pain as soon as it is felt and request medication prior to activities or painful treatments	B. Prevents anticipatory fear of pain and allows for more effective relief than to attempt to control severe pain

NURSING DIAGNOSES

Altered nutrition: Less than body requirements related to inability to ingest food (anorexia, nausea, vomiting, pain, oral inflammation), inability to absorb nutrients (use of antibiotics and loss of intestinal surface [mucositis]) all resulting from disease process, chemotherapy/external radiation therapy

High risk for fluid volume deficit related to excessive losses (vomiting, diarrhea), altered intake of fluids (weakness, oral pain, nausea) all resulting from chemotherapy/external radiation therapy

EXPECTED OUTCOMES

Adequate control of nausea, vomiting, diarrhea, anorexia with appropriate nutritional and fluid intake evidenced by ability to retain foods and liquids with daily ingestion of calculated caloric, protein, carbohydrate, fat, and fluid requirements, stable weight pattern, I&O and electrolytes in balance.

INTERVENTION	RATIONALE
I. Assess for:	
A. Weakness, fatigue, pain, and effect on interest and desire to eat, presence of anorexia, nausea, vomiting, diarrhea, dysphagia, oral mucositis, altered taste perception, weight loss (20% under ideal weight)	A. Provides data related to reduced intake resulting in risk for malnutrition and I&O imbalance; chemotherapeutics and antibiotics cause these signs and symptoms and intestinal changes that affect absorption; malignancy can increase need for additional nutrition as cells proliferate and use more energy reserves; the drugs stimulate vomiting center, and the destruction of taste buds can cause the loss of taste sensation
B. Nutritional status that includes daily caloric intake	B. Nutritional requirements that are not met by oral intake can be administered by enteral feedings or total parenteral nutrition (TPN)
C. Daily fluid intake and types of fluids preferred, ability to secure fluids as desired	C. Provides information about fluids and possible need for assistance or increases in intake

INTERVENTION	RATIONALE
D. Thirst, decreased skin turgor, dry skin and mucous membranes, decreased urinary output, concentrated urine, increased sodium level	D. Indicates fluid and electrolyte losses and possible dehydration as a result of diarrhea and reduced fluid intake

II. Monitor, describe, record:

A. I&O q4–8h that includes losses through vomiting and diarrhea	A. Indicates possible abnormal ratio associated with dehydration
B. Daily Wt on same scale, at same time, wearing same clothing and compared to baselines; weekly anthropometric measurements	B. Indicates weight loss caused by muscle wasting, poor intake, and decreased nutrients to cells
C. VS q4–8 hours as appropriate	C. BP decreases, P increased and weak associated with fluid deficit
D. Serum electrolyte (Na), albumin, transferrin, amino acids, iron, creatinine, BUN	D. Indicates fluid deficit and/or nutritional deficiency
E. Urinary Sp. gr. and osmolality for increases	E. Increases in Sp. gr. over 1.025 indicates fluid deficit as urine concentration increases

III. Administer:

A. Anti-emetic (prochlorperazine, benzquinamide) PO or IM 12 hours prior to therapy and continue q4–6h up to and following therapy	A. Acts by blocking chemoreceptor zone that affects vomiting center

INTERVENTION	RATIONALE
B. Gastrointestinal stimulant (metoclopramide) PO	B. Acts to stimulate motility and increase gastric emptying to decrease nausea and vomiting
C. Vitamins and minerals PO	C. Replaces lost or depleted body elements and substances necessary for proper functioning

IV. Perform/provide:

INTERVENTION	RATIONALE
A. Environment that is free of odors, unpleasant sights during meals	A. Prevents stimulation of vomiting
B. Rest and mouth care prior to and following meals	B. Reduces fatigue and enhances desire to eat
C. Low-residue, liquid, high-caloric and high-protein diet with supplements of Ensure or others as desired; allow to select preference in foods and fluids	C. Provides additional calories for increased metabolism and dietary restrictions if vomiting or diarrhea are present
D. Change of position and other movements slowly and deliberate	D. Prevents stimulation of the chemoreceptor trigger zone that controls vomiting
E. Small, frequent servings of gelatin, soda, custards, wine, or brandy, other soft foods	E. Prevents early satiety and stimulates appetite
F. Fluid intake of 500 mL more than output or 2 to 4 L/day, allow to sip beverages if nauseated	F. Replaces fluid loss and prevents dehydration and crystal formation as a result of chemotherapy

INTERVENTION	RATIONALE
G. Raise head of bed following meals	G. Reduces stimulation to vomiting center and assists in retaining food
H. Administration of chemotherapeutic agents slowly and at night if possible	H. Decreases stimulation of vomiting center and prevents opportunity for nausea to occur
I. Tube or intravenous feedings if appropriate	I. Alternate methods of providing fluids and nutrition if oral intake not tolerated
J. Suggest consult with nutritionist	J. Provides assistance with food and supplement selections and ideas to stimulate appetite, flavorings if taste is impaired

NURSING DIAGNOSES

Diarrhea related to medications (antimetabolite chemotherapy), external radiation therapy causing inflammation and ulceration of intestinal mucosa and increased motility

Constipation related to medications (vinca alkaloid chemotherapy), gastrointestinal obstructive lesions (invasion by tumor), less-than-adequate fluid, dietary, and bulk intake (mucositis, anorexia, nausea), less-than-adequate physical activity (weakness, immobility), emotional status (apathy, depression), all reducing bowel peristalsis

EXPECTED OUTCOMES

Baseline bowel elimination pattern established evidenced by bowel sounds within normal expectations and soft, formed, brown, feces q1–2 days

INTERVENTION	RATIONALE
I. Assess for: A. Bowel elimination frequency, consistency, urgency, abdominal cramping, increased or decreased bowel sounds, feeling of rectal fullness, straining during defecation	A. Provides data regarding diarrhea or constipation
III. Administer: A. Antidiarrheal (diphenoxylate/atropine, kaolin/pectate) PO	A. Acts by inhibiting mucosal receptors causing peristalsis resulting in decreased motility, acts to decrease fluid content of feces and as mucosal protectant
B. Laxative/stool softener (docusate calcium, docusate sodium, hydrophilic psyllium) PO	B. Acts by lowering surface tension that allows water to soften feces, acts to provide bulk to feces for easier passage
IV. Perform/provide: A. Low residue and fat content in small, frequent meals or liquid diet; restrict spicy, raw, gas-producing foods	A. Allows bowel to rest and controls diarrhea by reducing irritation and bowel motility
B. Foods high in fiber if bowel inflammation not severe	B. Provides bulk to feces and prevents constipation
C. Increased fluid intake and daily exercises and mobility	C. Promotes peristalsis to prevent or treat constipation, provides essential fluid to soften feces or replace fluid loss if diarrhea present

INTERVENTION	RATIONALE
D. Privacy, sitting position on commode or toilet for defecation as soon as the urge is present, bed in high position if bedpan is used	D. Enhances defecation by gravity in an accustomed position
E. Care of perianal area following each episode of diarrhea	E. Prevents skin irritation from body excretions that leads to skin breakdown
F. Retention or cleansing enema if oral or suppository medications are ineffective	F. Promotes bowel elimination and prevents impaction

NURSING DIAGNOSES

Impaired skin integrity related to external mechanical factor (radiation therapy), internal somatic factors of medication, altered metabolic state, immunologic deficit, altered pigmentation, excretions/secretions (chemotherapeutic agents)

Altered oral mucous membrane related to medications (chemotherapy), radiation (head and neck irradiation) causing oral mucositis/stomatitis, lack of salivation, decreased oral fluids and foods causing dryness

EXPECTED OUTCOMES

Skin and mucous membrane intact and integrity maintained evidenced by cleanliness, dryness, and freedom from irritation, inflammation, lesions, or disruption

INTERVENTION	RATIONALE
I. Assess for:	
A. Skin changes, including erythema, urticaria, darkened color of mouth, nail beds, gums, or teeth, dryness, rash, pruritis, or disruption, sensitivity to the sun	A. Results from chemotherapy effect on skin injection sites, sebaceous and sweat glands, radiation effect of desquamation at entry and exit sites

INTERVENTION	RATIONALE
B. Redness, peeling, and blistering of the skin	B. Results from chemotherapy administration following irradiation
C. Oral mucosa for lesions, ulcers, leukoplakia, xerostomia, pain or discomfort, stomatitis, dysphagia	C. Results from therapy that decreases saliva or destroys salivary glands, malnutrition, rapid destruction of cells
D. Pruritis, irritation, ulceration of perianal and/or vulvar areas	D. Results from persistent diarrhea, effect of therapy on mucous membranes
III. Administer:	
A. Emollients (cornstarch, baking soda) to bath water; skin lubricant (Lubriderm, Aquaphor) TOP to skin other than radiation sites	A. Acts to relieve itching, dry skin, and possible cracking and breakdown
B. Protectants (A&D ointment, Karaya gel) TOP to anal area	B. Protects perianal skin
C. Moisturizers (petroleum jelly, cocoa butter, lanolin) TOP to lips, artificial saliva (Ora-Lub) TOP to oral mucosa	C. Provides moisture to lips and oral mucosa
D. Astringent (chlorhexidine gluconate, Domboro solution) as cleansing agent or soak to wound	D. Acts to treat moist desquammation caused by external radiation

INTERVENTION	RATIONALE
E. Anesthesia/analgesia TOP applied with soft-tipped applicator	E. Promotes comfort and prevents injury to oral tissues
IV. Perform/provide:	
A. Gentle cleansing of skin with mild soap, tepid water; pat dry with soft cloth, avoid washing or removing radiation site markings	A. Avoids further skin irritation while cleansing and relieving pruritis
B. Exposure of irradiated areas to air if possible	B. Promotes return of skin integrity
C. Cool, moist compress to itchy areas and cool environment, apply pressure to areas	C. Promotes comfort and relieves pruritis without scratching skin
D. Occlusive or nonadherent dressing to skin disruption	D. Treatment for skin reaction to external radiation
E. Dry, clean, wrinkle-free linens, devices such as sheepskin, flotation pads	E. Promotes comfort and prevents possible irritants or pressure to skin surface
F. Cleanse and dry perianal area after each bowel elimination	F. Prevents irritation or excoriation
G. Gentle oral hygiene following meals and as needed, mouth wash q2–4h with saline, hydrogen peroxide, sodium bicarbonate solution, unwaxed floss; spray oral cavity with water q1–2h if unable to rinse	G. Decreases dryness and promotes comfort if stomatitis is present

H. Remove dentures if oral cavity is painful except at mealtime

H. Provides relief of pain caused by pressure of dentures

I. Restrict hot, spicy foods, citrus beverages from the diet, and include ice, ice cream, cool beverages, popsicles, soft foods; restrict alcohol and smoking; offer hard candy for dry mouth

I. Irritates oral mucosa; provides smoothing effect if oral pain is present, stimulates salivation by sucking on ice or candy

J. Avoid use of tape, lotions, deodorants, strong soaps on skin

J. Results in skin irritation and possible breakdown

V. Teach patient/family:
   A. Avoid scratching, sun exposure, application of harsh substances to skin during therapy

A. Results in irritation and sunburn

NURSING DIAGNOSES

Altered protection related to abnormal blood profile (leukopenia, thrombocytopenia, anemia), drug therapy (antineoplastics), disease (cancer)

High risk for infection related to inadequate primary defenses (skin moist desquamation or oral mucosa disruption), inadequate secondary defenses (leukopenia, neutropenia, immunosuppression), pharmaceutical agents (chemotherapy), invasive procedure (IV, infusion device, right atrial catheter administration of chemotherapy)

EXPECTED OUTCOMES

Risk for infection and bleeding tendency minimized or absent evidenced by VS and temperature within baseline levels, cultures of urine, sputum, vaginal, oral mucosa free of pathogens, laboratory tests (platelets, WBC, neurophils) within normal ranges except when lowest count can be expected following chemotherapy, urinary pattern and breath sounds within baseline parameters

INTERVENTION	RATIONALE
I. Assess for:	
A. Temperature of >100°F, chills, cough, chest pain, adventitious breath sounds, sore throat, oral pain, urine cloudiness and foul-smelling odor, urgency, burning, and frequency on urination	A. Indicates infectious process resulting from myelosuppression affecting lungs, urinary tract, and oral mucosa
B. Skin and mucous membranes for redness, irritation, drainage	B. Indicates possible infectious process resulting from chemotherapy/radiation
C. Skin for petechiae, ecchymosis, feces and urine for blood, hemarthrosis, gums for bleeding, hemoptysis, epistaxis, hematemesis	C. Indicates bleeding resulting from myelosuppression, malignant infiltration, and/or therapy
D. Fatigue, dizziness, pallor, tachycardia, dyspnea, palpitations	D. Indicates anemia resulting from persistent bleeding
II. Monitor, describe, record:	
A. VS and T, lung sound q4h	A. Elevated temperature indicates infection, increased pulse associated with temperature and anemia, respiratory changes and presence of adventitious sounds indicates pulmonary infection
B. WBC and absolute neutrophil count	B. Leukopenia and neutropenia resulting from myelosuppression predisposing to infection when absolute neutrophil count <1000 cells/mm^3

INTERVENTION	RATIONALE
C. Platelets	C. Thrombocytopenia resulting from platelet destruction, myelosuppression causing increased risk for bleeding when count <20,000/mm^3
D. RBC, Hct, Hb	D. Decreased by tumor infiltration, myelosuppression causing bleeding and resulting in anemia
E. Culture of urine, sputum, drainage of lesions	E. Identifies causative organisms of infection and antimicrobial sensitivities

III. Administer:

A. Broad-spectrum antibiotic PO or IV	A. Preventive measure if infection is suspected, or treatment if diagnosis of infection is made
B. Granulocyte colony-stimulating factor (filgrastim) PO	B. Acts to stimulate immature neutrophils and activate mature neutrophils to decrease infection in myelosuppressive states
C. Transfusion of platelet products, packed red blood cells IV	C. Treatment for thrombocytopenia or anemia

IV. Perform/provide:

A. Handwashing with antimicrobial product using appropriate technique prior to each contact or care activity	A. Prevents transmission of micro-organisms to decrease risk for infection

INTERVENTION	RATIONALE
B. All procedures using sterile technique and supplies, especially invasive ones	B. Prevents contamination and risk for infection
C. Increased fluid intake to 2500 mL/day if allowed	C. Promotes urination to prevent stasis and risk for urinary tract infection
D. Position change, cough, deep breathing q3–4h	D. Prevents respiratory tract stasis and risk for pulmonary infection
E. Assistance with perineal care following urination and defecation such as gentle cleansing, wiping from front to back for female, catheter care if needed	E. Prevents contamination with pathogens to skin, mucosa, and urinary tract
F. Meticulous skin and oral care to prevent or treat irritation, breakdown, especially infusion sites	F. Prevents infection via first line of defense
G. IV site, solution, and tubing changes per protocol	G. Prevents trauma and introduction of pathogens
H. Avoid rectal temperature, administration of enemas, catheterization, injections, or any other invasive procedures if possible	H. Prevents possible trauma, introduction of pathogens, and bleeding
I. Obtain cultures from appropriate site and send to laboratory	I. Provides for testing to identify pathogens responsible for infection and effective antimicrobials for therapy

INTERVENTION	RATIONALE
J. Use smallest-gauge needle for injections, apply firm pressure to site	J. Prevents excessive bleeding
K. Use electric razor for shaving, soft tooth brush for oral care	K. Prevents excessive bleeding in myelosuppression
L. Avoid blood pressure cuff overinflation	L. Prevents trauma and skin bruising
M. Adequate rest and moderate exercises, adequate nutrition	M. Protects against potential for infection

V. Teach patient/family:

A. Avoid straining during defecation and using force when blowing nose	A. Encourages bleeding as these activities traumatize mucosa
B. Wash hands after bathroom use, prior to eating and other activities	B. Reduces risk for infection
C. Avoid exposure to those with infections or who are ill, have recently been vaccinated, avoid contact with cat or dog feces or sharing utensils/clothing with others	C. Prevents transmission of pathogens from others

NURSING DIAGNOSES

Activity intolerance related to generalized weakness (destruction of cells by therapy regimen, increased metabolic rate), causing increasing use of energy and deconditioned state

Fatigue related to altered body chemistry (chemotherapy), overwhelming psychological or emotional demands (diagnosis of cancer, diagnostic tests and procedures), increased energy requirements to perform activities of daily living (ADL) (weakness, vulnerable state, neurotoxicity)

EXPECTED OUTCOME

Conservation of strength and endurance during therapy evidenced by verbalizations of feeling less fatigued and tired, participation in ADL within limitations (imposed or otherwise), improved rest/sleep pattern, general mental participation and interest shown in activities, procedures, and treatments

INTERVENTION	RATIONALE
I. Assess for: A. Ability to perform ADL, verbal complaints of fatigue, weakness, pain or other discomforts, lack of energy or desire to participate in care	A. Provides indications of limitations resulting from chemotherapy/internal radiation
B. Emotional lability of irritability, lethargy, disinterest	B. Nonverbal signs of fatigue
C. Rest/sleep pattern, bed rest status	C. Leads to deconditioning and weakness
IV. Perform/provide: A. Care and treatments at times most likely to support independent ADL such as following rest, and at optimal effectiveness of analgesia	A. Facilitates participation in ADL
B. Periods of rest or sleep with activities scheduled to avoid interruptions	B. Promotes needed rest to treat fatigue

INTERVENTION	RATIONALE
C. Articles needed placed within reach	C. Places objects for easy access to conserve energy
D. Environment that is noxious-free, comfortable, noise and activity-free	D. Reduces fatigue by promoting rest
E. Assistance when needed with encouragement and praise for all attempts at self-care	E. Maximizes interest in self-care
F. Active or passive ROM if on bed rest, progressive ambulation with or without assistance	F. Provides activity to increase tolerance and endurance
G. Assistance with plan to adjust daily changes that maintains activities, rest, nutritional, fluid, and elimination needs	G. Promotes activities within limitations to prevent fatigue and avoid those that increase fatigue
V. Teach patient/family:	
A. Inform that fatigue is common side effect of therapy and will subside and gradually disappear by 2 to 4 weeks following therapy	A. Provides reassurance that weakness and fatigue are temporary

NURSING DIAGNOSES

Body image disturbance related to biophysical and psychosocial factors (chemotherapy/external radiation), causing alopecia, skin and nail changes, weight loss

Diversional activity deficit related to environmental lack of diversional activity (protective isolation precautions), causing decreased stimulation and boredom

Impaired social interaction related to therapeutic isolation (internal radiation), causing barriers to communication, absence of family and/or significant other

EXPECTED OUTCOMES

Improved self-esteem evidenced by change in appearance brought about by use of wig and eventual return of hair growth, clothing to cover skin pigmentation, and weight gain to eventually reach baseline; social diversion and interaction provided evidenced by verbalizations that boredom decreased, and appropriate preparation of family to allow for visitation, participation in activities

INTERVENTION	RATIONALE
I. Assess for:	
A. Interests, hobbies, desire for specific activities, feelings of loneliness, changes in social involvement	A. Provides a selection of possible activities to remedy therapeutic isolation
B. Feelings regarding isolation procedures and effect on self-concept, family relationships	B. Prevents transmission of pathogens to patient during period of immunosuppression and causes negative feelings about imposed limitations
C. Remarks and feelings about temporary or permanent hair loss, skin changes (erythema, pigmentation, telangiectasia, roughness), weight loss, nail changes (thick, ridged, detached, dark color), changes in life-style and role function	C. Reflects devasting effect that consequences of therapy have on body image

INTERVENTION	RATIONALE
IV. Perform/provide:	
A. Radio, TV, newspaper, books, games, cards; arrange to have work brought from home	A. Provides diversion and stimulation, reinforces contact with the outside
B. Visits from family and friends, instruct in precautions to take to avoid exposure to radiation and prevent exposure of patient to pathogens	B. Reduces feelings of loneliness and displays interest and caring
C. Private room and bath with appropriate signs posted, limit contact to 1/2 hour and wear monitoring device, maintain a distance of 6 feet or 20 feet for longer interactions, limit linen change, flush toilet 2 to 3 times	C. Precautions taken in caring for patients treated with internal radiation
D. Encourage positive comments, interest in appearance, assist to identify inner resources and coping skills	D. Improves self-esteem and feelings of self-worth
E. Suggest early acquisition of a wig, hat, or scarf to wear, clothing that covers visible body parts and conceals thinness	E. Provides covering if complete or uneven hair loss occurs or skin becomes discolored
F. Suggest makeup and grooming ideas	F. Promotes adaptation to body image changes during therapy

INTERVENTION	RATIONALE
V. Teach patient/family:	
A. Use of mild shampoo, q1wk, avoid curlers, dryers, hot irons, hair spray, harsh brushing or combing	A. Prevents damage to hair and additional loss
B. Avoid exposure to sun and to use a sun screen	B. Photosensitivity can result in skin burn
C. Inform that hair growth usually returns following therapy with a change in color and texture and nails return to normal	C. Provides reassurance that hair loss is temporary

NURSING DIAGNOSIS
Sexual dysfunction related to altered body structure or function from gonadal dysfunction (chemotherapy), reduced testosterone and sexual activity (external radiation), impotence, infertility, vaginal mucositis

EXPECTED OUTCOME
Recognition and understanding of treatment effect on sexuality and sexual function evidenced by expression of possible resolution of these effects

INTERVENTION	RATIONALE
I. Assess for:	
A. Impotence, infertility, sterility; vaginal mucositis, weakness, fatigue	A. Results from chemotherapy/ external radiation to ovaries/testes causing physical discomfort and changes in sexual patterns
B. Feelings about changes in sexual function (temporary or permanent)	B. Changes brought about from chemotherapy/ external radiation cause psychological stress

INTERVENTION	RATIONALE
C. Impaired relationship, withdrawal from significant other	C. Results from changes in sexuality
D. Willingness to discuss sexual activities and concerns	D. Provides information about level of receptiveness to alternatives or basis for referral
IV. Perform/provide: A. Reinforce physician information about therapy effect and treatment options/methods for impotence and/or sterility	A. Promotes understanding and possible alternatives to resolve problems of sexuality
B. Information about sexual therapist referral that includes sexual partner	B. Promotes resolution of sexual dysfunction

NURSING DIAGNOSIS

Knowledge deficit related to information regarding ongoing chemotherapy protocol and physical/psychosocial care of all affected systems; preventive measures to avoid complications of therapy

EXPECTED OUTCOMES

Appropriate verbalizations and performance of care measures following instruction and information about life-style modifications, prevention of, and/or treatments for all side effects of chemotherapy evidenced by ongoing compliance with and successful completion of therapy

INTERVENTION	RATIONALE
I. Assess for: A. Knowledge and understanding of therapy protocol and rationale	A. Provides a basis for teaching plan and techniques to utilize

INTERVENTION	RATIONALE
B. Learning readiness and ability of patient and family to provide ongoing care and skills to perform procedures	B. Provides information about special needs to ensure compliance with and adaption to the therapy (nutritionist, social services, nursing services, resources for equipment and supplies)
IV. Perform/provide:	
A. Written medication protocol and care plan that includes preventive measures, signs and symptoms to report	A. Provides documentation for patient and family to remind and/or reinforce information needed to ensure compliance
B. Time for questions and explanations during instruction	B. Provides clarification of information given
V. Teach patient/family:	
A. Chemotherapeutic agents, how the drugs are administered (route), side effects and toxic effects of the drugs, expected outcome in regard to the cancer	A. Provides information about the drugs and expected effect of the therapy
B. Length of therapy and importance of keeping all appointments for medication administration and laboratory tests	B. Promotes compliance with protocol and identifies potential for severe side effects (immunosuppression, bleeding tendency)
C. Relaxation techniques such as deep breathing, imagery, music, and diversional activities	C. Reduces anxiety and assists to cope with illness, therapy, and effects

INTERVENTION	RATIONALE
D. Handwash technique, careful and gentle cleansing of skin and mucous membranes of oral cavity, perianal/rectal and genitalia areas, avoid exposure to crowds or people with infection, avoid douche and enema administration, maintain separate cleansing and other articles used for personal hygiene and meals	D. Prevents infection/inflammation when immunosuppression is present
E. Use of nontraumatic articles for personal hygiene such as soft toothbrush, electric razor, take axillary temperature, avoid straining at defecation, harsh blowing of nose, clothing that constricts; inform of method to control bleeding by pressure	E. Prevents bleeding from mucous membranes during immunosuppression
F. Administration of analgesia orally or by patient-controlled device, medications such as anti-emetics, antidiarrheals, stool softeners, antimicrobials, other prescribed drugs	F. Provides intermittent or continuous pain relief or control; nausea, vomiting, diarrhea, constipation, infection, or other medication regimens
G. Daily fluid and dietary intake and supplemental calories if needed, provide food lists and suggestions to improve appetite and control nausea and vomiting, inclusions and restrictions of food selections	G. Fulfills requirements to assist in maintaining health status and prevent complications related to infection, skin breakdown, malnutrition

INTERVENTION	RATIONALE
H. Care of venous catheter or implanted infusion device, Ommaya reservoir	H. Promotes patency of device and prevents infection at insertion site, displacement or dislodgement of device
I. Measures to conserve energy and aids to use; daily exercise routine within limitations	I. Maintains strength and endurance to prevent weakness and fatigue
J. Measures to preserve body image changes brought about by alopecia; skin and nail changes, thinness	J. Maintains self-esteem while visible effects of chemotherapy occur
K. Resources in the community for home care such as American Cancer Society, Hospice, others	K. Assists to secure additional information, care, and support

NURSING DIAGNOSIS
Knowledge deficit related to information regarding internal radiation therapy and physical/psychosocial care, preventive measures to avoid complications of therapy

EXPECTED OUTCOMES
Appropriate verbalizations of the internal radiation procedure and performance of preventive measures following instruction and information about postradiation care

INTERVENTION	RATIONALE
V. Teach patient/family:	
A. Type of radiation, organ to be treated, route or placement (oral, IV, surgical implantation, intracavitary injection)	A. Provides preradiation information regarding the procedure and what to expect

INTERVENTION	RATIONALE
B. Radionuclide is administered in water or a capsule and swallowed, that body fluids (saliva, urine, feces, other fluids) are considered contaminated for 4 days, and the radionuclide is metabolized and excreted in 2 weeks, to flush toilet two to three times following use, careful handwashing after contact with body fluids, to report nausea for first 4 hours following ingestion to prevent contamination and loss of radiation	B. Pre- and postinternal oral radiation information given to patient
C. Precautions such as sleeping alone, flushing toilet, refraining from kissing family members, storing used linens in plastic bag for 10 days before washing, wash linens and dishes separately, avoid sharing any personal hygiene articles	C. Provides information for home care for 14 days following oral radiation therapy to prevent exposure of radioactivity to others
D. Radionuclide is administered by surgical insertion; that essential care is given, fluids are encouraged, that body fluids are not contaminated, that activity is restricted to prevent displacement of the implant, and no precautions are needed following discharge except avoiding use of tampons, intercourse for 3 weeks	D. Pre- and post-internal intracavitary or interstitial radionuclide implantation information given to the patient

INTERVENTION	RATIONALE
E. Time and distance requirements postradiation	E. Provides precautions needed to protect personnel and visitors from radiation exposure
F. Report drainage, odor, bleeding or pain at radiation site, changes in urinary patterns, skin texture, appetite, bowel elimination, or other complaints	F. Signs and symptoms of complications of internal radiation, radiation cystitis, tissue fibrosis
G. Resources in the community for home care (educational, social, personal care)	G. Assists to secure additional information, care, and support

NURSING DIAGNOSIS
Knowledge deficit related to information regarding external radiation therapy and physical/psychosocial care, preventive measures to avoid complications of therapy

EXPECTED OUTCOMES
Appropriate verbalizations of the external radiation procedure and performance of preventive measures following instruction and information about postradiation care

INTERVENTION	RATIONALE
V. Teach patient/family:	
A. External radiation and site, how performed, expected response and outcome in regard to cancer, side effects of the therapy	A. Provides information about the therapy and its effect

INTERVENTION	RATIONALE
B. Length of therapy and importance of keeping all appointments for ongoing therapy	B. Promotes compliance with treatment and opportunity to observe for untoward effects
C. Skin changes at irradiated site such as peeling, pruritis, pigmentation and care procedures such as gentle cleansing with mild soap and warm water and avoiding markings, then pat dry, avoid rubbing or scratching, use of deodorant, constrictive clothing, exposure to sun, tape to skin, to apply skin lubricant, emollients, care of skin breakdown or desquamation response (wound care)	C. Skin responses to external radiation and care to prevent or minimize damage
D. Measures to take to protect the patient from invasion by infectious agents, blood loss, weight loss from anorexia, nausea, vomiting, and fatigue (see Knowledge Deficit nursing diagnosis for chemotherapy)	D. Prevents infection, bleeding, fatigue, fluid/nutritional deficits common with immunosuppression
E. Resources in the community for home care	E. Assists to secure additional information, care, and support

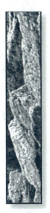

Cardiovascular
Systems Standards

cardiovascular systems data base

abdominal aortic aneurysm/resection and graft

acute venous insufficiency (thrombophlebitis/thrombosis)

chronic venous insufficiency (venous ulcer/varicose veins
and ligation)

coronary artery disease/angina pectoris

diminished arterial circulation to extremities/arterial bypass

heart failure/pulmonary edema

hypertension

inflammatory heart disease (endocarditis/myocarditis/pericarditis)

myocardial infarction

permanent pacemaker

cardiovascular systems data base

HISTORICAL DATA REVIEW

Past Events:

1. Acute and/or chronic cardiac, arterial, or venous disease or disorders, presence of other diseases that affect the cardiovascular system (diabetes, anemia, renal disorders, chronic obstructive pulmonary disease, coagulation disorders)
2. Chronic signs and symptoms related to cardiac or vascular disorders (pain, dyspnea, orthopnea, palpitations, edema, fatigue, syncope, color change, or coldness and numbness of extremities)
3. Cardiovascular disease, diabetes, asthma of family members
4. Childhood diseases (rheumatic fever, streptococcus infections) that can be related to cardiac conditions
5. Anxiety, personality traits, stressors, dietary restrictions, exercise routine, tobacco/alcohol/caffeine use
6. Treatments, oxygen, rehabilitation associated with cardiovascular system, presence of pacemaker
7. Medications (prescription and over-the-counter) for cardiovascular and non-cardiovascular conditions, use of recreational/athletic enhancement drugs
8. Hospitalizations and feelings about care, surgery associated with or affecting heart or blood vessels

Present Events:

1. Medical diagnoses associated with or affecting cardiac function, vascular patency and function
2. Pulse rate/minute, rhythm, amplitude, pulse characteristics (bounding, strong, weak), apical pulse, apical-radial pulse
3. Blood pressure (systolic/diastolic) both arms in sitting, standing, lying, and paradoxical blood pressure, pulse pressure
4. Pain in chest (substernal, precordial) radiating to jaw, neck, shoul-

ders, arms and severity, pain in leg calf or in legs during ambulation or standing, aching in legs, headache; factors that precipitate and alleviate pain
5. Dyspnea, exertional dyspnea, orthopnea, tachypnea, fatigue, edema and weight gain, vertigo, level of consciousness and mentation
6. Redness, pallor, cyanosis of extremity skin, varicosities or scars
7. Activities of daily living and effect on cardiovascular status and vital signs, activity intolerance, insomnia, fatigue, restlessness, preferences in positioning for rest and sleep

PHYSICAL ASSESSMENT DATA REVIEW

1. Symmetry of chest, pulsations in aortic area, pulmonary area, ventricular areas, and point of maximal intensity (PMI)
2. Cyanosis of lips, ear lobes, oral mucosa
3. Symmetry and skin color/texture of arms, legs, hands, and feet, color changes when extremity dangling or elevated, temperature of extremities
4. Eruptions, ulcers, or exudate on extremities, hair distribution, calf pain, Homan's sign
5. Venous enlargement, smooth, dilated, tortuous in legs, distension of neck veins, dependent or pitting edema in legs
6. Femoral, popliteal, carotid, temporal, and dorsalis pedis pulses and characteristics, capillary refill
7. Carotid artery pulsations and bruits
8. Heart sounds for extra heart sounds, apical pulse, murmurs and characteristics, clicks, snaps and characteristics, friction rub
9. Lung sounds for rales or crackles

NURSING DIAGNOSES CONSIDERATIONS

1. Activity intolerance
2. Altered tissue perfusion (renal, cardiopulmonary, cerebral, gastrointestinal, peripheral)
3. Anxiety
4. Decreased cardiac output
5. Fluid volume excess
6. Risk for infection
7. Risk for injury

8. Impaired gas exchange
9. Knowledge deficit
10. Pain

GERIATRIC CONSIDERATIONS

The pumping action of the heart and the transporting function of the vascular system are affected by organic changes (reduced stroke volume and cardiac output, atherosclerosis) associated with the aging process. Normally the aging cardiovascular system adapts to the reduction in activities of the older adult, but these changes can result in difficulty to adapt if an illness is present that can increase the workload of this sytem. Cardiovascular changes associated with aging that should be considered when assessing the geriatric patient include:

1. Reduced heart size caused by decreased activity or immobility, heart displacement by kyphosis or scoliosis
2. Hemodynamic stress resulting in thickening and sclerosing of endocardium, rigidity of valves, increased resistance to blood flow
3. Gradual increased connective tissue with decreased elastin resulting in stiffness and increased size of veins and large arteries in muscle, thicker heart valves, endocardium and left ventricle muscles, increased resistance to compression when taking pulse
4. Atherosclerosis resulting in calcification, reduced lumen size, and circulation abnormalities
5. Decreased venous valve effectiveness resulting in decreased blood return to the heart, reduction in activity causing distended superficial veins and varicosities
6. Decreased left ventricle work resulting in reduced cardiac output, reduced cardiac reserve resulting in poor reaction to stress
7. Decreased blood flow through coronary arteries by 35 percent by age 60, muscle fiber loss resulting in reduced contractility and filling capacity
8. Decreased ability of heart to utilize oxygen resulting in ischemia and pain
9. Decreased capillary permeability resulting in ineffective transport of nutrients and oxygen to tissues and removal of waste products
10. Increased systolic and diastolic blood pressures with widening of pulse pressure, longer time needed for systolic to return to baseline following exercise
11. Increased peripheral resistance resulting in an increase in blood pressure and workload of the heart

12. Increased pulse variability and vagal tone resulting in decreased pulse rate
13. Decreased sensitivity to pressure changes by baroreceptors in aorta and carotid arteries resulting in slow response to postural changes
14. Cellular changes, conduction system changes, neurogenic effect that can impair vasomotor response of vessels resulting in electrocardiography (ECG) changes

DIAGNOSTIC LABORATORY TESTS AND PROCEDURES

1. Electrocardiography (ECG), Holter monitoring, signal averaged ECG, exercise ECG (stress test), nuclear scans such as thallium stress tests and gated blood pool imaging, His bundle electrophysiology, chest x ray (CXR), cardiac catheterization, cardiac angiography, echocardiography, transesophageal echocardiography, phonocardiography, magnetic resonance imaging (MRI), positron emission tomography (PET), Doppler ultrasonography, computeriezd tomography (CT), plethysmography, contrast arteriography and venography, vascular endoscopy, venous and arterial Doppler and duplex imaging studies, ankle-brachial index
2. Complete blood count (CBC), cardiac enzymes such as creatine kinase (CK) and isoenzyme CK-MB, lactic acid dehydrogenase (LDH) and cardiac associated isoenzymes, coagulation tests such as prothrombin time (PT), partial thromboplastin time (PTT), erythrocyte sedimentation rate (ESR), lipid tests such as cholesterol, triglycerides, high- and low-density lipoproteins (HDL, LDL), electrolytes such as potassium (K), sodium (Na), calcium (Ca), blood urea nitrogen (BUN), creatinine, arterial blood gases (ABGs), routine urinalysis

MEDICATIONS

1. Anti-arrhythmics: bretylium tosylate, quinidine sulfate, verapamil, propranolol hydrochloride, tocainide hydrochloride, moricizine, acebutolol, lidocaine
2. Anticoagulants: warfarin, heparin
3. Antihypertensives: vasodilators (hydralazine), beta-adrenergic blockers (propranolol hydrochloride, metoprolol tartrate, nadolol), alpha-adrenergic blockers (prazosin hydrochloride, phentolamine mesylate), central-adrenergic blockers (clonidine hydrochloride, methyldopa), peripheral-adrenergic blockers (reserpine combined with a diuretic), calcium-channel blockers (nicardipine hydrochlo-

ride, nifedipine, verapamil hydrochloride, diltiazem hydrochloride), angiotensin-converting enzyme inhibitors (captopril, enalapril maleate, lisinopril, ramipril)
4. Antimicrobials: penicillin, streptomycin
5. Beta-adrenergic blockers: propranolol hydrochloride, metroprolol tartrate, atenolol, isoproterenol, dobutamine
6. Calcium-channel blockers: diltiazem hydrochloride, nifedipine, verapamil hydrochloride
7. Diuretics: furosemide (loop), chlorothiazide (thiazide), spironolactone (potassium-sparing)
8. Fibrinolytics: streptokinase, urokinase, anistreplase
9. Inotropics: digoxin, digitoxin, dopamine, amrinone
10. Lipid-lowering agents: cholestyramine, colestipol, lovastatin, pravastatin
11. Oxygen: delivered via nasal cannula or face mask
12. Vasodilators: nitroglycerin, isosorbide dinitrate

abdominal aortic aneurysm/resection and graft

DEFINITION

The abnormal dilatation of the abdominal portion of the aorta most commonly caused by atherosclerosis and associated hypertension. This results in a degeneration and weakness of the wall of this large artery, and a segment gradually becomes permanently dilated. This plan includes specific care related to the risk of rupture and the surgical repair of an abdominal aortic aneurysm. The surgery is similar to any abdominal procedure and this plan can be used in association with the PREOPERATIVE CARE, POSTOPERATIVE CARE, and HYPERTENSION care plans for general medical and surgical care.

NURSING DIAGNOSES

Anxiety related to threat of death (sudden rupture of aneurysm preoperatively or rupture of bypass graft postoperatively)

Risk for injury related to possible complications from aneurysm (impending aneurysm rupture preoperatively, risk of bypass graft rupture postoperatively, or distal embolism pre- and postoperatively)

EXPECTED OUTCOMES

Anxiety decreased and within manageable limits evidenced by verbalization that anxiety has been reduced following information about signs and symptoms of aneurysm expansion or indication of rupture to monitor and report; risk of rupture prevented and embolism absent evidenced by vital signs, peripheral pulse and color and skin temperature of extremities within baseline determinations

INTERVENTION	RATIONALE
I. Assess for:	
A. Level of anxiety, verbal expression of concerns and reasons for it such as fear, uncertainty, apprehension	A. Anxiety ranges from mild to severe, some anxiety is normal when an individual feels a threat as a result of an illness
B. Nonverbal expression of anxiety such as restlessness, irritability	B. May not be able to communicate feelings but reveal responses that assist in identifying level of anxiety
C. Flank, groin, or lumbar pain, lower extremity changes in sensation and movement, feeling of abdominal fullness, pulsating mass in abdomen	C. Indicates expansion in size of aneurysm by pressure on spinal nerves and abdominal organs
D. Increased flank pain radiating to lower abdominal, groin, or genital area, abdominal distention with an increasing abdominal girth, decreased peripheral pulses, reduction in blood pressure in thigh	D. Indicates leakage and impending rupture of aneurysm that is >5 cm in diameter
E. Severe flank and back pain, light-headed feeling, pulsating abdominal mass, ecchymosis in flank and perineal area, nausea, sudden drop in blood pressure (<100) and increased pulse (>100)	E. Indicates shock associated with ruptured abdominal aortic aneurysm (or graft postoperatively)
F. Diminishing peripheral pulses, extremities cool with pallor, extremities, groin, or abdominal pain, numbness in extremities	F. Indicates distal embolism caused by thrombus from the aneurysm preoperatively or from the graft site postoperatively

INTERVENTION	RATIONALE
II. Monitor, describe, record:	
A. VS, apical pulse, peripheral pulses q2–4h or as appropriate, and compare to baselines	A. Changes can be caused by hypovolemic shock following rupture or arterial embolism in extremity
B. RBC, Hct, Hb, for decreases, increases in WBC	B. Occurs as a result of aneurysm rupture and hemorrhage to various sites
C. Abdominal ultrasonography every 6 months	C. Monitors changes in the size of the aneurysm
III. Administer:	
A. Antihypertensives PO	A. Acts to control blood pressure as long-term exposure of the aortic wall to high pressure results in dilatation
IV. Perform/provide:	
A. Environment that promotes trust and calm attitude of caring and acceptance of behaviors	A. Provides support and reduces anxiety, enhances rapport and nurse–patient relationship
B. Allow for expression of fears and concerns, listen and provide feedback to clarify behavior	B. Assists in identifying and acknowledging anxiety and fear
C. Limit activity, lifting or pulling heavy objects, or straining during defecation, place on bed rest if appropriate	C. Reduces risk of aneurysm rupture preoperatively and graft rupture postoperatively by preventing rise in blood pressure

D. Position of legs in straight position without use of knee gatch or bending knees when sitting

D. Reduces risk of rupture by decreasing restriction of blood flow causing increasing pressure at aneurysm or graft site

E. Prepare for emergency care for hypovolemic shock, or prepare for embolectomy if appropriate

E. Complications of aortic aneurysm that require immediate medical or surgical intervention

NURSING DIAGNOSIS
Knowledge deficit related to identification of risk factors and care associated with abdominal aortic aneurysm, postoperative follow-up care, and prevention of complications associated with aneurysm resection and graft

EXPECTED OUTCOMES
Appropriate verbalizations of signs and symptoms to report and care regimen to prevent increased risk for aneurysm rupture and performance of postoperative care following instruction and information about life-style modifications, and prevention of graft rupture or wound infection

INTERVENTION

RATIONALE

V. Teach patient/family:
   A. Importance of weight control, daily exercise routine, low cholesterol dietary intake, limited alcohol intake, need to cease smoking and to reduce stress

A. Risk factors associated with hypertension, vascular disease predisposing to aortic aneurysm

   B. Report increased pain in flank, abdominal, or groin, weakness, pale and cool extremities, ecchymosis of perineum or scrotum

B. Signs and symptoms of impending or actual aneurysm rupture or graft leakage

INTERVENTION	RATIONALE
C. Report change in urinary pattern, decreased libido/impotence, bloody diarrhea	C. Indicates complications of surgical resection of aneurysm and graft (bowel ischemia, renal function impairment)
D. Wound care using sterile technique, report redness, swelling, drainage	D. Indicates wound infection
E. Rest periods during the day, moderation of activities	E. Recommendations to prevent weakness and fatigue
F. Avoid sitting for long periods, crossing legs, straining during defecation, lifting or pulling heavy objects	F. Restricts blood flow to extremities causing increased pressure on aneurysm or graft site, prevents rupture or leakage
G. Administration of stool softeners, antihypertensives	G. Prevents constipation and straining, controls blood pressure and persistent systolic pressure against wall of aorta
H. Fluid intake of eight to ten glasses/day, low-calorie and -cholesterol diet, offer sample menus and food lists	H. Provides appropriate fluid/nutritional intake to prevent constipation and reduce weight if needed
I. Reinforce information about resumption of sexual activity, alternatives or options available to improve sexual activity or reduce fear associated with the activity	I. Provides information about sexual dysfunction or activity following surgery

INTERVENTION	RATIONALE
J. Resources in the community for equipment and supplies, social services, nursing services, rehabilitation services, support group	J. Adjuncts to home care available for specific needs

acute venous insufficiency
(thrombophlebitis/thrombosis)

DEFINITION
Acute venous conditions include thrombosis (clot in a superficial or deep vein) and its associated condition, thrombophlebitis (inflammation of the wall of the vein with thrombosis). The causes of thrombus formation are venous stasis (immobility, obesity, surgery), hypercoagulability (dehydration, hematologic conditions), and vein wall trauma (IV injections, fractures, Buerger's disease). It can result in obstruction of venous flow and pulmonary embolism. This plan, which includes care specific to thrombus and thrombophlebitis, can be used in association with CHRONIC VENOUS INSUFFICIENCY and PULMONARY EMBOLISM care plans.

NURSING DIAGNOSES
Pain related to physical injuring agent of thrombophlebitis in an extremity causing inflammation and decreased blood flow

   Altered peripheral tissue perfusion related to interruption of venous flow in an extremity (obstruction, immobility) causing venous stasis

   Risk for impaired skin integrity related to external factor of immobilization (bed rest to prevent emboli), internal factor of altered nutritional state (obesity) and altered circulation (venous stasis)

EXPECTED OUTCOMES
Pain controlled, improved venous blood flow, prevention of emboli and bleeding associated with therapy, skin free of pressure and disruptions all evidenced by verbalizations that pain is well managed with medications, progressive resolution of thrombophlebitis (reduced edema, redness, warmth, pain) in affected extremity, maintenance of blood flow and tissue perfusion, absence of signs and symptoms of pulmonary emboli

INTERVENTION	RATIONALE
I. Assess for:	
A. Swelling, redness, induration, warmth along a vein at an IV site	A. Indicates phlebitis of a superficial vein caused by trauma of IV catheter insertion and improper IV site care
B. Calf tenderness, redness, edema, warmth, vein dilation, positive Homan's sign, heavy feeling in extremity	B. Indicates deep-vein thrombosis in one or both extremities causing reduced venous flow to the area
C. Skin for redness, irritation, or pallor on bony and pressure areas	C. Indicates risk for breakdown as a result of immobility from imposed bed rest
D. Skin and mucous membranes for ecchymoses, petechiae, prolonged bleeding from puncture sites, epistaxis, hemoptysis, oral bleeding, hematuria, hematemesis, blood in feces, heavy menstrual flow	D. Indicates bleeding response to anticoagulant therapy
E. Chest pain, restlessness, tachycardia, dyspnea, tachypnea	E. Signs and symptoms of pulmonary emboli caused by thrombi dislodgement
II. Monitor, describe, record:	
A. PT (warfarin therapy), PTT (heparin therapy)	A. Measures therapeutic effect of anticoagulants
B. Venous duplex scan, Doppler flowmeter, plethysmography and impedance plethysmography	B. Visualizes the vein for thrombus; measures blood flow, patency, and velocity of deep veins to evaluate venous obstruction, reveals venous filling and emptying, and maximal venous filling

INTERVENTION	RATIONALE
C. Lung scan	C. Evaluates pulmonary embolism
III. Administer: A. Anticoagulant IV for thrombo-embolic disease, PO to treat thrombosis, SC as prophylaxis preoperatively and for immobility	A. Acts by inhibiting the synthesis of clotting factors or conversion of fibrinogen to fibrin depending on the drug
B. Analgesic PO	B. Acts to relieve pain caused by inflammation
IV. Perform/provide: A. Bed rest and activity restrictions (can be for a week)	A. Improves venous flow and decreases risk for thrombus dislodgement
B. Elevate extremities above level of the heart, foot of the bed 6 inches	B. Promotes venous blood flow return, relieves venous stasis, edema, and pain
C. Avoid moving bed, support extremity when moving, assist when moving in bed	C. Protects extremity from movement and reduces pain
D. Avoid using pillows under knees and the knee gatch on the bed	D. Compromises blood flow
E. Bed cradle and footboard	E. Relieves pain caused by pressure of linens on affected area
F. Pad or protect pressure areas, especially the feet	F. Prevents excessive pressure leading to skin breakdown

INTERVENTION	RATIONALE
G. Continuous warm wet packs to affected extremity	G. Decreases inflammation and vasospasms, relieves pain
H. Elevation of extremity and small warm pack to IV site	H. Reduces inflammation and pain of superficial thrombophlebitis
I. Rotate IV sites q72 hours, dilute medications as recommended	I. Prevents irritation and trauma to veins
J. Calf measurement daily	J. Indicates reduction or increase in edema
K. Elastic wrapping from groin to toe when appropriate and rewrap as needed, assess skin when removed	K. Promotes venous circulation and reduces venous pressure
L. Use small-gauge needles and apply pressure to punctures, avoid overinflation of BP cuff, rectal temperature	L. Prevents bleeding during anticoagulant therapy
M. Limited range of motion, progressive ambulation when allowed with elastic hose applied	M. Promotes venous flow following acute stage of thrombophlebitis

NURSING DIAGNOSIS

Knowledge deficit related to discharge follow-up care to maintain venous blood flow and prevent deep-vein thrombosis, administration and monitoring of anticoagulant therapy

EXPECTED OUTCOMES

Maintenance of venous blood flow with reduced risk for chronic venous insufficiency, compliance with anticoagulant therapy and prevention of complications evidenced by correct medication administration and precautions identified to prevent bleeding and manifestations to report, precautions to prevent compromised venous blood flow (elastic hose, exercise and mobility measures, nutritional/fluid restrictions and inclusions)

INTERVENTION	RATIONALE
V. Teach patient/family:	
A. Measure and apply elastic hose from groin to toe, allow to practice application and removal, inform to wear all day until otherwise notified	A. Promotes venous flow and prevents venous stasis following deep-vein thrombosis
B. Avoid sitting or standing for prolonged periods, crossing legs when sitting, wearing garters, girdles	B. Compromises venous flow
C. Avoid rubbing or massaging extremity	C. Prevents possible dislodgement of thrombus
D. Daily exercise routine such as walking, bicycling, treadmill within recommended limits	D. Promotes venous circulation
E. Elevate legs when sitting and perform ROM on feet daily	E. Promotes venous return
F. Fluid intake of 2500 mL/day, low-calorie diet if overweight, refer to nutritionist if appropriate	F. Reduces blood viscosity, maintains ideal weight to prevent circulatory problems

INTERVENTION	RATIONALE
G. Anticoagulants to include name, action, route, dosage, frequency, side effects with written instructions, and importance of laboratory tests to monitor for drug effect and need for possible dosage adjustment	G. Maintains therapeutic levels to prevent recurrence of thrombus
H. Inform physician of other drugs taken, prescription and OTC, avoid use of alcohol	H. Desired effect of therapy can be altered by some drugs
I. Use electric razor, soft toothbrush, avoid blowing nose hard and straining during defecation, activities that could traumatize tissue such as contact sports, walking without shoes, strenuous exercises	I. Minimizes bleeding associated with anticoagulant therapy
J. Report bleeding from skin or mucous membranes, or blood in urine, feces, and sputum	J. Indicates side effect of anticoagulant and prevents excessive loss by early readjustment of medication dosage
K. Report return of pain, swelling in extremity, respiratory changes and chest pain	K. Indicates possible recurrence of thrombosis or pulmonary embolus
L. Importance of follow-up appointments with physician	L. Monitors condition and allows for reinforcement or change in activities, medications, treatments
M. Wear identification bracelet indicating anticoagulant therapy	M. Provides information useful in emergency situations

chronic venous insufficiency
(venous ulcer/varicose veins and ligation)

DEFINITION

Chronic venous insufficiency usually follows acute deep-vein thrombosis that can eventually lead to damaged veins and compromised venous circulation. As valves become incompetent, venous pressure increases and the veins become distended and distorted (varicose veins). The surgical procedure performed to treat varicose veins involves the ligation and stripping of the saphenous vein and ligation of as many of its affected smaller veins that result in additional incisions of an extremity. Long-term elevated pressure and continued insufficiency can finally cause venous stasis ulcer as the small superficial veins rupture resulting in a prolonged difficult healing process and risk for infection of the open wound. This plan includes care specific to varicose veins with ligation/stripping and venous stasis ulcer. It can also be used with the individual plan developed for THROMBOPHLEBITIS/THROMBOSIS, the acute conditions associated with venous insufficiency, and the PREOPERATIVE CARE and POSTOPERATIVE CARE plans for general surgical care if vein ligation/stripping is done

NURSING DIAGNOSES

Chronic pain related to chronic physical disability of long-term venous insufficiency causing preoperative varicose veins and venous stasis ulcer discomfort

 Pain related to physical injury of surgical procedure causing postoperative incisional discomfort

 Altered peripheral tissue perfusion related to interruption of venous flow (flow from both directions, surgical excision of veins) causing increased venous pressure, venous stasis, stasis dermatitis and venous ulceration, diminished flow to operative extremity postoperatively

EXPECTED OUTCOMES

Pain managed or controlled evidenced by verbalizations of ability to perform activities, compliance with preventive measures to minimize discomfort of varicose veins; improved venous circulation and decreased venous pressure evidenced by increased blood return and compliance with treatment regimen (elastic support hose, position of legs above heart level, exercise program)

INTERVENTION	RATIONALE
I. Assess for:	
A. Leg pain or aching, swelling, feeling of heaviness, itching, cramping relieved by walking or elevating legs	A. Indicates signs and symptoms of varicosities that appear as dilated, bulging subcutaneous veins or valve incompetence that increased venous pressure
B. Skin for brownish or rusty color, reddish or purplish color	B. Indicates changes that occur with varicosities and changes in circulation
C. Pain of venous ulcer, changes such as drainage, swelling at site	C. Pain associated with treatment, infection of ulcer
II. Monitor, describe, record:	
A. Peripheral pulses, capillary refill in toes q4h	A. Diminished pulses, slow refill indicates inadequate blood flow postoperatively
B. Doppler flowmeter, plethysmography, venography	B. Measures deep and peripheral blood flow for venous patency/incompetency, size and vein dilation
III. Administer:	
A. Analgesic (opiate or nonopiate) PO or IM	A. Acts to relieve chronic or acute post-operative pain

INTERVENTION	RATIONALE
IV. Perform/provide:	
A. Elevate extremities 20 degrees above heart level, elevate foot of bed 6 inches, elevate operative extremity	A. Promotes venous return flow in legs and relieves pain and aching caused by venous insufficiency and surgical vein ligation
B. Encourage to walk and maintain activities; ambulate 1 to 2 days for 5 minutes q2h and foot and leg exercises q1–2h for 5 minutes post-operatively	B. Promotes venous blood flow and relieves pain caused by varicosities; promotes circulation and prevents venous stasis following surgery
C. Elastic anti-embolic hose of proper width and length, pneumatic leggings with pressure applied at intervals of 1 minute, elastic bandage from groin to foot postoperatively, remove and reapply as needed for dressing change	C. Provides even compression to the superficial veins and increased blood flow and minimal venous pressure; provides compression and prevents bleeding following vein ligation
D. Bed cradle over extremities when in bed	D. Prevents pressure of linens on limb
E. Discourage from sitting for long time, crossing legs or placing pressure on popliteal area with use of knee gatch or pillows under knees	E. Prevents constriction that can compromise circulation and cause venous stasis

NURSING DIAGNOSIS

Impaired skin integrity related to internal factor of altered circulation causing venous stasis ulcer

EXPECTED OUTCOMES
Skin integrity maintained evidenced by intactness and freedom from lesions, infection, and progressive healing/reduced size of stasis ulcer

INTERVENTION	RATIONALE
I. Assess for: 　A. Breaks in skin, size and location, presence of any disruption or lesion, color changes, texture, presence of discolored and scarred area(s) from healed ulcer	A. Indicates changes caused by venous insufficiency and risk for or presence of stasis ulcer most commonly in malleolar area
B. Dry, cold, thin, shiny feel and appearance of skin	B. Predisposes to skin breakdown
C. Drainage and odor, swelling, pain at ulcer site	C. Indicates infection or cellulitis
III. Administer: 　A. Antimicrobials specific to culture and sensitivity findings PO	A. Acts to inhibit cell wall synthesis and destroy micro-organisms
IV. Perform/provide: 　A. Gentle skin and feet cleansing with mild soap and warm water, pat dry	A. Prevents trauma to skin and feet; dry, scaly skin
B. Use padding in vulnerable areas such as between toes, bony areas	B. Protects from trauma or pressure that can cause breaks in skin
C. Debride, irrigate wound/ulcer with saline or antiseptic solution, and apply dressings that are permeable to moisture	C. Treatment to promote healing

INTERVENTION

RATIONALE

D. Application of Unna boot wrapping around the ulcer area and changes q1–2 weeks as needed, Duoderm compression wrap

D. Dressing that contains zinc oxide, calamine, and glycerin provides compression and allows for drainage from the ulcer to enhance healing

E. Obtain culture for laboratory analysis

E. Monitors for early detection of infectious agent

NURSING DIAGNOSIS

Knowledge deficit related to discharge follow-up care to enhance venous circulation, continued treatment of venous stasis ulcer, and vein ligation postoperative care

EXPECTED OUTCOMES

Maintenance of venous blood flow, progressive healing of ulcer, and prevention of complications evidenced by compliance with treatment regimen (extremity elevation, leg exercises, elastic pressure on extremity, ulcer care and dressing change)

INTERVENTION

RATIONALE

V. Teach patient/family:
  A. Maintain walking and routine activities; leg exercise and walking regimen postoperatively

  A. Enhances blood flow and reduces venous pressure and pain caused by varicosities or surgery

  B. Avoid sitting or standing for prolonged periods, crossing legs when sitting

  B. Prevents venous stasis and compromised blood flow

  C. Elevate legs when sitting and following ambulation

  C. Promotes venous return

INTERVENTION	RATIONALE
D. Application, removing and washing of elastic support hose, application of postoperative elastic compression bandages from foot to groin	D. Maintains circulatory patency and prevents edema in legs
E. Avoid wearing tight clothing such as garters, girdles, tight shoes	E. Prevents constriction of blood flow
F. Avoid heat applications, trauma to feet and legs by going barefoot, bumping against furniture	F. Prevents burns, possible breaks in skin that can lead to ulcer formation
G. Care of stasis ulcer, including wet to dry dressings, home visit or appointment for compression boot or wrap application and removal	G. Promotes continuous assessment and care for healing stasis ulcer
H. Report any skin color changes, dermatitis, skin breaks, incisional bleeding or drainage, resumption of heavy feeling or pain in legs, swelling of leg	H. Indicates possible complication of compromised circulation or vein ligation
I. Importance of keeping appointments for suture removal, monitoring of ulcer and varicose veins treatments	I. Provides ongoing medical and postoperative follow-up care

coronary artery disease/angina pectoris

DEFINITION
Coronary artery disease (CAD), or ischemic heart disease, is a progressive disease characterized by deposits of atherosclerotic plaques within the large- and medium-size arteries supplying the heart. This results in a reduced flow of blood or obstruction of blood flow to the myocardium causing hypoxia, ischemia, and pain. Angina pectoris is the precordial chest pain that results from the imbalance between oxygen demand of the myocardium (activity or exertion, stress, cold exposure, large meals, hypertension) and the ability of the atherosclerotic coronary arteries to supply oxygen to the myocardium when these conditions exist. A common surgical procedure performed to treat CAD is percutaneous transluminar coronary angioplasty (PTCA). This involves the insertion of a balloon-tipped catheter into the coronary artery and inflation of the balloon to apply pressure to the plaque and open the occluded area or the use of a laser to remove the plaque

NURSING DIAGNOSES
Anxiety related to change in health status, threat of death causing inability to manage stress, angina attacks and associated symptoms

    Ineffective individual coping related to multiple life changes causing chronic anxiety, worry, emotional tension, and inability to cope with long-term illness and uncertainty about future and life-style changes

EXPECTED OUTCOMES
Anxiety within manageable levels, development of coping skills evidenced by verbalizations that anxiety is decreasing, ability to problem solve and modify life-style to meet needs brought about by disease

INTERVENTION	RATIONALE
I. Assess for:	
A. Level of anxiety, use of coping mechanisms, stated fears of uncertainty of disease outcome, life-style changes, and feelings of impending doom or death	A. Anxiety can range from mild to severe and increase oxygen consumption, assists in identifying inappropriate use of coping skills
B. Restlessness, diaphoresis, complaining, joking, withdrawal, talkativeness, increased P and R	B. Nonverbal expressions of anxiety when not able to communicate feelings
C. Personal resources to cope with stress, anxiety, and interest in learning to problem solve	C. Support systems and personal strengths assist to develop coping skills
IV. Perform/provide:	
A. Environment conducive to rest, expression of fears and anxiety, avoid anxiety-producing situations	A. Decreases stimuli that cause stress/anxiety, venting of feelings decreases anxiety
B. Suggest new methods to enhance coping skills and problem solving, allow to externalize and identify those that help	B. Offers alternative coping strategies that allow for release of anxiety and fear
C. Information about all diagnostic tests and procedures, treatment regimen, equipment such as ECG	C. Reduces fear and anxiety about unfamiliar environment
D. Inform that angina is not a heart attack and that ischemia is reversible	D. Relieves concern about threat of death

INTERVENTION	RATIONALE
E. Diversional activities such as relaxation exercises, TV, radio, music, reading	E. Reduces anxiety and promotes comfort

NURSING DIAGNOSIS

Pain related to physical factor of reduced coronary blood flow (atherosclerosis) causing decreased myocardial oxygenation and ischemia (angina attack)

EXPECTED OUTCOMES

Pain episodes reduced and controlled evidenced by less frequent need for medications, verbalizations that pain is relieved, relaxed muscles and facial expressions, able to participate in modified activities

INTERVENTION	RATIONALE
I. Assess for:	
A. Onset of pain, location and if radiating to arms, neck, mandible, maxilla, teeth, severity and length of time it lasts, if increased over time, if occurs at rest or during exercise, strong emotions, after meals, during sexual activity or during exposure to temperature extremes	A. Symptoms and causes associated with angina episode, pain usually moderate lasting less than 5 minutes and is usually precipitated by exertion or emotion and can occur only during the day or night or both
B. Clenched fist over sternum, dyspnea, pallor, diaphoresis, restlessness, tachycardia, elevated BP	B. Nonverbal manifestations of angina attack

INTERVENTION	RATIONALE
III. Administer: A. Vasodilator, SLG or TOP	A. Acts to improve mycardial blood to reduce oxygen consumption and pain by relaxing smooth muscle of coronary and peripheral vessels
IV. Perform/provide: A. Bed rest in calm, quiet environment, avoid stressful situations	A. Stress increases oxygen consumption and pain
B. Position of comfort during angina pain in semi- or high-Fowler's	B. Decreases oxygen requirement
C. Speak slowly in low voice, remain during pain episode	C. Provides support and caring attitude, reduces anxiety associated with pain
D. Offer medication prior to activity, repeat sublingual medication up to three doses 5 to 10 minutes apart if pain not relieved	D. Administered to prevent pain or if pain unrelieved by rest and medication
E. Report unrelieved pain lasting 15 minutes or more or worsening of pain	E. Can lead to or indicate myocardial infarct

NURSING DIAGNOSES

Altered cardiac tissue perfusion related to interruption in coronary arterial blood flow (atherosclerosis) to myocardium causing myocardial ischemia, angina attack, and risk for myocardial infarction

  Activity intolerance related to imbalance between oxygen supply and demand causing myocardial ischemia and angina attack

EXPECTED OUTCOMES

Adequate oxygenation of myocardium and optimal level of activity achieved evidenced by VS within baseline parameters and ability to carry out activities without fatigue, pain or increases in pulse or respirations, verbalizations that excessive activities are avoided or modified

INTERVENTION	RATIONALE
I. Assess for: A. Precordial or substernal pain, dyspnea, tachycardia, irregular pulse	A. Indicates decreased cardiac perfusion
B. Type of activities that initiate attack, level of fatigue or weakness, dizziness and dyspnea during activities, need to modify activities	B. Exertion can precipitate angina as oxygen consumption is increased
II. Monitor, describe, record: A. VS, especially BP with aministration of vasodilators; 5 minutes before, during, and after activity for increases in P and R	A. Vasodilation reduces BP and can cause hypotension, VS changes can increase demands of myocardium for oxygen
B. ECG during angina attack, nuclear scan, coronary angiography, exercise stress test	B. Identifies ischemia and cardiac muscle involved, coronary arterial obstruction; risk for presence of CAD
III. Administer: A. Vasodilator SLG, TOP	A. Acts to prevent or treat attacks by coronary vasodilation causing a reduction of pain and work of the heart

INTERVENTION	RATIONALE
B. Beta-adrenergic blockers PO	B. Acts to reduce oxygen requirement and work of the heart by slowing the rate, increases tolerance for activity
C. Calcium-channel blockers PO	C. Acts to reduce oxygen requirement and work of the heart by increasing the heart contractions
D. Anticoagulant/antiplatelet PO	D. Prevents thrombus formation in coronary arteries
E. Oxygen via nasal cannula	E. Improves oxygenation to myocardial tissue

IV. Perform/provide:

A. Schedule periods of activity and alternate with rest periods according to imposed restrictions	A. Maintains activity level below angina threshold level
B. Increase activities while assessing for signs of intolerance	B. Allows activities while preventing increased work of heart and fatigue
C. Avoid activities after meals or during stressful situations	C. Prevents angina attack
D. Avoid smoking and beverages containing caffeine	D. Stimulates cardiac activity that increases oxygen consumption, causes vasoconstriction of vessels and results in decreased oxygen availability

NURSING DIAGNOSES

Knowledge deficit related to disease process, medications, reduction of risk factors (stress, obesity, nicotine, hypertension, atherosclerosis), life-style changes (dietary, exercise, health practices), signs and symptoms to report, discharge follow-up care

Noncompliance related to health beliefs and cultural influences causing resistance to modification of life-style, acceptance of treatment regimen, and increased risk for myocardial infarction

EXPECTED OUTCOMES

Knowledge and understanding of disease and care with life-syle modified to reduce angina attacks and risk for myocardial infarction evidenced by BP and lipid panel within normal parameters, weight and stress reduced, fewer angina attacks experienced, compliance with medication, activity, and dietary regimens, smoking abstinence, ongoing physician monitoring of cardiac status

INTERVENTION	RATIONALE
I. Assess for:	
A. Educational, developmental levels, knowledge of diagnosis and treatment regimen	A. Provides information about teaching strategies to use and prevents rejection of medical regimen
B. Readiness and willingness to learn	B. Learning cannot take place during periods of high anxiety, stress, or denial
C. Health practices, health beliefs, ethnic identity (religion, diet, language), value orientations, family interactions	C. Factors to incorporate into teaching plan to facilitate compliance
D. Degree of motivation to change life-style, behaviors that indicate resistance in making life-style changes	D. Necessary to reduce risk factors, although refusal to change habits is a right and should be respected

INTERVENTION	RATIONALE
E. Overweight, smoking habit, sedentary and stressful life-style, high-fat and -cholesterol dietary intake	E. Risk factors associated with CAD, angina, and possible heart attack
F. Hypertension, diabetes mellitus, other chronic diseases	F. Predisposes to risk for angina, and possible heart attack
IV. Perform/provide:	
A. Acknowledgment of patient perceptions with nonjudgmental attitude	A. Establishes nurse–patient relationship in an accepting environment
B. Explanations that are clear, accurate in understandable terms, small amount of information over time	B. Prevents misconceptions, erroneous attitudes and beliefs about disease
C. Environment conducive to learning with space, lighting, and proper equipment and supplies	C. Distractions will interfere with learning
D. Treatment regimen that is acceptable and suitable to life-style	D. Promotes compliance
E. Teaching aids (pamphlets, video tapes, pictures, written instructions)	E. Reinforces learning and ensures compliance
F. Team of resource personnel	F. Nutritionist, social worker, counselor can assist in teaching specific care and providing support for changes

INTERVENTION	RATIONALE
V. Teach patient/family:	
A. Pathophysiology, process, and effect of CAD and angina	A. Promotes understanding of disease that facilitates compliance and prevent complications
B. Risk factors such as obesity, stress, smoking, diet, exercise deficit	B. Contribute to cardiovascular disease but can be modified with changes in lifestyle
C. Avoid strenuous exercise, extreme cold temperatures, large meals, extreme stress, smoking, excessive alcohol intake	C. Factors that precipitate angina attack
D. Identify stressors and how to reduce them by planning rest periods, avoid excessive work hours, rushing, tenseness, impatience, time watching	D. Reduces stress that precipitate angina attacks
E. Monitoring of hypertension by BP and dysrhythmias by P, allow to return demonstration and practice	E. Identifies increase or decrease in blood pressure and irregularities in pulse
F. Develop daily activity program to include walking, swimming, bicycling, three times/week; avoid activities that include lifting heavy objects, pulling or pushing	F. Reduces risk factor of sedentary life-style

INTERVENTION	RATIONALE
G. Cease activities that cause pain, fatigue, dyspnea, dizziness	G. Indicates possible strain on cardiac function
H. Dietary changes with sample menus for 1200 to 1400 calorie, high-fiber diet, low salt intake of <4 g/day, cholesterol intake of <300 mg/day, list of foods to restrict and include to maintain nutritional status and explain rationale for dietary changes	H. Reduces risk factors associated with CAD, angina, and hypertension
I. Administration of vasodilator to include route, action, dosage, expected results, frequency and when to take, how to take, possible side effects; to take 5 to 10 minutes prior to activities, repeat dosage at 5-minute intervals for up to three doses to relieve pain	I. Acts to increase oxygen to myocardium during angina attack and relieve pain
J. Rationale, administration of other medications prescribed such as antilipemics, calcium-channel blockers, beta-adrenergic blockers, expected responses such as decreased P rate, dizziness when changing from a lying position	J. Promotes compliance of complete prescribed medication regimen

INTERVENTION	RATIONALE
K. Report pain that is not relieved, slow, irregular P, headache, dizziness, notify physician prior to using any other medications	K. Can indicate possible complication of cardiac disorder
L. Contact support groups for stress and weight reduction, stop smoking program	L. Provides assistance to reduce risk factors

diminished arterial circulation to extremities/arterial bypass

DEFINITION

Diminished peripheral arterial occlusive conditions are characterized by a progressive narrowing of the lumen and damage to the lining of the vessels. It is most commonly caused by atherosclerosis (arteriosclerosis obliterans), thrombosis/inflammation (Buerger's disease or thrombo-angiitis obliterans), vasospasm (Raynaud's disease), or trauma. All affect the arterial circulation to the extremities. Surgical resection of the affected segment and graft, or bypass of the segment with a graft, are procedures performed to correct inadequate circulation to an extremity caused by arterial occlusion. The site most occluded and treated surgically is the femoropopliteal arterial segment, although other affected segments can be surgically constructed. This plan includes care specific to diminished arterial circulation and the surgical reconstruction of arterial occlusion. It can be used in association with PREOPERATIVE CARE, and POSTOPERATIVE CARE for general surgical care

NURSING DIAGNOSES

Chronic pain related to chronic physical disability of impaired circulation to extremities causing continuous or intermittent pain over period of 6 months or more

Pain postoperatively related to physical injury of surgery to correct arterial occlusion

High risk for activity intolerance related to circulatory problem causing pain during walking

EXPECTED OUTCOMES

Chronic or acute pain managed or controlled in extremities or surgical site evidenced by verbalizations that pain managed by pharmacological and/or nonpharmacological methods, activities maintained with minimal pain (sleep, walking, personal care)

INTERVENTION	RATIONALE
I. Assess for:	
A. Intermittent claudication with pain or aching in legs during ambulation, burning or aching at rest or in recumbent position during sleep	A. Indicates verbal descriptors of the effects of atherosclerosis as oxygenated blood is decreased by diminished arterial circulation to extremities
B. Frequency of claudication and effect on walking/exercises	B. Decreases activity tolerance over time when claudication occurs more often with less exertion
C. Intermitten pallor followed by cyanosis with numbness, coldness and pain, then redness with tingling and throbbing in fingers and toes	C. Indicates arteriospastic episode of Raynaud's disease with symptoms caused by vasoconstriction when digits are exposed to cold or during emotional stress
D. Intermittent claudication in legs or rest pain in one or more digits with sensitivity to cold	D. Indicates Buerger's disease at varying stages of the disease
E. Restlessness, guarded movements, facial grimace, communication of pain site, type, and severity	E. Indicates verbal and nonverbal descriptors of postoperative pain
III. Administer:	
A. Mild analgesic PO, narcotic analgesic IM postoperatively	A. Acts to relieve chronic or acute pain

INTERVENTION	RATIONALE
B. Vasodilator PO	B. Acts to increase blood flow to peripheral vessels to reduce rest pain in Buerger's disease
C. Calcium-channel blocker PO	C. Acts to decrease vasospastic episodes and associated pain in Raynaud's disease

IV. Perform/provide:

A. Maintain bed rest if pain severe and ischemia is present	A. Rest reduces muscle contractions and increased ischemia in extremities
B. Cease walking or activity prior to pain or before pain becomes severe	B. Intermittent claudication can be predicted and prevented
C. Allow to rest periodically during ambulation	C. Prevents pain caused by impaired arterial circulation
D. Position legs below the heart level such as dangling or elevate head of bed or use recliner, avoid elevating legs	D. Increases arterial flow to the lower extremities by gravity
E. Change position for comfort postoperatively and support body parts when moving in bed	E. Reduces pain by relieving stress on incisional area
F. Protect extremity or digits from cold and trauma	F. Prevents pain caused by cold temperatures and injury to vulnerable areas

INTERVENTION	RATIONALE
G. Walking program or Buerger-Allen exercises	G. Provides exercise program to promote circulation and prevent progressive intolerance to activity

NURSING DIAGNOSES

Altered peripheral tissue perfusion related to interruption of arterial flow in extremities and digits (atherosclerosis, inflammation, arteriospasms) causing changes in vessels, vasoconstriction, and possible occlusion, ischemic lesions; related to postoperative reduction in blood flow to extremity (edema, inflammatory response, use of femoral vein for graft reconstruction and possible occlusion of graft)

Risk for impaired skin integrity related to external factor of environmental temperature (cold) and internal factor of altered circulation (ischemic lesions)

EXPECTED OUTCOMES

Maintenance of arterial blood flow and tissue perfusion evidenced by absence of pain that results from compromised circulation, peripheral pulses, capillary refill time, and skin intactness, color and temperature of extremity, and/or digits within baseline determinations

INTERVENTION	RATIONALE
I. Assess for: A. Intermittent claudication or rest pain, weak/absent peripheral pulse and increased capillary refill time, rubor when extremity is in dependent position, sudden onset of coldness, pallor followed by cyanosis when extremity elevated	A. Indicates reduction of arterial blood flow to extremities, intermittent claudication is the result of hypoxia and accumulation of waste products in muscle tissue during walking

INTERVENTION	RATIONALE
B. Sensory and motor function, hematoma, edema, pedal pulse of the operative extremity	B. Postoperative observations to determine tissue perfusion and graft patency
C. Skin for intactness, healed areas, ulceration, or infection, rubbed area, scratches, calluses	C. Chronic diminished arterial blood flow can result in tissue damage and poor healing as tissues do not receive oxygen, nutrients, and anti-infectious agents (WBC)

II. Monitor, describe, record:

A. Peripheral pulses, capillary refill q4h or as appropriate	A. Indicates status of arterial circulation
B. Doppler pressure and pedal pulse q1h for 24 hours then q8h	B. Monitors postoperative arterial blood flow
C. Doppler plethysmography, ankle/arm blood pressure index, magnetic resonance imaging, arteriography (preoperatively)	C. Procedures to measure arterial blood flow, level and severity of diminished circulation, or visualization of arterial lumen prior to surgery

IV. Perform/provide:

A. Place extremities in position lower than heart or with feet flat on floor when in sitting position, elevate head of bed 6 inches on blocks	A. Allow blood to flow to legs and feet

INTERVENTION	RATIONALE
B. Warm environmental temperature, cover extremities with warm socks or gloves, or cover with blanket	B. Prevents chilling by insulating from cold that reduces blood flow
C. Avoid using pillows under knees, knee gatch, prolonged sitting or crossing legs while sitting	C. Compromises blood flow to extremities
D. Avoid smoking, caffeine-containing beverages, stressful situations	D. Prevents vasoconstriction caused by nicotine and caffeine, stimulation of sympathetic nervous system
E. Leg exercises q2h, maintain leg in slightly elevated position with knee slightly flexed, allow for short, frequent walking, limit positioning of leg in a dependent position	E. Promotes tissue perfusion in operative extremity
F. Careful foot care and cleansing with mild soap and warm water, pat dry	F. Cleansing and gentle care prevent trauma to feet
G. Encourage to wear hose and adequate shoes that are not tight, avoid bumping feet, walking barefoot	G. Protects the feet from trauma or breaks that can lead to ulceration
H. Trim toenails straight across, use padding on corns and between toes	H. Protects skin from friction and possible cuts or damage

NURSING DIAGNOSIS

Knowledge deficit related to discharge follow-up care to enhance arterial circulation, continued prevention of complications of chronic and post-operative impaired tissue perfusion and skin breakdown

EXPECTED OUTCOMES

Maintenance of arterial blood flow, compliance with preventive and treatment regimen evidenced correct foot care, control of factors that affect arterial circulation (warmth, smoking, proper positioning of extremity, weight reduction, progressive walking/exercise with pain control)

INTERVENTION	RATIONALE
V. Teach patient/family:	
A. Pathophysiology, process, and effect of diminished arterial circulation on health status	A. Promotes understanding of disease that facilitates compliance and prevents complications
B. Risk factors such as obesity, smoking, sedentary life-style, dietary intake of sodium, cholesterol, fat, conditions such as diabetes, hypertension, coronary artery disease	B. Contribute to vascular disease but can be modified with changes in life-style
C. Daily walking routine exercises with increases in distances and rest periods scheduled as needed; foot and leg exercises q1h	C. Maintains blood flow to extremities by increasing collateral blood supply in intermittent claudication and ensures postoperative bypass or graft patency
D. Avoid smoking, wearing tight restrictive clothing, sitting or standing for prolonged periods, compressing the popliteal area by crossing legs or using pillows under knees	D. Causes vasoconstriction and diminished blood flow to extremities

INTERVENTION	RATIONALE
E. Dietary reduction of cholesterol and fat, calories if weight loss needed, written list of foods to avoid, purchasing and cooking information and sample meal plans	E. Prevents continued development of atherosclerosis that affects blood flow to extremities
F. Administration of antilipemics if ordered to include action, dose, frequency, route, side effects	F. Promotes compliance with drug regimen to reduce atherosclerosis
G. Daily foot care, including cleansing, recommended lubrication and shoes/socks, padding areas, cutting nails straight or see podiatrist for nail and callus/corn care	G. Prevents arterial ulcers or infection
H. Signs and symptoms to report to physician such as increasing pain, coldness, pallor or cyanosis, edema, numbness, at operative site or extremity	H. Allows for early intervention to prevent or treat postoperative complications
I. Community resources to assist in weight reduction, special dietary therapy, program to stop smoking	I. Provides information, support to implement life-style changes

heart failure/pulmonary edema

DEFINITION

Heart failure is the manifestations resulting from a chronic or acute abnormal state of cardiac pumping performance causing heart rate and volume that are insufficient to meet metabolic requirements to the tissues. This results in systemic (right-sided failure) and pulmonary circulatory congestion (left-sided failure) with signs and symptoms depending on the side of the ventricular failure. Conditions that predispose to heart failure are cardiac muscle dysfunction (myocardial infarction, cardiomyopathy, myocarditis), preload disorders (hypervolemia, valvular septal defects, valvular regurgitation), afterload disorders (valvular stenosis, hypertension, peripheral vascular resistance), or diseases (hyper- or hypothyroidism, chronic obstructive pulmonary disease, systemic infection, anemia). This plan includes care specific to cardiac failure and follow-up care to maintain cardiac status. It can be used in association with HYPERTENSION, MYOCARDIAL INFARCTION, and INFLAMMATORY HEART DISEASE (MYOCARDITIS) care plans

NURSING DIAGNOSES

Anxiety related to threat to or change in health status causing inability to manage feelings of uncertainty and apprehension regarding situation crisis and outcome of illness

Ineffective individual coping related to situational crisis of illness, possible recurrence, inability to cope with long-term chronic illness and future life-style changes

EXPECTED OUTCOMES

Anxiety within manageable levels, development of coping and problem-solving skills evidenced by verbalizations that anxiety is decreasing, participation in care activities and receptive to planning for ongoing care needed to manage disease

INTERVENTION	RATIONALE
I. Assess for:	
A. Level of anxiety, use of coping mechanisms, stated fears of uncertainty of disease outcome, life-style changes, and feelings of impending doom or death	A. Anxiety can range from mild to severe and increase oxygen consumption, assists to identify inappropriate use of coping skills; high level of anxiety associated with dyspnea
B. Restlessness, diaphoresis, complaining, joking, withdrawal, talkativeness, increased P and R	B. Nonverbal expressions of anxiety when not able to communicate feelings
C. Personal resources to cope with stress, anxiety, and interest in learning to problem-solve	C. Support systems and personal strengths assist to develop coping skills
III. Administer:	
A. Anti-anxiety agent/sedative PO	A. Acts to reduce anxiety level and provides calming effect and rest, depresses subcortical levels of CNS, limbic system
IV. Perform/provide:	
A. Environment conducive to rest, expression of fears and anxiety, avoid anxiety-producing situations	A. Decreases stimuli that cause stress/anxiety, venting of feelings decreases anxiety
B. Suggest new methods to enhance coping skills and problem solving, allow to externalize and identify those that help	B. Offers alternative coping strategies that allow for release of anxiety and fear

INTERVENTION	RATIONALE
C. Positive feedback regarding progress made, focus on abilities rather than inabilities	C. Provides support for adaptive behavior, promotes self-worth and responsibility
D. Diversional activities such as relaxation exercises, TV, radio, music, reading	D. Reduces anxiety and promotes comfort
E. Limit visitors according to condition, avoid stressful situations	E. Eliminates unnecessary stimuli that increases anxiety
F. Allow to participate in planning of care to maintain usual activities when possible	F. Allows for some control over situations

NURSING DIAGNOSES

Decreased cardiac output (CO) related to inotropic changes in the heart, alteration in rate and rhythm causing decreased contractility, ventricular hypertrophy, dysrhythmias, and congestive heart failure

Altered cardiopulmonary, gastrointestinal, and peripheral tissue perfusion related to interruption of arterial flow or reduced blood flow to the organs and extremities as a result of decreased CO and vasoconstriction causing hemodynamic/respiratory/digestive changes (fluid in alveoli or pulmonary congestion with ventilation perfusion imbalance, systemic venous congestion of organs with peripheral edema, nausea and vomiting with poor perfusion to gastrointestinal tract)

Fluid volume excess related to compromised regulatory mechanism (renal dysfunction resulting from decreased blood flow and increased antidiuretic secretion) causing sodium and water retention

EXPECTED OUTCOMES

Adequate cardiac output and tissue perfusion evidenced by available hemodynamic measurements (CO, CVP, PAP) within normal ranges, P, BP, R, peripheral pulses, and capillary refill time within normal baseline ranges, absence of dysrhythmias; peripheral, cardiopulmonary perfusion adequate with absence of signs and symptoms indicating systemic circulatory insufficiency (hepatomegaly, nausea, dependent edema) or pulmonary edema (dyspnea, tachypnea, crackles, wheezes, pallor or cyanosis); resolution of fluid volume excess evidenced by I&O ratio in balance, weight and edema reduced with therapy, lung sounds within normal parameters

INTERVENTION	RATIONALE
I. Assess for: A. P rate and rhythm (irregular of <60 or >100/bpm), reduced or increased BP depending on compensation, rapid and labored respirations (>20), apical pulse (<60/bpm), ECG tracings for dysrhythmias	A. Identifies changes associated with decreased CO caused by heart failure
B. Lung sounds for crackles, rhonchi, abnormal heart sounds, gallop auscultated, dyspnea, jugular vein distention, cyanosis, decreased mental alertness or thought processes, dependent edema in legs or sacrum, urinary output of <30 mL/hr, coolness and pallor to extremities with decreased pulses, capillary refill of <3 seconds	B. Identifies changes associated with reduced CO and perfusion problems in other system functions that result in hypoxia and organ dysfunction
C. Severe dyspnea, orthopnea with crackles and gallop auscultated, distended neck veins, oliguria, peripheral edema, cough with blood-tinged sputum, gurgling respirations, fatigue and weakness, and sense of doom	C. Indicates cardiac failure with pulmonary edema (left-sided)

INTERVENTION	RATIONALE
II. Monitor, describe, record: A. VS, CO, CVP, PAP q1–2h as appropriate for CO <4 L/minute, wedge pressure >18 mm Hg	A. Indicates hemodynamic stability to determine cardiac function status and potential for failure
B. ECG single or continuous for dysrhythmias	B. Indicates ventricular abnormalities that decrease CO leading to serious dysrhythmias that reduce filling time and myocardial contractility, and increase need for oxygen
C. I&O q1h or as appropriate for greater intake than output with fluid excess, and increased output with diuretic therapy	C. Indicates kidney perfusion and function, effect of diuretic therapy
D. Weight daily at same time, on same scale, wearing same clothing	D. Monitors degree of fluid excess and effectiveness of therapy
E. ABGs, liver enzymes, electrolytes (Na, K), pulse oximetry, BUN, creatinine, glucose, digitalis level	E. Indicates impact of condition on organ and system functions (liver, kidneys), electrolytes can be affected by medications with hypokalemia leading to dangerous dysrhythmias, decreases in oxygen level (arterial or saturation) indicates need for supplemental oxygen, digitalis level reveals therapeutic or toxicity levels that can lead to life-threatening dysrhythmias

INTERVENTION	RATIONALE
F. Echocardiography, chest x-ray	F. Procedures performed to assist in diagnosis of cardiac function and possible pulmonary edema
III. Administer:	
A. Vasodilator SLG while monitoring hemodynamic status	A. Acts to decrease afterload by improving blood flow to myocardium and reduce workload of heart
B. Inotropic PO	B. Acts to improve myocardial contractility and CO
C. Diuretic PO, IV while monitoring electrolyte imbalance, with potassium replacement if needed	C. Acts to increase water, sodium, and potassium excretion depending on type administered
D. Bronchodilator PO, IV	D. Acts to dilate airways to facilitate breathing if dyspneic
E. Anti-emetic PO, IV	E. Acts to control nausea and prevent vomiting
F. Oxygen via nasal cannula	F. Provides oxygen for hypoxia as a result of decreased CO
IV. Perform/provide:	
A. Bed rest with activity restrictions as ordered, decrease activity level if symptoms appear	A. Reduces cardiac workload to improve CO

INTERVENTION	RATIONALE
B. Place in semi- or high Fowler's position with periodic change to a flat position	B. Increases tidal volume and facilitates breathing with less effort, or promotes venous return in presence of edema
C. Calm, quiet, comfortable environment	C. Promotes environment with minimal stimuli that can increase stress and secretion of catecholamines and cardiac workload
D. Avoid straining during defecation or holding the breath	D. Increases venous return and preload causing increased cardiac workload
E. Small, more frequent meals, assist or feed if needed, rest period prior to and following meals, odor-free environment	E. Minimizes myocardial workload with need for additional blood flow to gastrointestinal system needed for digestion, prevents stimuli to vomiting center
F. Mouth care prior to and following meals, avoid foods that are irritating to gastrointestinal tract	F. Promotes comfort and prevents nausea
G. Warmth to extremities and maintain extremities in dependent position, passive or assistive ROM	G. Decreases preload by increasing vasodilation, the dependent position to decrease venous return and ROM to decrease venous pooling leading to thrombophlebitis
H. Cautious administration of IV solutions, avoiding Na if fluids are retained	H. Improves preload

INTERVENTION	RATIONALE
I. Fluid and sodium oral intake restrictions as ordered in beverages and foods	I. Reduces fluid volume and retention

NURSING DIAGNOSES

Ineffective breathing pattern related to anxiety (deteriorating health status), decreased lung expansion and musculoskeletal impairment (weakness, pressure of fluid accumulation in lungs)

Impaired gas exchange related to alveolar-capillary membrane changes (fluid accumulation in alveoli and interstitium), altered oxygen supply (reduced perfusion from reduced CO)

EXPECTED OUTCOMES

Respiratory function (rate, depth, rhythm, ease) and breath sounds within baseline parameters, tissues oxygenated evidenced by ABGs within normal ranges, skin and mucous membranes pink and warm

INTERVENTION	RATIONALE
I. Assess for:	
A. Respiratory rate, depth, ease, dyspnea, orthopnea, breath sounds for crackles and wheezes or diminished breath sounds auscultated, dry or productive cough	A. Changes indicate impaired function associated with pulmonary edema
B. Cyanosis, air hunger, confusion, irritability, restlessness, lethargy	B. Indicates decreasing oxygen levels and hypoxemia
II. Monitor, describe, record:	
A. R and breath sounds q2–4h	A. Indicates changes in respiratory status caused by congestion
B. ABGs, pulse oximetry	B. Measures arterial oxygen and saturation levels to determine hypoxemia

INTERVENTION	RATIONALE
III. Administer:	
A. Bronchodilator PO, IV	A. Acts to dilate the airways to enhance movement of air in and out of lungs
B. Diuretic PO, IV	B. Acts to decrease fluid accumulation in the lungs
C. Mucolytic INH	C. Liquefies secretions for easy removal by cough or suctioning
D. Oxygen via nasal cannula, face mask	D. Acts to provide supplemental oxygen based on ABGs and oximetry results
IV. Perform/provide:	
A. Place in semi-Fowler's or orthopneic position	A. Facilitates chest expansion and air movement
B. Change position from side to side, cough and deep-breathing exercises or incentive spirometer q2h as appropriate	B. Improves ventilation and clears airways of obstructive substances
C. Request to breathe slowly, demonstrate breathing pattern to mimic	C. Prevents hyperventilation
D. Tracheal suctioning if unable to cough up secretions	D. Removes mucus from large bronchi
E. Avoid smoking and environmental odors that are strong and irritating to respiratory tract	E. Results in bronchospasm and reduces oxygen inflow

INTERVENTION	RATIONALE
F. Prepare for intubation and mechanical ventilation	F. Measure to prevent or treat respiratory failure

NURSING DIAGNOSES

Activity intolerance related to imbalance between oxygen supply and demand (fluid accumulation in lungs) causing tissue hypoxia, weakness, fatigue, and increased energy requirements to perform ADL

Sleep pattern disturbance elated to internal factors of illness (nocturnal dyspnea) and psychological stress (anxiety) causing insomnia or disruption of sleep

Fatigue related to psychological demands (stress of life-threatening illness) causing anxiety and sleep disturbance, and altered physical abilities (dyspnea, hypoxia, immobility) causing reduced energy, endurance

EXPECTED OUTCOMES

Progressive increase in activity tolerance and return to sleep and rest pattern with reduction in fatigue level evidenced by increased performance of ADL with decreased dyspnea, increased energy and endurance, VS stable before, during, and after activity, uninterrupted sleep with verbalizations that feeling more rested and less anxious

INTERVENTION	RATIONALE
I. Assess for:	
A. Level of fatigue, weakness, and potential for activity progression, effect of dyspnea on activities and sleep	A. Provides baseline and allows for planning activities and need for assistance
B. Interest and ability in performing ADL with or without assistance	B. Readiness and increased energy level necessary for successful program
C. Sleep/rest pattern, wakefulness during night	C. Optimal rest and sleep necessary to reduce fatigue and perform activities

INTERVENTION	RATIONALE
D. R >20/minute, P >120/ bpm and not returning to pre-activity level within 3 minutes, palpitations, dyspnea, dizziness, chest pain, weakness, and stopping activity if symptoms appear	D. Signs and symptoms of activity intolerance leading to fatigue
III. Administer:	
A. Sedative PO, unless respirations <12/minute	A. Acts on limbic and subcortical levels of CNS and increases sleep time
IV. Perform/provide:	
A. Bed rest during acute state in a position of comfort with body parts supported such as arms resting on pillows	A. Conserves energy and provides needed rest to reduce cardiac workload
B. Perform or assist in ADL and other activities as needed, place all articles and call light within reach to use as desired	B. Conserves energy while preserving as much control and independence as possible
C. Increase activities gradually from sitting up in bed, in chair, walking in room, to bathroom, and in hall with daily increase in distance and ADL activities	C. Progressive change in activities increases with endurance and energy level and prevents rapid changes in work of the heart

INTERVENTION	RATIONALE
D. Place bed in low position and clear pathways if ambulating independently with a walker or cane, inform to get out of bed slowly and take time needed for slow progress in ambulation	D. Prevents falls if weak until endurance returns
E. Organize activities around rest periods in a quiet, calm, dimly lit, stimuli-free environment	E. Permits rest without interruptions
F. Assist to assume preferred position for sleep, offer backrub, oral care, extra pillows, other activities based on sleep pattern	F. Provides for usual bedtime rituals to ensure comfort and sleep

NURSING DIAGNOSES

Knowledge deficit related to disease process, medications, life-style changes (dietary, exercise, nicotine, stress, health practices), signs and symptoms to report, discharge follow-up care

Noncompliance related to health beliefs and cultural influences causing resistance to modification of life-style, acceptance of treatment regimen, and increased risk of acute heart failure

EXPECTED OUTCOMES

Knowledge and understanding of disease and care with life-style modified to reduce risk for decompensated heart failure evidenced by BP and lipid panel within normal parameters, weight and stress reduced, compliance with medication, activity, and dietary regimens, smoking abstinence, ongoing physician monitoring of cardiac status

INTERVENTION	RATIONALE
I. Assess for:	
A. Educational, developmental levels, knowledge of diagnosis and treatment regimen	A. Provides information about teaching strategies to use and prevents resistance to medical regimen
B. Readiness and willingness to learn	B. Learning cannot take place during periods of high anxiety, stress, or denial
C. Health practices, health beliefs, ethnic identity (religion, diet, language), value orientations, family interactions	C. Factors to incorporate into teaching plan to facilitate compliance
D. Degree of motivation to change life-style, behaviors that indicate resistance in making life-style changes	D. Necessary to reduce risk factors, although refusal to change habits is a right and should be respected
E. Overweight, smoking habit, sedentary and stressful life-style, high-fat, -cholesterol, -sodium diet	E. Risk factors that need modifications to prevent progression of cardiac failure
F. Economic resources to carry out therapeutic regimen	F. Lack of financial assistance can prevent compliance
IV. Perform/provide:	
A. Acknowledgment of patient perceptions with nonjudgmental attitude	A. Establishes nurse–patient relationship in an accepting environment

INTERVENTION	RATIONALE
B. Explanations that are clear, accurate in understandable terms, small amount of information over time	B. Prevents misconceptions, erroneous attitudes and beliefs about disease
C. Environment conducive to learning with space, lighting, and proper equipment and supplies	C. Distractions will interfere with learning
D. Treatment regimen that is acceptable and suitable to life-style	D. Promotes compliance
E. Teaching aids (pamphlets, videotapes, pictures, written instructions)	E. Reinforces learning
F. Team of resource personnel	F. Nutritionist, social worker, counselor can assist in teaching specific care and providing support for changes
V. Teach patient/family: A. Pathophysiology, process, and causes of heart failure	A. Promotes understanding of disease that facilitates compliance and prevents complications
B. Importance of following a planned regimen and that all treatments must become part of daily routine	B. Promotes compliance of continued long-term care to prevent complications
C. Risk factors such as obesity, stress, smoking, diet, exercise deficit	C. Contribute to cardiovascular disease that can lead to heart failure

INTERVENTION	RATIONALE
D. Avoid strenuous exercise, large meals, extreme stress, smoking, excessive alcohol intake	D. Factors that can be modified to reduce cardiac workload and maintain cardiac status
E. Rest periods prior to and after activities, small meals six times/day	E. Prevents fatigue and additional work of the heart
F. Reinforce physician information regarding resumption of sexual activity and suggest changes to make	F. Changes in sexual pattern reduces cardiac workload
G. Monitoring of P prior to inotropic for decreases of <60/bpm or increases >120/bpm, allow to return demonstration and practice	G. Identifies P rate prior to medication administration for possible withholding and reporting to physician
H. Develop daily progressive activity program, avoid activity if tolerance decreases, dizziness, fatigue, dyspnea occur	H. Reduces risk factor of sedentary life-style while avoiding strain on cardiac function
I. Dietary changes with sample low salt intake of <4 g/day or as ordered, high-potassium foods, list of foods to restrict, and include to maintain nutritional status and explain rationale for dietary requirements and changes	I. Reduces risk factors associated with cardiac failure and resulting fluid retention, replaces potassium lost if diuretic administered

INTERVENTION	RATIONALE
J. Administration of inotropic, vasodilator, and diuretic to include route, action, dosage, expected results, frequency, when to take, how to take, possible side effects	J. Acts to decrease and strengthen ventricular contractility and emptying, increase CO; acts to excrete water and sodium by preventing absorption; a vasodilator increases blood flow to the myocardium
K. Weigh three times/week or as ordered and maintain a log for future evaluation during physician visit	K. Indicates weight gain caused by fluid retention or weight loss caused by diuretic therapy
L. Report weight gain of >2 lb/day, edema in extremities, weight loss of >5 lb/week, cough, dyspnea: nausea, vomiting, diarrhea, visual changes, mental confusion, pulse of <60/bpm	L. Signs and symptoms of possible heart failure, digitalis toxicity, or electrolyte imbalance to allow early treatment
M. Contact support groups for stress and weight reduction, stop smoking/alcohol programs	M. Provides assistance to reduce risk factors

hypertension

....

DEFINITION
The sustained or intermittent elevation of blood pressure of >140 mm Hg systolic and >90 mm Hg diastolic. It can be primary, the most common, or secondary, associated with renal disease, endocrine disorders, neurological disorders, and some drug therapy. It is known to cause increased peripheral vascular resistance that results in an increased workload on the heart and large and small vascular changes that results in circulatory deficits to the eyes, brain, kidneys, and heart. It is generally related to atherosclerosis, renal pathology, peripheral vascular disease, aortic aneurysm, and heart failure. Age, sex, and ethnicity are risk factors associated with hypertension that cannot be altered, however overweight, dietary intake, and stress are risk factors that can be changed. This plan includes interventions specific to an acute episode of hypertension, prevention of complications, and the reduction of risk factors and future complications of this long-term disorder. It can be used in association with HEART FAILURE/PULMONARY EDEMA, CORONARY ARTERY DISEASE/ ANGINA PECTORIS, and MYOCARDIAL INFARCTION care plans

NURSING DIAGNOSES
Pain related to physical injuring agent of increased cerebrovascular pressure or cardiac ischemia causing headache or chest pain

Altered peripheral tissue perfusion related to vascular resistance associated with atherosclerosis causing hypertension

Risk for activity intolerance related to circulatory problem causing inadequate organ or tissue perfusion, generalized weakness or fatigue

EXPECTED OUTCOMES
Pain absent or minimized and activity tolerance and endurance increased evidenced by verbalizations that feeling more relaxed and more rested with less fatigue, no requests for analgesic, able to participate in ADL, adequate tissue perfusion evidenced by BP readings within baseline lev-

els, normal mental status maintained, peripheral pulses and capillary refill time within normal parameters

INTERVENTION	RATIONALE
I. Assess for:	
A. Headache severity, location, time, associated dizziness and tightness in the head	A. Provides pain data to determine need for analgesia, headache usually occurs in the morning from increased cerebral spinal fluid pressure
B. BP elevations and continued increases regardless of treatments, angina pain, oliguria, cool and pallor of extremity skin, diminished peripheral pulse and capillary refill	B. Indicates reduced tissue perfusion to organs and tissues
C. Chest pain, dyspnea, dizziness, increased P and BP with activity, complaints of weakness and fatigue	C. Indicates reduced activity tolerance
II. Monitor, describe, record:	
A. BP and P q4h or as appropriate in sitting, lying, standing position as ordered, prior to and following activities	A. Indicates increases or decreases in BP or P to allow for interventions to normalize levels or rates
B. I&O q1–4h as appropriate	B. Indicates renal perfusion and effect on output, monitors use of diuretics

INTERVENTION	RATIONALE
III. Administer:	
A. Mild to moderate analgesic PO	A. Acts to block pain impulses to reduce headache pain
B. Antihypertensives PO such as beta-adrenergic blocker, alpha-adrenergic blocker, central-acting adrenergic blocker, calcium-channel blocker, angiotensin-converting enzyme blocker prescribed singly or in combination	B. Acts to reduce BP by reducing peripheral resistance with vasodilation, increase, decrease, or maintain cardiac output, block entry of calcium into smooth muscle, blocks conversion of angiotensin I to angiotensin II
C. Diuretic PO such as thiazide, loop, potassium-sparing	C. Acts to increase excretion of water, sodium, potassium or promote water and sodium excretion and retain potassium
D. Vasodilator PO	D. Acts to decrease peripheral vascular resistance by arterial dilation
IV. Perform/provide:	
A. Calm, quiet, nonstressful environment, well-ventilated and dimmed	A. Decreases stimuli that increases headache
B. Avoid bumping into bed, elevate head of bed to height of comfort	B. Decreases or relieves headache
C. Activity restrictions as ordered, rest between activities, assist with ADL when needed, and place all articles within reach for easy access	C. Promotes rest and conserves energy

INTERVENTION	RATIONALE
D. Limit visitors and length of visit	D. Promotes rest and prevents stimuli that causes fatigue
E. Inform to report headache that is not relieved by analgesic; dyspnea, dizziness, chest pain during activity	E. Allows for interventions to prevent complications caused by impaired blood perfusion of organs
F. Modified dietary regimen	F. Restricts fat, cholesterol, sodium intake, calories

NURSING DIAGNOSES

Risk for injury related to internal factor of increased cerebral vascular pressure causing stroke, increased vascular resistance affecting work of the heart causing angina/myocardial infarct/heart failure, impaired renal perfusion causing fluid volume excess

Anxiety related to threat of change in health status or death as a result of cardiac or cerebral complications of sustained hypertension

EXPECTED OUTCOMES

Risk of complications by hypertension and associated anxiety reduced or controlled evidenced by absence or resolution of abnormal signs and symptoms indicating heart or cerebral dysfunction, blood pressure maintained at baseline level with therapy, verbalizations that anxiety is within manageable levels with return of usual muscle relaxation and sleep pattern

INTERVENTION	RATIONALE
I. Assess for: A. Headache, dizziness, changes in visual acuity or mentation, motor and sensory changes, nausea, vomiting, seizures	A. Signs and symptoms of cerebral edema or ischemia or cerebrovascular accident

INTERVENTION	RATIONALE
B. Chest pain, dyspnea, nausea, tachycardia, distended neck veins, edema or fluid volume excess, abnormal heart and lung sounds auscultated, weakness, fatigue, diaphoresis, oliguria	B. Signs and symptoms of impending or presence of cardiac ischemia or heart failure
C. Restlessness, irritability, insomnia, tachycardia, tachypnea, tremor	C. Signs and symptoms of anxiety that can increase blood pressure

II. Monitor, describe, record:

A. BP for increases regardless of therapy q4h or as indicated	A. Sustained increases are predisposing to complications
B. I&O q1h or as appropriate	B. Indicates impaired renal function or dehydration associated with diuretic therapy, possible fluid volume excess
C. Daily weight, same time, scale, and clothing	C. Fluid retention causes weight gain, fluid loss from diuretic therapy causes weight loss
D. ECG for Q, T wave changes or ST segment changes	D. Indicates cardiac ischemia
E. Cardiac enzymes (CPK-MB, AST, LDG) for increases, BUN, creatinine	E. Elevations indicate cardiac damage or renal impairment
F. Chest x ray	F. Indicates effusion associated with heart failure

INTERVENTION	RATIONALE
III. Administer:	
A. Vasodilator IV	A. Acts to decrease work of the heart and oxygen requirements
B. Inotropic SLG	B. Acts to strengthen cardiac contractions in heart failure
C. Diuretic IV	C. Acts to decrease cerebral and peripheral edema
D. Beta-adrenergic blocker IV	D. Acts to decrease cardiac contractions and rate in cardiac ischemia
E. Potassium replacement IV	E. Treats or prevents hypokalemia with diuretic therapy
F. Oxygen via nasal cannula	F. Acts to supplement oxygen to tissues
IV. Perform/provide:	
A. Bed rest in semi- or high Fowler's position	A. Promotes comfort and reduces oxygen demands and fatigue
B. Restrict activities that cause any straining such as defecation or holding breath	B. Affects cardiac workload and output
C. Quiet, calm environment with assistance as needed, rest periods before and after activity	C. Provides emotional and physical support and conserves energy

NURSING DIAGNOSIS

Knowledge deficit related to disease process, medications, life-style changes, follow-up care, and reduction of risk factors (dietary, exercise, stress, smoking, overweight)

Noncompliance related to health beliefs and practices, cultural influences causing resistance to modification of life-style, acceptance of treatment regimen, and increased risk for cerebrovascular accident

EXPECTED OUTCOMES

Knowledge and understanding of disease and ongoing care with life-style modified to reduce risk factors associated with hypertension evidenced by verbalizations and understanding of and compliance with medication and dietary regimen, activity routine and restriction with participation in cardiac rehabilitation, signs and symptoms to report to physician and ongoing physician monitoring of cardiac/vascular status

INTERVENTION	RATIONALE
I. Assess for: 　A. Readiness, willingness, and motivation to learn about hypertension, discharge care, and life-style changes	A. Learning can best take place if client is receptive and compliance is more likely to occur
B. Health practices, health beliefs, ethnic identity (religion, diet, language), value orientations, family interactions and cooperation	B. Factors to incorporate into teaching plan to facilitate learning and compliance
IV. Perform/provide: 　A. Acknowledgment of perceptions with a nonjudgemental attitude	A. Establishes nurse–patient relationship in an accepting environment

INTERVENTION	RATIONALE
B. Explanations that are clear, accurate in understandable terms, small amount of information over time	B. Prevents misconceptions, erroneous attitudes and beliefs about disease
C. Environment conducive to learning with space, lighting, and proper equipment and supplies	C. Distractions or discomfort will interfere with learning
D. As much control over lifestyle change decisions as possible	D. Allows power to be given or retained by patient
E. Teaching aids (pamphlets, videotapes, pictures, written instructions)	E. Reinforces learning
F. Team of resource personnel/professionals	F. Nutritionist, social worker, counselor, rehabilitation therapist, and others can assist in teaching specific care and in providing support for desired changes
V. Teach patient/family: A. Anatomy, pathophysiology of hypertension, and effect of sustained hypertension on other organs (heart, eyes, kidneys, brain), and possible complications (myocardial infarction, stroke)	A. Promotes understanding of disease that facilitates compliance of lifetime therapy

INTERVENTION	RATIONALE
B. Risk factors such as over-weight, stress, smoking, fat, cholesterol, and sodium in diet, exercise deficit, alcohol intake; assist to formulate a realistic plan to avoid risk factors	B. Contributes to information about factors that can be modified with life-style changes
C. Dietary modification with sample menus for restriction in cholesterol, saturated fat, sodium content, calories, beverages containing caffeine, list of foods to include and restrict, tips on purchasing and preparing foods, amount of alcohol intake to allow/day	C. Reduces risk factors associated with hypertension
D. Administration and rationale of all prescribed medications (antihypertensives, antilipemics, diuretics, electrolyte replacement), written schedule of times and amounts, side effects to expect and to report, list of drugs that affect blood pressure or effectiveness of antihypertensives	D. Promotes compliance of complete medication regimen even when normal blood pressure levels are maintained

INTERVENTION	RATIONALE
E. Inform of common side effects of diuretic therapy such as dry mouth, frequent voiding, weakness, muscle fatigue, irregular pulse, paresthesia, lethargy, insomnia, and suggest to chew gum or candy, take diuretic in evening instead of morning; effects of antihypertensives such as orthostatic hypotension (getting up slowly and sitting at side of bed before standing), bradycardia, syncope, tachycardia, fatigue, dizziness, light-headedness and to avoid alcohol, driving or operating machinery when dizzy	E. Provides information and adjustments to make while taking medications
F. Procedure to take blood pressure, allow to demonstrate and practice in arm while sitting or standing, how to take weight once or twice a week and to maintain records of both for physician review during follow-up visits	F. Determines systolic and diastolic blood pressures, report increases or decreases
G. Progressive activity routine allowing for restrictions (lifting, strenuous exercises), rest periods when needed during activity, take steps to arrange for cardiac rehabilitation program if ordered	G. Supports life-style change (aerobic activities such as walking, swimming to a maximum of three times/ week for 30 minutes)

INTERVENTION	RATIONALE
H. Avoid stressful situations, consider counseling or stress reduction program to assist in development of coping and problem-solving skills	H. Prevents risk factor associated with hypertension
I. Report steady increases in BP, headache, nausea, vomiting, edema of ankles, changes in pulse or respirations or vision, muscle weakness or cramping to physician	I. Indicates increased risk for stroke, myocardial infarction, congestive heart failure, electrolyte imbalance
J. Importance of having laboratory tests such as lipid panel, electrolyte panel, and physician appointments as scheduled, notify physician prior to using any other medications	J. Evaluates effect of diet, medications, or other therapy for adjustment if needed
K. Contact support groups to stop smoking, for weight reduction, alcoholism, American Heart Association for information/educational materials	K. Provides assistance to reduce risk factors

inflammatory heart disease
(endocarditis/myocarditis/pericarditis)

DEFINITION

Infective endocarditis is the inflammation of the inner layer of the heart chambers and can result in defective valves causing blood flow and pressure changes. These changes eventually cause the formation of vegetations and valve dysfunction. Endocarditis usually occurs in those with known cardiac conditions. Myocarditis is the inflammation of the middle layer of the heart or heart muscle that results from microbial invasion (viral, bacterial, parasitic), radiation therapy, or chemicals such as alcohol. It usually affects both ventricles and can lead to cardiac enlargement, dysrhythmias, and heart failure. Pericarditis is the inflammation of the fibroserous sac that covers and supports the heart. It can be caused by infectious agents (viral, bacterial, parasitic, fungal), cardiac injury from trauma or surgery, radiation therapy, or drug reactions. Dry pericarditis results in adhesions that can obliterate the pericardial sac, exudative pericarditis results in accumulation of fluid in the sac that restricts ventricular filling and emptying and affects cardiac output. This plan includes interventions specific to these conditions but can be used in association with the HEART FAILURE/PULMONARY EDEMA care plan

NURSING DIAGNOSES

Pain related to physical injuring agent of microbial invasion of cardiac muscle or tissue inside or outside of the heart

   Hyperthermia related to illness of inflammation/infectious process

EXPECTED OUTCOMES

Relief or control of pain and temperature reduced and within baseline parameters evidenced by verbalizations that pain absent and rest and comfort increased following analgesic, temperature in range of 98.6°F (37°C) maintained

INTERVENTION	RATIONALE
I. Assess for:	
A. Chest pain, descriptors that include site, severity, frequency, or whether continuous, presence of palpitations, backache, headache, joint pain	A. Symptom associated with endocarditis, myocarditis, pericarditis
B. Elevated temperature in 102°F (38.9°C) range, chills, malaise, sweats, diaphoresis	B. Indicates signs and symptoms of acute or subacute infectious process
II. Monitor, describe, record:	
A. VS and temperature q4h	A. Increased pulse and respirations associated with temperature elevation
B. WBC, ESR	B. Normal or slight elevation of WBC in myocarditis and pericarditis, high elevation of 15,000 to 20,000 cu/mm in endocarditis; increases in ESR of >20 mm/hr for female, >13 mm/hr for male
C. Blood, throat cultures and sensitivities	C. Identifies causative organism and sensitivity to antibiotic therapy
III. Administer:	
A. Antipyretic PO	A. Acts to reduce temperature and promote comfort while reducing workload of heart in presence of fever
B. Analgesic IM	B. Acts to reduce chest pain that is severe, usually morphine

INTERVENTION	RATIONALE
C. Corticosteroid PO	C. Acts to reduce inflammatory process in pericarditis
D. Antimicrobial PO or IV in acute conditions; prophylactic therapy in endocarditis prior to invasive procedures (dental, surgery)	D. Acts to interfere with cell wall synthesis and cause death of pathogens

IV. Perform/provide:

A. Calm, restful environment with optimal warm temperature and ventilation, warm blankets and change of damp linens or clothing	A. Prevents stimuli that increases pain and chilling associated with fever
B. Bed rest if pain present or rest periods before and after activity	B. Exertion and fatigue increase pain perception
C. Semi-Fowler's, upright, leaning forward position, whichever enhances comfort	C. Reduces pain and promotes comfort
D. Backrub, sponge bath	D. Cooling measures to decrease temperature
E. Fluid intake of 2 to 3 L/day as permitted	E. Replaces fluid lost from diaphoresis as temperature increases or persists

NURSING DIAGNOSES

Decreased cardiac output related to factor of structural valvular changes causing heart failure in endocarditis, dysrhythmias, dilated cardiomyopathy, and heart failure in myocarditis, cardiac tamponade, heart failure in pericarditis or pericarditis with effusion

Activity intolerance related to imbalance between oxygen supply and demand (decreased cardiac output), generalized weakness (bed rest in presence of pain, inflammatory process)

EXPECTED OUTCOMES
Adequate cardiac output and progressive increase in activity tolerance and endurance within imposed limitations evidenced by hemodynamic parameters within baseline determinations (respirations, pulse, blood pressure, ECG strips), participation in ADL with partial or without assistance, and verbalizations that weakness and fatigue are disappearing and energy level increasing during activities

INTERVENTION	RATIONALE
I. Assess for:	
A. Stable pulse rate and rhythm, blood pressure, ECG tracings for dysrhythmias, urinary output of >30 mL/hr, dyspnea, clear lung sounds and absence of murmur, friction rub on auscultation	A. Identifies changes associated with reduced cardiac output
B. Activity level, extent of fatigue and cause, ability to participate in ADL, presence of pain, dyspnea, tachycardia, vertigo, weakness during activity	B. Indicates degree of activitiy intolerance and need to cease
II. Monitor, describe, record:	
A. VS, ECG as appropriate depending on acuteness of condition	A. Provides information about cardiac output complication and risk of activity intolerance
B. I&O q1h or as appropriate	B. Provides information about cardiac output as it affects renal function

INTERVENTION	RATIONALE
C. Cardiac enzymes	C. Increased enzyme levels associated with myocarditis, possibly pericarditis
D. Chest x ray, echocardiography	D. Procedures that assist with diagnosis of endocarditis, myocarditis
III. Administer:	
A. Oxygen via nasal cannula	A. Provides supplemental oxygen in presence of low cardiac output
IV. Perform/provide:	
A. Bed rest only when pain, temperature, or signs of heart damage are present	A. Reduces oxygen consumption and workload of the heart
B. Activities with scheduled rest periods	B. Prevents fatigue when in weakened state
C. Reduce or cease activity if weakness, tachycardia, dyspnea, increased BP, vertigo, diaphoresis occur	C. Identifies physical response to activity and prevents possible dysrhythmia
D. Assistive ROM and position change in bed q2h	D. Maintains muscle and joint function
E. Place articles within reach, commode at bedside, assist with care when needed	E. Conserves energy and promotes self-care within limitations
F. Encouragement and praise for attempts and participation in activity	F. Increases motivation to progress

NURSING DIAGNOSES

Anxiety related to change in health status (cardiac inflammatory process, risk of life-threatening dysrhythmia, heart failure, possible long-term treatment) causing ineffective coping and problem solving

Knowledge deficit related to follow-up treatment regimen and measures to prevent recurrence or complications of a cardiac inflammatory disease

EXPECTED OUTCOMES

Anxiety within manageable limits, development of coping skills, and compliance with discharge teaching evidenced by verbalizations that anxiety is decreasing and ability to continue self-monitoring and to carry out measures to prevent complications

INTERVENTION

I. Assess for:
   A. Level of anxiety, fear, and presence of insomnia, agitation, focus of anxiety, stated feelings about disease and possible outcome, ability to problem-solve

   B. Misconceptions about disease and willingness to follow discharge care plan

V. Teach patient/family:
   A. Environment conducive to rest, expression of fears and anxiety, and conducive to learning with space and privacy without distractions, avoid anxiety-producing situations

RATIONALE

A. Indicates range of anxiety that can be used as a basis for psychological support

B. Allows for clarification to reduce anxiety and ensure correct information

A. Decreases stimuli that cause stress/anxiety, venting of feelings decreases anxiety

INTERVENTION	RATIONALE
B. Explanation about the disease and the cause, all treatments in clear, understandable terms	B. Reduces concern about threat to health status and possible life-style changes
C. Inform that chest pain subsides in a few days	C. Reduces anxiety and fear of a serious heart disease
D. Relaxation techniques such as exercises, music, feedback, TV, reading, and others	D. Reduces anxiety and provides diversional activities
E. CPR techniques if appropriate	E. Promotes feeling of knowing what to do in an emergency
F. Activity routine that progresses following a period of convalescence of 2 to 4 weeks as advised, report increased pulse, weakness, vertigo	F. Resumes former life-style activities
G. Self-administration of antibiotic therapy IV for 6 weeks; prophylactic antibiotic therapy PO prior to dental or surgical procedures	G. Continues therapy if discharge takes place prior to completion; precautions taken to prevent sequela of endocarditis
H. Take temperature, and allow to return demonstration and practice, report any elevation, chills, malaise, increased fatigue, colds, chest pain	H. Indicates the presence of infection or other complication
I. Maintain nutritional and fluid daily intake	I. Promotes positive health practices

INTERVENTION	RATIONALE
J. Management of Holter telemetry and ECG checks by telephone or visit to technician/physician	J. Monitors continuous heart function for dysrhythmias
K. Avoid contact with persons with URI or infections	K. Prevents transmission of infection that can lead to heart involvement
L. Importance of keeping follow-up appointments	L. Provides ongoing monitoring to identify effectiveness of medication therapy and signs and symptoms of complications for early intervention

myocardial infarction

DEFINITION
Myocardial infarction (MI), also called heart attack, is the destruction and subsequent formation of necrosis of a segment of the myocardium resulting from an occlusion in a coronary artery causing a change or cessation of blood flow to this muscle. It usually occurs as a result of coronary artery disease with the ischemia causing angina and eventual damage to the myocardium. It can occur at various sites of the myocardium depending on specific coronary arterial insufficiency. This plan includes interventions specific to MI prior to open heart surgical and other invasive procedures (coronary bypass) and can be used in association with HEART FAILURE/PULMONARY EDEMA care plan

NURSING DIAGNOSES
Pain related to physical factor of myocardial ischemia as coronary blood flow is reduced causing metabolism end-products to accumulate that irritates nerve endings in heart muscle

Anxiety related to threat of death (heart attack), change in health status (unspecified consequences, multiple changes in life-style) causing inability to control pain episodes and to cope with uncertainty about future

EXPECTED OUTCOMES
Pain and anxiety reduced and controlled evidenced by verbalizations that pain is relieved and anxiety within manageable limits, relaxed muscles and facial expressions, restful sleep, less frequent request for analgesic, and successful use of coping mechanisms and relaxation techniques

INTERVENTION	RATIONALE
I. Assess for:	
A. Substernal pain, pressure, or feeling of heaviness, pain radiating to left arm, pain in shoulder, back, neck, jaw, palpitations, duration of 5 minutes or more, what precipitates or relieves pain	A. Pain typical of MI resulting from myocardial ischemia
B. Clutching at chest, pallor, restlessness, diaphoresis, nausea	B. Nonverbal associated symptoms of pain caused by infarction
C. Increases in BP, P, and R that are shallow, dyspnea, palpitations	C. Results from pain, unrelieved pain, or anxiety
D. Fear, feeling of suffocation, restlessness, irritability, withdrawal, tachycardia, tachypnea, hostility, grieving behaviors	D. Identifies level of anxiety associated with pain, fear of possible death
E. Internal and external stressors related to acute illness and personal resources with stress, anxiety	E. Assists to develop coping skills that are constructive using personal strength and support systems in place
II. Monitor, describe, record:	
A. VS and characteristics q2–4h	A. Increases with pain and anxiety and catecholamine release by stress increases BP and P
B. ECG strip during pain episode, or serial ECG readings	B. Identifies location of infarction and ischemic area causing the pain

INTERVENTION	RATIONALE
III. Administer:	
A. Analgesic, usually morphine IV, IM	A. Drug of choice for pain reduction in MI, acts by inhibiting pain pathways in CNS
B. Vasodilator SLG	B. Acts as coronary vasodilator increasing blood flow to myocardium to reduce pain
C. Antianxiety agent/sedative PO	C. Acts to reduce anxiety level and provides calming effect and rest, depresses subcortical levels of CNS, limbic system
IV. Perform/provide:	
A. Calm, quiet, comfortable environment that is supportive and allows for questions and verbalizations of concerns	A. Minimal stimuli reduce pain and anxiety
B. Remain until pain is relieved and maintain a calm, caring attitude	B. Provides support and reassurance to decrease anxiety and fear
C. Place on bed rest in semi-Fowler's position	C. Reduces pain by promoting comfort and respiratory effort
D. Relaxation techniques and diversional activities such as music, TV, reading	D. Reduces anxiety and distress
E. Limit visitors according to condition, avoid stressful situations	E. Eliminates unnecessary stimuli that increases pain and anxiety

INTERVENTION	RATIONALE
F. Encourage to report any pain at onset and any recurrence of pain before, during, or after therapy, pain unrelieved by vasodilator and lasting longer than 20 minutes	F. Extreme pain increases workload of heart, recurrence can indicate extension of infarction with decreasing ventricular function

NURSING DIAGNOSES

Decreased cardiac output (CO) related to inotropic changes in the heart (ischemia and infarction), alteration in rate, rhythm, and conduction (ischemia and infarction) causing decreased contractility, stroke volume, and dysrhythmias

   Altered cardiopulmonary tissue perfusion related to interruption of arterial flow to myocardial tissue (occlusion, infarct) causing reduced blood supply, cardiac output, and hemodynamic/respiratory changes

EXPECTED OUTCOMES

Adequate cardiac output and tissue perfusion evidenced by available hemodynamic measurements (CO, CVP, PAP) within normal ranges, P, BP, and R, within normal baseline ranges, dysrhythmias controlled or eliminated, cerebral, renal, peripheral, cardiopulmonary perfusion adequate with absence of signs and symptoms indicating circulatory insufficiency or pulmonary edema

INTEVENTION	RATIONALE
I. Assess for: A. P rate and rhythm (irregular of <60 or >100/bpm), reduced BP (<80 mm Hg), rapid and labored respirations(>20), apical pulse (<60/bpm), ECG tracings for dysrhythmias	A. Identifies changes associated with decreased CO caused by changes in heart rate, rhythm, and conduction

INTERVENTION	RATIONALE
B. Lung sounds for crackles, rhonchi, heart sounds for murmur, friction rub auscultated, dyspnea, jugular vein distention, cyanosis, decreased mental alertness, dependent edema, urinary output of <30 mL/hr, coolness and pallor to extremities with decreased pulses, capillary refill of <3 seconds	B. Identifies changes associated with reduced CO and perfusion problems in other system functions that result in organ dysfunction and hypoxia
C. Severe dyspnea, orthopnea with crackles and gallop auscultated, distended neck veins, oliguria, peripheral edema, gurgling respirations, and sense of impending doom	C. Indicates cardiac failure with pulmonary edema as pumping action of the heart is affected by the infarction

II. Monitor, describe, record:

INTERVENTION	RATIONALE
A. VS, CO, CVP, PAP q2–4h as appropriate for CO <4 L/minute, wedge pressure >18 mm Hg	A. Indicates hemodynamic stability to determine cardiac function status and potential for MI extension or heart failure
B. ECG single or continuous for T-wave changes, QRS segments, premature ventricular contractions (PVC)	B. Indicates myocardial tissue hypoxia, ventricular abnormalities that decrease CO leading to serious dysrhythmias

INTERVENTION	RATIONALE
C. ABGs, cardiac enzymes (AST, CPK-MB, LDH), pulse oximetry, PT (PO anticoagulant), PTT (IV anticoagulant)	C. Increases in CPK-MB indicates cardiac muscle damage and returns to normal in 3 to 4 days, LDH returns to normal within 10 days, decreases in oxygen indicates need for supplemental oxygen
D. Echocardiography, nuclear scan	D. Procedures performed to assist in diagnosis of cardiac function and MI
III. Administer: A. Vasodilator SLG	A. Acts to dilate coronary arteries and peripheral vessels to improve blood flow and reduce workload of heart
B. Beta-adrenergic blocker PO	B. Acts by decreasing myocardial contractility and heart rate and oxygen need
C. Inotropic PO	C. Acts to improve myocardial contractility and CO
D. Calcium-channel blocker PO	D. Acts to increase cardiac blood flow and reduce afterload and contractility of the heart resulting in decrease in work of the heart

INTERVENTION	RATIONALE
E. Antiarrhythmic PO, IV	E. Acts to delay the rate of depolarization, prolong repolarization and conduction, increase heart rate if bradycardia noted, selection depending on specific need
F. Anticoagulant PO, IV, antiplatelet agent PO	F. Acts to prevent thrombosis causing occlusion of coronary arteries, route dependent on acuteness of condition
G. Thrombolytic agent IV	G. Acts to relieve obstruction caused by thrombosis and improve CO
H. Oxygen via nasal cannula	H. Provides oxygen for hypoxia as a result of decreased CO

IV. Perform/provide:

A. Bed rest with activity restrictions as ordered, decrease activity level if symptoms appear	A. Reduces cardiac workload to improve CO
B. Place in semi- or high Fowler's position	B. Increases tidal volume and facilitates breathing with less effort
C. Calm, quiet, comfortable environment	C. Promotes environment with minimal stimuli that can increase stress and secretion of catecholamines and cardiac workload

INTERVENTION	RATIONALE
D. Avoid straining during defecation or holding breath	D. Increases venous return and preload causing increased cardiac workload
E. Restrict fluids as ordered if edema is present	E. Prevents excess fluid volume and retention
F. Prepare for intubation and mechanical ventilation, injection of thrombolytic agent, percutaneous transluminal coronary angioplasty, insertion of pacemaker	F. Ensures proper oxygenation of tissues, treats thrombosis to improve coronary arterial blood flow, controls irregular heart rhythm
G. Have cart with emergency equipment and supplies available	G. Provides for CPR and defibrillation if needed

NURSING DIAGNOSES

Hyperthermia related to illness (destruction and inflammation of myocardium)

 Altered nutrition: Less than body requiremens related to inability to ingest food (pain) causing nausea and vomiting

EXPECTED OUTCOMES

Return of temperature to normal in 3 to 7 days following acute onset of MI, resolution of pain with return to nutritional intake gradually to general diet within specific restrictions

INTERVENTION	RATIONALE
I. Assess for:	
A. Temperature elevation, chills, diaphoresis, malaise	A. Response to myocardial damage precipitating inflammatory process

INTERVENTION	RATIONALE
B. Nausea, vomiting, factors that influence or cause these, characteristics, frequency, and amount of vomiting	B. Occurs as a result of anxiety or pain from vagal reflex affecting the gastrointestinal tract

II. Monitor, describe, record:
A. Temperature q4h

A. Increases in 24 hours of >100°F (37.5°C) for up to a week, begins to decrease as healing takes place and scar tissue forms

B. WBC, ESR

B. Leukocytosis resulting from inflammation caused by MI with return to normal in 2 weeks, ESR increased during acute inflammation following damage to the myocardium

III. Administer:
A. Antipyretic PO

A. Acts to reduce temperature by inhibiting heat-regulating center

B. Antiemetic PO, IM

B. Acts to control vomiting by blocking chemoreceptor acting on vomiting center

IV. Perform/provide:
A. Fluid intake of 2,500 mL/day if allowed, liquid diet for the first 24 hours

A. Replaces fluid lost if diaphoretic with temperature elevation, liquid diet reduces the need for increased CO and oxygen consumption for digestive process

INTERVENTION	RATIONALE
B. Environment with optimal temperature and ventilation, free from odors and unpleasant sights	B. Promotes comfort at a time when feeling warm from temperature or nauseated as environment can stimulate vomiting center
C. Light-weight clothing, sponge bath if not chilled	C. Promotes comfort and reduces temperature
D. Small servings of food six times/day when diet advances to solids	D. Reduces volume of gastric contents and cardiac workload that can result in bradycardia or ectopic beats
E. Dietary inclusion of bulk and fiber	E. Prevents constipation and enhances bowel elimination without straining (Valsalva decreases CO and causes bradycardia)
F. Oral care prior to meals, following emesis, and rest periods after meals	F. Enhances appetite and promotes comfort while decreasing stimulation to vomiting center

NURSING DIAGNOSES

Activity intolerance related to imbalance between oxygen supply and demand (reduced CO and hypoxia, pain), weakness, and fatigue (enforced bed rest)

Sleep pattern disturbance related to internal factors of illness and psychological stress (fear and anxiety, sleep interrupted by treatments) causing weakness and fatigue, insomnia

EXPECTED OUTCOMES

Improved activity tolerance and endurance, and optimal rest/sleep patterns achieved evidenced by progressive participation in ADL with or without assistance and stable VS, verbalizations that fatigue is reduced and energy increased, and feeling rested with progressive increases in length of sleep periods

INTERVENTION	RATIONALE
I. Assess for:	
A. Level of fatigue, weakness, dyspnea, pallor, changes in VS following activity, potential for activity progression	A. Indicates activity status and allows for progressive return to activities and rehabilitation planning
B. Heart rate of >20/bpm of rest rate and not returning to pre-activity level within 3 minutes, BP increased 15 mm Hg during activity, cyanosis, diaphoresis, pain, dizziness, palpitations during activity	B. Indicates activity intolerance and risk for oxygen deprivation leading to change in exercise regimen
C. Interest and ability in performing ADL and other activities	C. Indicates readiness for program to ensure success of rehabilitation
D. Variation from usual sleep pattern, irritability, orientation changes, lethargy, yawning, tremors, listlessness	D. Interruptions in sleep are caused by multiple monitoring and treatments and result in sensory and psychological changes
III. Administer:	
A. Oxygen via nasal cannula	A. Increases oxygen for organs during periods of activity
B. Sedative PO	B. Acts to promote relaxation and induce sleep
IV. Perform/provide:	
A. Vital signs before, following, and 3 minutes following activity	A. Indicates response to activity and possible need for change in activity level or medications

INTERVENTION	RATIONALE
B. Bed rest or restricted activity as ordered, adequate rest periods during acute stage (3 days) and later between activities	B. Allows for healing and reduces oxygen demand and promotes rest
C. Quiet, temperature controlled and ventilated environment	C. Promotes rest and sleep
D. Organized care within limitations of fatigue and need for rest	D. Reduces frequency of interruptions that interfere with rest
E. Assist with ADL as needed, place articles within reach and anticipate needs	E. Conserves energy while allowing some control over care
F. ROM, assistive or passive TID	F. Promotes muscle and joint movement, enhances circulation
G. Limit visitors and length of stay if advisable	G. Promotes rest and conserves energy
H. Increase activities as tolerated within imposed limitations beginning with sitting at side of bed for 5 minutes three to five times/day, sitting in chair three times/day for 15 minutes, ambulating for 5 minute periods as tolerated, and praise all attempts at meeting these goals	H. Provides for slow, progressive program to prevent rapid increase in cardiac workload

INTERVENTION	RATIONALE
I. Allow to void and perform usual rituals prior to sleep (teeth brushing, snack, reading), avoid care during sleep	I. Promotes sleep by following established routines, treatments should allow for completion of sleep cycles (90 minutes for each complete cycle) to replenish mental and physical fatigue

NURSING DIAGNOSIS

Knowledge deficit related to disease process, medications, life-style changes and follow-up care (dietary, exercise, health practices, reduction of risk factors such as stress, smoking, overweight, hypertension)

EXPECTED OUTCOMES

Knowledge and understanding of disease, and ongoing care with life-style modified to reduce risk factors associated with recurrence of MI evidenced by verbalizations of and understanding and compliance with medication and dietary regimen, activity routine and restrictions with participation in cardiac rehabilitation, signs and symptoms to report to physician and ongoing physician monitoring of cardiac status

INTERVENTION	RATIONALE
I. Assess for:	
A. Readiness, willingness, and motivation to learn about MI, discharge care and life-style changes	A. Learning can best take place if client is receptive and compliance is more likely to occur
B. Health practices, health beliefs, ethnic identity (religion, diet, language), value orientations, family interactions and cooperation	B. Factors to incorporate into teaching plan to facilitate learning and compliance

INTERVENTION	RATIONALE
IV. Perform/provide:	
A. Acknowledgment of perceptions with a nonjudgmental attitude	A. Establishes nurse–patient relationship in an accepting environment
B. Explanations that are clear, accurate in understandable terms, small amount of information over time	B. Prevents misconceptions, erroneous attitudes and beliefs about MI
C. Environment conducive to learning with space, lighting, and proper equipment and supplies	C. Distractions or discomfort will interfere with learning
D. As much control over lifestyle change decisions as possible	D. Allows power to be given or retained by patient
E. Teaching aids (pamphlets, videotapes, pictures, written instructions)	E. Reinforces learning
F. Team of resource personnel/professionals	F. Nutritionist, social worker, counselor, sex therapist, rehabilitation therapist, and others can assist in teaching specific care and providing support for desired changes
V. Teach patient/family:	
A. Anatomy, function of the heart, pathophysiology of MI, and the healing process that takes about 6 to 8 weeks	A. Promotes understanding of disease that facilitates compliance

INTERVENTION	RATIONALE
B. Risk factors such as over-weight, stress, smoking, fat and cholesterol in diet, exercise deficit, alcohol intake, sodium intake, hypertension	B. Contributes to information about factors that can be modified with life-style changes
C. Dietary modification with sample menus for restriction in cholesterol, saturated fat, sodium content, beverages containing caffeine, list of foods to include and restrict, tips on purchasing and preparing foods, amount of alcohol intake to allow/day	C. Reduces risk factors associated with vessel changes predisposing to MI
D. Administration and rationale of all prescribed medications (vasodilators, antilipemics, beta-adrenergic blockers), written schedule of times and amounts, side effects to expect and to report	D. Promotes compliance of complete medication regimen
E. Procedure to take pulse, allow to demonstrate and practice	E. Determines heart rate and any irregularities to report
F. Progressive activity routine allowing for restrictions (lifting, pushing, jogging, after eating), rest periods when needed during activity, to cease activity if dizzy, dyspneic or has pain; take steps to arrange for cardiac rehabilitation program if ordered	F. Supports post–MI life-style change to accommodate healing heart muscle

INTERVENTION	RATIONALE
G. Resumption of sexual activity after time advised by physician with restrictions in positions, if fatigued, following bathing or meals, inform to take vasodilator prior to intercourse	G. Supports life-style changes needed to manage this activity without dyspnea or pain
H. Avoid stressful situations, consider counseling or stress reduction program to assist in development of coping and problem-solving skills	H. Prevents risk factor associated with heart attack
I. Guidelines for home activities such as housework, driving car, recreational activities, others that patient requests	I. Provides support for role performance
J. Report pain that is not relieved, dyspnea, pulse irregularity, edema, activity intolerance to physician	J. Indicates possible MI recurrence
K. Importance of having laboratory tests done and physician appointments as scheduled, notify physician prior to using any other medications	K. Anticoagulant or other therapy can be evaluated and adjusted if needed
L. Contact support groups to stop smoking, for weight reduction, alcoholism, American Heart Association for information/educational materials	L. Provides assistance to reduce risk factors

permanent pacemaker

DEFINITION

Permanent pacemakers are surgically inserted battery-powered devices (pulse generator) that control the beating of the heart when the conduction system develops problems or fails. They deliver rhythmic electric stimuli via an electrode (pacing catheter) placed in one or more chambers of the heart. They are utilized in long-term management to control serious dysrhythmias. This plan includes interventions specific to this procedure and can be used in association with PREOPERATIVE CARE and POSTOPERATIVE CARE for general surgical care

NURSING DIAGNOSIS

Decreased cardiac output related to electrical factor of alteration in conduction, alteration in rate and rhythm (dysrhythmias) prior to pacemaker insertion

EXPECTED OUTCOMES

Cardiac output maintained with adequate perfusion to all organs evidenced by blood pressure, pulse rate, respirations, peripheral pulses, and capillary refill within baseline determinations, oriented with normal mentation, skin pink and warm, and urinary output of >30 mL/hour

INTERVENTION	RATIONALE
I. Assess for: A. Decreased BP, increased and irregular P, weakness and vertigo, diminished peripheral pulses, skin pallor and cool to touch, restlessness, tachypnea	A. Indicates low cardiac output caused by dysrhythmias

INTERVENTION	RATIONALE
II. Monitor, describe, record:	
A. VS and ECG q4h or as appropriate	A. Indicates presence and status of dysrhythmias
B. I&O q1h for urinary output of at least 30 mL/hour	B. Indicates poor renal perfusion from low cardiac output
C. Electrolytes (K, Mg), CBC, BUN, ABGs	C. Cardiac function affected by K level, laboratory results indicate effect of low cardiac output on organs
III. Administer:	
A. Antiarrhythmics PO, IM, IV	A. Acts to suppress dysrhythmias by decreasing myocardial excitability and conduction velocity
B. Inotropics PO, IV	B. Acts to increase and strengthen heart rate
C. Oxygen via nasal cannula	C. Therapy to ensure oxygen to organs and reduces workload of the heart
IV. Perform/provide:	
A. Calm, quiet environment conducive to rest	A. Promotes rest by decreasing stimuli and reducing anxiety prior to surgery
B. Maintain bedrest in semi- or high Fowler's position	B. Reduces work of the heart to maximize cardiac output
C. Restrict activities, smoking, holding the breath, or straining during defecation, assist with ADL as needed	C. Reduces work of the heart and prevents vagal stimulation and sudden changes in cardiac output

INTERVENTION	RATIONALE
D. Small frequent feedings with restriction in caffeine-containing beverages	D. Reduces stimulation and work of the heart during digestion
E. Prepare for temporary pacing as ordered	E. Emergency measures if dysrhythmia worsens or becomes life-threatening

NURSING DIAGNOSIS

Risk for injury related to internal factor of postoperative complications of permanent pacemaker (malfunction of sensor or pulse generator), perforation of myocardium by catheter

EXPECTED OUTCOMES

Pacemaker in proper position and functioning within normal parameters postoperatively evidenced by stable BP, P, and ECG for correct pacing set during insertion, absence of catheter displacement causing possible dysfunction, perforation, and cardiac tamponade

INTERVENTION	RATIONALE
I. Assess for:	
A. Type of pacing and rate set by physician during surgery	A. Provides a basis for determining deviation from set rate or malfunction
B. Decreased BP, apical pulse less than preset rate with changes in ECG pacer spikes, dyspnea, palpitations, syncope	B. Indicates pacemaker malfunction that can result from failure to fire, sense, or capture and possible need to replace pacemaker or leads
C. Intercostal muscle spasms, hiccoughs, dyspnea, muffled heart sounds on auscultation, narrowing pulse pressure as BP declines	C. Indicates myocardial perforation and possible cardiac tamponade

INTERVENTION	RATIONALE
IV. Perform/provide:	
A. Activity restrictions and limited movement of the shoulder and arm (extension and abduction) on the insertion side for 2 days	A. Prevents catheter break or displacement or myocardial perforation in the immediate postoperative period
B. Reposition on side, check function with a pacemaker magnet	B. Corrects catheter displacement and monitors pacemaker function
C. Record the type and serial numbers of pulse generator and leads, date of surgery and the programmed rate and other functions	C. Provides information for future use as needed
D. Prepare for chest x ray and surgical replacement of pacemaker or catheter and repair of perforation if appropriate	D. Actions to diagnosis and correct catheter placement or malfunctioning pacemaker
E. Prepare for pericardiocentesis	E. Emergency treatment for cardiac tamponade

NURSING DIAGNOSIS

Knowledge deficit related to postoperative follow-up care of permanent pacemaker insertion and function

EXPECTED OUTCOMES

Appropriate care and management of pacemaker achieved evidenced by verbalizations of actions and precautions to take such as administration of prescribed medications, activities and dangers to avoid that can affect function, ongoing monitoring, and follow-up appointments to the physician

INTERVENTION	RATIONALE
V. Teach patient/family:	
A. Care of incisional site and to report redness, swelling, pain; inform to avoid wearing constrictive clothing near the pacemaker insertion site	A. Indicates possible infection of wound and prevents pressure to surgical site
B. Taking the pulse (radial) and report if slower than the set rate, allow to return demonstration and practice	B. Monitors pulse for decreases and possible malfunction
C. Range of motion exercises to arm and shoulder slowly at least three times/day	C. Promotes joint mobility and muscle strength while preventing displacement of the catheter
D. Avoid activities involving the arm and shoulder or lifting heavy objects (>5 pounds), sexual activity for 6 weeks	D. Prevents displacement of the catheter
E. Avoid contact sports or activities that include contact with surgical site	E. Prevents trauma to pulse generator and possible malfunction
F. Avoid areas of high voltage, magnetic fields, microwave ovens, airport detectors, radiation areas, devices to discourage theft in stores	F. Prevents pacemaker malfunction and can cause return of dysrhythmia, distances and precautions vary with specific risk for exposure
G. Medication administration, including action, dosage, route, side effects, and what to report	G. Promotes compliance of correct medication regimen

INTERVENTION	RATIONALE
H. Report changes in pulse regularity, fatigue and weakness, chest pain, dizziness, dyspnea	H. Indicates possible complications of pacemaker insertion
I. Carry a pacemaker card with all necessary information, wear a medical alert identification bracelet	I. Provides emergency information if needed
J. Monitoring of ECG by telephone and when and how performed	J. Provides information about routine pacemaker check or if symptoms occur
K. Importance of visiting physician periodically as instructed	K. Evaluates pacemaker function and need for change in programming

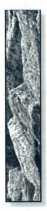

Respiratory System Standards

respiratory system data base

chronic obstructive pulmonary disease (emphysema/chronic bronchitis/asthma)

laryngectomy/neck dissection

pleuritis/pleural effusion

pneumonia

pneumothorax/hemothorax

pulmonary embolism

pulmonary resection (lobectomy/segmental/pneumonectomy)

rhinoplasty/septoplasty

tonsillitis/tonsillectomy

respiratory system data base

HISTORICAL DATA REVIEW
Past events:
1. Acute and/or chronic lung and airway disease or disorders
2. Signs and symptoms related to upper (nose, throat) or lower (bronchi, lungs) respiratory disorders (nasal discharge, epistaxis, postnasal drip, nasal congestion, headache in upper respiratory system and dyspnea, cough, sneezing, wheezing, sputum and characteristics, hemoptysis in lower respiratory system)
3. Pulmonary disease, allergies of family members
4. Allergies and effect on respirations, nasal mucosa
5. Childhood immunizations and immunization for flu and pneumonia
6. Anxiety, tobacco use, occupational/environmental irritants, multiple colds, exercise routine and tolerance, anorexia and weight loss
7. Treatments, oxygen, desensitization therapy, rehabilitation associated with respiratory system, chest physiotherapy
8. Medications (prescription and over-the-counter) for respiratory conditions
9. Hospitalization and feelings about care, surgery associated with upper or lower respiratory tract

Present events:
1. Medical diagnoses associated with or affecting respiratory function, airway patency, and ventilation
2. Respiratory rate, depth, ease, changes with exertion
3. Abnormal pattern, dyspnea, orthopnea, tachypnea, wheezing, stridor, and accessory muscles used
4. Presence of artificial airway and/or mechanical ventilation
5. Chest or pleuritic pain, throat pain, sinus headache
6. Productive or nonproductive cough and color, consistency, and amount of sputum, epistaxis, hoarseness
7. Cyanosis or pallor of skin and mucous membranes

8. Activities of daily living and effect on respirations; activity intolerance, weakness, fatigue, insomnia, anxiety level
9. Preference in positioning, daily exercises/treatments for optimal breathing

PHYSICAL ASSESSMENT DATA REVIEW

1. Symmetry of chest shape, chest contour, anterior/posterior chest expansion, and movements during inspiration and expiration
2. Nasal shape, symmetry, edema, drainage, septal alignment, throat redness or edema
3. Nasal/airway patency and breathing pattern
4. Clubbing of fingers and toes
5. Hypoxemia with cyanosis (lips, face, nailbeds), confusion, restlessness
6. Crepitus, vocal and tactile fremitus palpated
7. Resonant sounds, pitch and intensity of lung fields on percussion
8. Breath sounds auscultated for crackles, wheezes, rhonchi, diminished or absent and areas involved

NURSING DIAGNOSES CONSIDERATIONS

1. Activity intolerance
2. Altered nutrition: less than body requirements
3. Altered tissue perfusion (cardiopulmonary)
4. Anxiety/fear
5. Dysfunctional ventilatory weaning process
6. Risk for aspiration
7. Risk for infection
8. Impaired gas exchange
9. Inability to sustain spontaneous ventilation
10. Ineffective airway clearance
11. Ineffective breathing pattern
12. Knowledge deficit
13. Sensory/perceptual alteration (olfactory)

GERIATRIC CONSIDERATIONS

Pulmonary changes in geriatric patients depend on the aging process and the environment and affect lung structure and function, gas exchange and pulmonary circulation, homeostasis, and ventilatory control. These changes are continuous and long term and result in reduced ventilation and alteration in ventilation/perfusion of the lungs. Respiratory changes associated with aging that should be considered when assessing the geriatric patient include:

1. Reduced bronchopulmonary movement and strength of muscles with an increased use of accessory muscles and diaphragm in breathing
2. Increased stiffness and rigidity of rib cage, calcification of cartilage at rib articulation areas with a decreased chest expansion
3. Reduced cough reflex and ciliary movement, sensitivity to stimuli, increased drying/atrophy of mucosa resulting in decreased broncho-elimination
4. Loss of lung elasticity, compliance and air retention in bases of lungs, shallow and more rapid respiratory rate with a decreased amount of air taken in, reduced respiratory excursion with difficulty in breathing deeply
5. Loss of blood vessel and lung elasticity, decreased number of alveoli and lung recoil with decreased alveoli perfusion and rate of movement of gases, greater risk for impaired gas exchange

DIAGNOSTIC LABORATORY TESTS AND PROCEDURES

1. Chest x ray (CXR), pulmonary function tests, bronchoscopy, bronchography, lung biopsy, thoracentesis with fluid examination, computerized tomography (CT), nuclear scan (Gallium), angiography, pulmonary stress test and body plethysmography, ultrasonography if fluid is present, fluoroscopy, thoracoscopy, transillumination, tissue biopsy, and skin tests
2. Arterial blood gases (ABGs), hemoglobin (Hb) and hematocrit (Hct), sputum studies (culture/stain), nose/throat cultures, therapeutic drug levels (theophylline), complete blood count (CBC), pulse oximetry

MEDICATIONS

1. Antiasthmatics: cromolyn sodium
2. Antihistamines: terfenadine, diphenhydramine hydrochloride, promethazine hydrochloride
3. Antimicrobials: penicillins, erythromycin, cephalosporins, aminoglycosides, tetracyclines
4. Antituberculars: isoniazid, rifampin, streptomycin, ethambutol, pyrazinamide

5. Antitussives: dextromethorphan hydrobromide, guaifenesin with codeine, benzonatate, hydrocodone bitartrate
6. Bronchodilators: theophylline, albuterol, ipratropium bromide, isoproterenol, epinephrine
7. Corticosteroids: prednisone, flunisolide, beclomethasone
8. Decongestants: ephedrine sulfate, phenylephrine hydrochloride
9. Expectorants: guaifenesin
10. Mucolytics: acetylcysteine, glyceryl gualacolate
11. Oxygen: delivered via nasal cannula or face mask

chronic obstructive pulmonary disease
(emphysema/chronic bronchitis/asthma)

DEFINITION

Chronic obstructive pulmonary disease (COPD) encompasses respiratory disorders characterized by increased airway resistance affecting the movement of air in and out of the lungs. The resistance is caused by edema or contractions (bronchospasms), or decrease in elastic recoil preventing the emptying of air from the lungs. Included in this grouping are asthma, chronic bronchitis, and emphysema. The most important risk factors involved in these diseases are smoking and environmental pollution. Although all three conditions can be present to some degree at the same time with any obstructive airflow limitation, one usually predominates with its specific subjective and objective diagnostic signs and symptoms

NURSING DIAGNOSES

Ineffective airway clearance related to tracheobronchial secretion resulting from inflammation and mucus accumulation in airways causing bronchospasms, and decreased energy and fatigue with decreased ability to cough causing stasis of secretions

Ineffective breathing pattern related to decreased lung expansion, energy and fatigue resulting from pain and inflammatory process causing anxiety, inadequate ventilation

Impaired gas exchange related to alveolar-capillary membrane changes and altered oxygen supply resulting from overdistention and destruction of alveoli and obstruction of smaller airways causing a reduction of airflow and tissue for gas exchange

EXPECTED OUTCOMES

Improved and adequate respiratory function, ventilation, and tissue oxygenation evidenced by respiratory rate, ease, depth, and breath sounds within baseline parameters, effective removal of secretions with airway clearance and patency, ABGs within normal range

INTERVENTION	RATIONALE
I. Assess for:	
A. Respiratory rate, depth, ease, noting dyspnea at rest or with exertion, tachypnea, prolonged expiration, wheezing, use of accessory muscles, sternal and intercostal retractions	A. Provides data baselines and changes indicating airway resistance, bronchospasms and narrowing of bronchi, presence of environmental irritants
B. Chronic cough with or without sputum production and ability to cough and expectorate increasing amounts of or tenacious secretions	B. Sputum production results from increasing goblet cells and irritant response
C. Decreased breath sounds, wheezing on expiration on auscultation, hyperresonance on percussion, decreased fremitus	C. Results from damage to bronchioles and indicates severity of disease
D. Changes in mental status (restlessness, confusion, lethargy), cyanosis, fatigue, air hunger	D. Indicates decreases in oxygenation and hypoxemia
E. Increased AP chest diameter and barrel chest appearance	E. Results from hyperinflation and pressure against chest wall
II. Monitor, describe, record:	
A. VS with R and breath sounds q2–4h or as needed	A. Indicates airway movement, resistance, changes indicating increasing severity of disease and possible complication of respiratory failure

INTERVENTION	RATIONALE
B. ABGs, pulse oximetry	B. Indicates need for supplemental oxygen if hypoxemia (hypoventilation) present, or prepresence of hypercapnia (chronic respiratory acidosis)
C. Chest x ray	C. Reveals hyperinflation, flattened diaphragm, bronchovascular markings
D. Pulmonary function studies	D. Reveals reduced diffusion capacity, increased residual volume and capacity, other changes depending on specific disease

III. Administer:

A. Antitussive/expectorant PO	A. Acts on bronchial cells to increase fluid production and promote expectoration, reduces surface tension of secretions, both to relieve nonproductive cough
B. Bronchodilator PO, INH	B. Acts to dilate bronchi, relieve bronchospasms in reversible airway obstruction
C. Oxygen via nasal cannula	C. Supplemental oxygen to maintain optimal level for tissue oxygenation

INTERVENTION	RATIONALE
IV. Perform/provide:	
A. Place in semi- or high Fowler's position on bed rest with restricted activities, orthopneic position using overbed table and pillow if needed	A. Provides needed rest and reduced need for oxygenation, facilitates comfort and ease of breathing to assist ventilation and air exchange
B. Assist in deep breathing, coughing exercises with pursed lip breathing, abdominal breathing with emphasis on prolonged expiratory phase q2h	B. Improves ventilation and coughing to reduce airway collapse and remove secretions, coughing clears the airways by propelling secretions to mouth, abdominal and pursed lip breathing uses stronger muscles to prolong expiratory phase and reduce carbon dioxide retention and lips act as retard valves, both maintain patency of compliant or floppy airways
C. Increased fluid intake to 2 L/day if permitted and if cough dry and hacking	C. Liquefies secretions for easier removal
D. Humidified air via cool mist vaporizer, postural drainage if condition warrants this procedure four times/day	D. Facilitates the removal of secretions, moistens mucous membranes
E. Orotracheal suctioning as appropriate and if ordered	E. Removes secretions when other methods have failed
F. Oral care after expectoration and provide tissues and bag for proper disposal	F. Promotes comfort and prevents transmission of organisms

NURSING DIAGNOSES

Anxiety related to threat to or change in health status and outcome of illness causing inability to manage feelings of uncertainty and apprehension regarding situation crisis, change in breathing pattern and inability to sleep

Ineffective individual coping related to inability to cope with long-term chronic illness, change in appearance, and future life-style changes

Fear related to hospitalization and treatments causing increased apprehension and tension

EXPECTED OUTCOMES

Anxiety and fear within manageable levels, development of coping and problem-solving skills evidenced by breathing with ease, sleeping 6 to 8 hours/night, verbalizations that anxiety is decreasing, fear reduced, participation in care activities and receptive attitude to planning for ongoing care needed to manage disease and chronic anxiety

INTERVENTION	RATIONALE
I. Assess for:	
A. Level of anxiety, use of coping mechanisms, stated fears of uncertainty of disease outcome, life-style changes, fear of suffocation and death	A. Anxiety can range from mild to severe and respiratory rate, rest will be affected accordingly, assists to identify inappropriate use of coping skills; high level of anxiety associated with dyspnea
B. Restlessness, diaphoresis, complaining, joking, withdrawal, talkativeness, increased P and R	B. Nonverbal expressions of anxiety when not able to communicate feelings
C. Personal resources to cope with stress, anxiety, and interest in learning to problem-solve	C. Support systems and personal strengths assist to develop coping skills

INTERVENTION	RATIONALE
D. Feelings and response to change in appearance, chest shape, progressive weight loss and cachexia, declining ability to carry out role and participate in activities	D. Changes in body image and self-concept are common problems associated with long-term respiratory disorders

III. Administer:
A. Anti-anxiety agent PO	A. Acts to reduce anxiety level and provides calming effect and rest, depresses subcortical levels of CNS, limbic system

IV. Perform/provide:
A. Environment conducive to rest, expression of fears and anxiety, avoid anxiety-producing situations	A. Decreases stimuli that cause stress/anxiety, venting of feelings decreases anxiety
B. Mimic slower respiratory rate, remain during dyspneic episodes to provide support	B. Allows to focus on breathing pattern with slowing rate and improves depth; results in reduced fear and anxiety
C. Suggest new methods to enhance coping skills and problem solving, allow to externalize and identify those that help	C. Offers alternative coping strategies that allow for release of anxiety and fear
D. Positive feedback regarding progress made, focus on abilities rather than inabilities	D. Provides support for adaptive behavior, promotes self-worth and responsibility

INTERVENTION	RATIONALE
E. Diversional activities such as relaxation exercises, TV, radio, music, reading, tapes, guided imagery	E. Reduces anxiety and promotes comfort
F. Limit visitors according to condition, avoid stressful situations	F. Eliminates unnecessary stimuli that increases anxiety
G. Allow to participate in planning of care to maintain usual activities when possible	G. Allows for some control over situations
H. Support grieving for loss of life-style and restrictions in activities, changes in physical appearance	H. Provides assistance in adaptation to changes imposed by disease

NURSING DIAGNOSES

Activity intolerance related to imbalance between oxygen supply and demand (inflammatory process) causing tissue hypoxia, weakness, decreased endurance, fatigue, and increased energy requirements to perform ADL

Sleep pattern disturbance related to internal factors of illness (dyspnea, coughing, insomnia from medication regimen) and psychological stress (anxiety) causing disruption of sleep, fatigue

EXPECTED OUTCOMES

Progressive increase in activity tolerance and return to sleep and rest pattern with reduction in fatigue level evidenced by increased performance of ADL with decreased dyspnea, increased energy and endurance, VS stable before, during, and after activity, uninterrupted sleep with verbalizations that feeling more rested and less anxious

INTERVENTION	RATIONALE
I. Assess for:	
A. Level of fatigue, weakness, and potential for activity progression, effect on respirations, dyspnea with activities	A. Provides baseline and allows for planning activities and need for assistance
B. Interest and ability in performing ADL with or without assistance	B. Readiness and increased energy level necessary for successful program
C. Sleep/rest pattern, wakefulness during night, irritability, lethargy	C. Optimal rest and sleep necessary to reduce fatigue and perform activities
D. R >20/min, P >120/bpm and not returning to preactivity level within 3 minutes, palpitations, dyspnea, dizziness, weakness, and stopping activity if symptoms appear	D. Signs and symptoms of activity intolerance leading to fatigue
III. Administer:	
A. Sedative PO, unless respirations <12/minute	A. Acts on limbic and subcortical levels of CNS and increases sleep time
B. Oxygen via nasal cannula	B. Supplements oxygen during daily activities or sleep as needed
IV. Perform/provide:	
A. Bed rest during acute state in a position of comfort with body parts supported with pillows	A. Conserves energy and provides needed rest

INTERVENTION	RATIONALE
B. Perform or assist in ADL and other activities as needed, place all articles and call light within reach to use as desired, utilize self-care aids as appropriate	B. Conserves energy while preserving as much control and independence as possible
C. Increases activities gradually from sitting up in bed, in chair, walking in room, to bathroom, and in hall with daily increase in distance and ADL activities, suggest deep breathing and pursed-lip breathing during activities	C. Progressive change in activities increases with endurance and energy level and prevents symptoms of activity intolerance
D. Organize activities around rest periods in a quiet, calm, dimly lit, environment free of stimuli and respiratory irritants	D. Permits rest without interruptions
E. Assist to assume preferred position for sleep, offer backrub, oral care, extra pillows, other activities based on sleep pattern	E. Provides for usual bedtime rituals to ensure comfort and sleep
F. Restrict visitors and limit time of visit	F. Prevents additional stimuli that interferes with rest, causes fatigue

NURSING DIAGNOSES

Risk for infection related to inadequate primary defenses (decrease in ciliary action, stasis of pulmonary secretions), chronic disease, and failure to avoid exposure to pathogens

Hyperthermia related to illness (infectious process of pneumonia or acute bronchitis)

EXPECTED OUTCOMES
Complication of chronic pulmonary disease prevented evidenced by temperature, respirations, WBC within normal range, negative sputum culture, absence of chest/tracheobronchial discomfort

INTERVENTION	RATIONALE
I. Assess for: A. Dyspnea or other respiratory changes, decreased breath sounds and crackles auscultated, pleuritic pain, cough with yellowish to greenish sputum and increased tenaciousness	A. Signs and symptoms of pulmonary infection, upper or lower tract
B. Temperature elevation, chills	B. Indicates presence of infection
II. Monitor, describe, record: A. Temperature q4h and PRN	A. Elevations indicate infection
B. WBC	B. WBC of >12,000/cm indicates infectious process
C. Sputum culture	C. Identifies infectious agent and evaluates antimicrobial therapy
D. Chest x ray	D. Reveals areas of consolidation in diagnosis of pneumonia
III. Administer: A. Antibiotic PO, IV	A. Acts to prevent cell wall synthesis to destroy microorganisms in the treatment of acute infection

INTERVENTION	RATIONALE
B. Corticosteroid PO, IV	B. Acts as an anti-inflammatory agent to reduce inflammation and increase body defenses in acute infection
C. Antipyretic PO	C. Acts to reduce temperature

IV. Perform/provide:

INTERVENTION	RATIONALE
A. Environment with optimal temperature, humidity, and ventilation, free of smoking or other irritants	A. Promotes comfort and respiratory ease
B. Avoid exposure to visitors or staff with upper respiratory infection	B. Prevents transmission of infectious agents
C. Calm, restful environment with warm blankets and change of damp linens or clothing	C. Prevents stimuli that decreases rest and prevents chilling associated with fever
D. Backrub, sponge bath, relaxation techniques	D. Cooling measures to decrease temperature and promote comfort
E. Fluid intake of 2 to 3 L/day as permitted, warm fluids if chilled	E. Replaces fluid lost from diaphoresis as temperature increases or persists
F. Cleansing and disinfection of equipment used in treatments	F. Prevents inhalation of infectious agents

NURSING DIAGNOSIS

Altered nutrition, less than body requirements related to inability to ingest food because of biologic factors (dyspnea, fatigue, anorexia) causing weight loss and decreased energy reserves

EXPECTED OUTCOMES

Nutritional status maintained evidenced by weight range within baseline determinations, Hb and albumin within normal ranges, fatigue reduced as appetite and food intake increase

INTERVENTION	RATIONALE
I. Assess for:	
A. Weight loss, skinfold thickness, anorexia, 24-hour recall of food intake with calorie count	A. Signs and symptoms of possible malnutrition state caused by need for increased calories for work of breathing
B. Effect of breathing pattern on appetite and amount of food intake	B. Dyspnea, coughing, and resulting fatigue cause decreased food intake
II. Monitor, describe, record:	
A. Weight on same scale, same time of day, same clothing q2days or as appropriate	A. Indicates weight changes that can reveal malnutrition
B. Transferrin, albumin, Hb	B. Indicates nutritional status
III. Administer:	
A. Vitamin/minerals PO	A. Supplements diet to ensure adequate intake of these requirements
B. Oxygen via nasal cannula	B. Relieves dyspnea during meals

INTERVENTION	RATIONALE
IV. Perform/provide: A. Non-anxiety-producing environment free of odors	A. Prevents stimuli that affects breathing pattern and appetite
B. Place in high Fowler's or sitting position	B. Relieves dyspnea during meals
C. Small, frequent meals instead of three large meals, allow time needed to eat slowly and not feel rushed	C. Feeling of fullness can place pressure on diaphragm and affect breathing
D. Oral care and rest period prior to meals	D. Promotes comfort of mucous membranes and appetite
E. Dietary high-calorie supplements with or between meals	E. Supplies needed extra caloric intake
F. Consult with nutritionist for meal planning	F. Provides assistance for high-calorie dietary intake according to personal preferences

NURSING DIAGNOSES

Knowledge deficit related to disease process, medications, life-style changes, and follow-up care (dietary requirements, exercise program, respiratory health practices, reduction of risk factors such as stress, smoking), measures to prevent infection, signs and symptoms to report to physician

Noncompliance related to health beliefs, cultural values evidenced by inability to implement proposed therapeutic regimen and failure to maintain health status

EXPECTED OUTCOMES

Knowledge and understanding of disease and ongoing care with life-style modified to reduce risk factors associated with COPD evidenced by verbalizations of and understanding and compliance with medication, immunization, and dietary regimen, activity routine and restrictions with participation in pulmonary rehabilitation, signs and symptoms to report and ongoing physician monitoring of respiratory status

INTERVENTION	RATIONALE
I. Assess for: A. Readiness, willingness, and motivation to learn, discharge care and life-style changes	A. Learning can best take place if client is receptive and compliance is more likely to occur
B. Health practices, health beliefs, ethnic identity (religion, diet, language), value orientations, family interactions and cooperation	B. Factors to incorporate into teaching plan to facilitate learning and compliance with long-term care
IV. Perform/provide: A. Acknowledgement of perceptions with a nonjudgmental attitude	A. Establishes nurse–patient relationship in an accepting environment
B. Explanations that are clear, accurate in understandable terms, small amount of information over time	B. Prevents misconceptions, erroneous attitudes and beliefs about disease
C. Environment conducive to learning with space, lighting, and proper equipment and supplies	C. Distractions or discomfort will interfere with learning

INTERVENTION	RATIONALE
D. As much control over life-style change decisions as possible, include in discharge planning	D. Allows power to be given or retained by patient
E. Teaching aids (pamphlets, videotapes, pictures, written instructions)	E. Reinforces learning
F. Team of resource personnel/professionals	F. Nutritionist, social worker, counselor, pulmonary rehabilitation therapist, and others can assist in teaching specific care and providing support for desired changes
V. Teach patient/family:	
A. Anatomy, function of the lungs, pathophysiology, and progressive nature of the disease, age-related factors causing deterioration	A. Promotes understanding of disease that facilitates compliance
B. Risk factors such as malnutrition, stress, smoking, exercise deficit, effect on body image and independence in self-care activities	B. Contributes to information about factors that can be modified with life-style changes
C. Dietary modification with sample menus for additional calories, list of foods to include and measures to take to improve appetite (oral care, frequent feedings, supplements)	C. Reduces risk factor associated with weight loss

INTERVENTION	RATIONALE
D. Administration and rationale of all prescribed medications (antibiotics, bronchodilators, anti-inflammatory), written schedule of times and dosages, side effects to expect and to report, demonstrate use of hand-held inhalers and small-volume nebulizer as well as care of equipment and allow to return demonstration	D. Promotes compliance of complete medication regimen
E. Fluid intake of 10 to 12 glasses/day with inclusion of high-calorie liquids	E. Maintains daily fluid needs
F. Environment free of smoking, pollutants, change filters monthly, remove cooking and other odors (plants, perfume)	F. Provides air free of irritants that provoke changes in breathing pattern
G. Continue coughing and deep-breathing exercises, inform of resources to obtain small-volume nebulizer, incentive spirometer, oxygen and equipment if needed (instruct in safety measures to follow in use of oxygen)	G. Maintains respiratory health status and prevents complications or safety hazards

INTERVENTION	RATIONALE
H. Progressive activity routine allowing for restrictions, rest periods when needed during activity, to cease activity if dizzy, dyspneic; take steps to arrange for pulmonary rehabilitation program if ordered	H. Supports life-style change to maintaining respiratory status
I. Suggest home modifications to support energy and endurance level	I. Conserves energy while maintaining control of self-care
J. Avoid stressful situations, consider counseling or stress-reduction program to assist in development of coping and problem-solving skills	J. Prevents risk factor associated with chronic pulmonary disease
K. Encourage to avoid groups or persons with upper respiratory disease or during flu season	K. Prevents transmission of infectious agents to already compromised respiratory system
L. Report temperature elevation, chills, dyspnea, pulse irregularity, activity intolerance, continued fatigue, chest pain, change in cough and sputum characteristics (yellow, rust colored), irritability, restlessness to physician	L. Indicates possible recurrence or complication of pneumonia (pleural effusion, atelectasis)

INTERVENTION	RATIONALE
M. Importance of having pneumovax and flu immunization, keeping appointments as scheduled, notify physician prior to using any other medications	M. Protects against bacterial pneumonia and influenza
N. Contact support groups to stop smoking, for financial counseling, American Lung Association for information/educational materials	N. Provides assistance to reduce risk factors

laryngectomy/neck dissection

DEFINITION
Laryngectomy is the surgical removal of the larynx performed to treat a malignant tumor. It can be partial (supraglottic, vertical) or total depending on the site and extent of tumor and may or may not involve loss of the voice and tracheostomy. Radical neck dissection can be done with laryngectomy to treat metastatic neck masses to remove cervical lymph nodes and drainage channels, muscle, spinal accessory nerve, and vessels on the tumor side. It is also done to treat oral malignancy and is accompanied by a tracheostomy. A modified neck dissection procedure leaves the nerve, muscle, and jugular vein in place. Finally, a procedure to allow for the postoperative insertion of a voice prosthesis can be performed if a complete loss of voice is anticipated. This plan, which includes interventions specific to these procedures, can be used in association with NEOPLASM (CHEMOTHERAPY/EXTERNAL AND INTERNAL RADIATION), PREOPERATIVE CARE, and POSTOPERATIVE CARE plans

NURSING DIAGNOSES
Ineffective airway clearance postoperatively related to tracheobronchial secretion or obstruction resulting from irritation of respiratory tract, presence of tracheostomy tube, and inability to cough, trauma of surgery causing edema, bleeding

    Risk for aspiration related to presence of tracheostomy tube, nasogastric tube, and trauma from neck surgery resulting in absence of normal protective mechanisms causing possible entry of secretions or feedings into tracheobronchial passages

EXPECTED OUTCOMES
Postoperative adequate respiratory function, ventilation, with proper tracheostomy placement and patency evidenced by respiratory rate, ease, depth, and breath sounds within baseline parameters, effective removal of secretions by coughing or suctioning, and absence of aspiration of secretions, liquid nutritional formula into airways and lungs leading to aspiration pneumonia

INTERVENTION	RATIONALE
I. Assess for: A. Respiratory rate, depth, ease, via normal passages or tracheostomy, chest expansion symmetry, decreased breath sounds	A. Provides data baselines and changes caused by postoperative obstruction of airways or tube (bleeding into the airway, edema, or plugged or dislodged tube)
B. Coughing ability with amount and viscosity of secretions, ability to expectorate or remove via the tube immediately postoperatively, color of secretions	B. Secretions can be copious with a tracheostomy tube in place, coughing removes secretions that can be aspirated, secretions are usually blood-tinged 48 hours following surgery
C. Type of tracheostomy tube, presence of laryngectomy tube, tube placement, and patency	C. Provides temporary airway that bypasses surgical area(s), tube can be cuffed or not cuffed, fenestrated speaking tube
II. Monitor, describe, record: A. R rate and ease, breath sounds q2–4h or as needed	A. Indicates airway movement, change in status and possible adventitious sounds or decreased breath sounds associated with mucus accumulation or aspiration
III. Administer: A. Mucolytic/bronchodilator INH	A. Acts to dilate airways and provide moisture to liquefy the secretions for easier removal

INTERVENTION	RATIONALE

IV. Perform/provide:

A. Place in semi- or high Fowler's position on bed rest; sidelying with head turned to one side if comfortable

A. Provides needed rest and facilitates comfort and ease of breathing, drainage of secretions

B. Cleanse and change inner cannula with hydrogen peroxide and pipe cleaners, rinse with water q2–4h, replace tube according to agency policy, change and secure ties properly as needed with another person to assist in stabilizing the neckplate and tube during these procedures

B. Maintains patency by removing secretions and crusting that obstructs tube causing narrowing of airway, ensures effective clearance while preventing tube dislodgement

C. Assist in deep-breathing, coughing exercises during deflation of tube, support head and neck when performing these exercises

C. Improves ventilation and coughing reduces accumulation of secretions, strenuous coughing should be discouraged

D. Humidified air via cool mist vaporizer or place a thin moist gauze bandage over stoma

D. Facilitates the removal of secretions, moistens mucous membranes

E. Suctioning of ostomy tube during cuff deflation with oropharyngeal to follow using sterile techniqe for 24 to 48 hours, instill 1 to 3 mL saline into tube immediately prior to suctioning; reinflate cuff during inspiration

E. Removes secretions immediately following surgery when not able to cough, and remove secretions, secretions accumulate above the cuff and need to be removed to prevent aspiration

INTERVENTION	RATIONALE
F. Oxygen as needed between suction passes	F. Ensures continuous oxygenation of tissues
G. Oral care after expectoration when able and provide tissues and bag for proper disposal	G. Promotes comfort and prevents transmission of microorganisms
H. Have ventilator bag and extra tracheostomy tube at bedside	H. Provides necessary equipment in an emergency and during tube change
I. Remove tacheostomy tube as edema is reduced and replace with smaller uncuffed tube and capped if tolerated and able to swallow, cough and remove secretions without use of suction	I. Removes artificial airway as ability to breathe improves for 24 hours with stoma covered with an occlusive dress dressing

NURSING DIAGNOSES

Anxiety related to threat to or change in health status causing inability to manage feelings of uncertainty and apprehension regarding uncertain prognosis, disfigurement, and possible reconstruction surgery

Ineffective individual coping related to inability to cope with long-term treatment regimen/rehabilitation, change in appearance (body image), and future life-style changes

Body image disturbance related to biophysical factor of change in structure and function of body part (laryngectomy especially with voice loss) and face and neck disfigurement with a permanent stoma and facial scarring resulting from surgical dissection procedure

EXPECTED OUTCOMES

Anxiety and fear within manageable levels, development of coping and problem-solving skills evidenced by verbalizations that anxiety is decreasing, fear reduced, participation in care activities and receptive to planning for ongoing stoma care and management of chronic anxiety

INTERVENTION	RATIONALE
I. Assess for:	
A. Level of anxiety, use of coping mechanisms, stated fears of uncertainty of disease outcome, life-style changes, fear of suffocation and of death	A. Anxiety can range from mild to severe and respiratory rate, rest will be affected accordingly, assists to identify inappropriate use of coping skills, high level of anxiety associated with tracheostomy
B. Restlessness, diaphoresis, complaining, joking, withdrawal, talkativeness, increased P and R	B. Nonverbal expressions of anxiety when not able to communicate feelings
C. Personal resources to cope with stress, anxiety, and interest in learning to problem-solve	C. Support systems and personal strengths assist to develop coping skills
D. Feelings and response to change in appearance, permanent stoma, voice loss and use of artificial devices, ability to carry out role and participate in activities	D. Changes in body image and self-concept a common and serious problem with disfigurement caused by throat and neck surgery
III. Administer:	
A. Anti-anxiety agent PO	A. Acts to reduce anxiety level and provides calming effect and rest, depresses subcortical levels of CNS, limbic system

INTERVENTION	RATIONALE
IV. Perform/provide:	
A. Environment conducive to rest, expression of fears and anxiety, avoid anxiety-producing situations	A. Decreases stimuli that cause stress/anxiety, venting of feelings decreases anxiety
B. Suggest new methods to enhance coping skills and problem solving, allow to externalize and identify those that help	B. Offers alternative coping strategies that allow for release of anxiety and fear
C. Positive feedback regarding progress made, focus on abilities rather than inabilities	C. Provides support for adaptive behavior, promotes self-worth and responsibility
D. Wipe and remove mouth of excess fluid or mucus	D. Reduces drooling in presence of circumoral paresthesia and inability to swallow
E. Privacy when dressings removed or changed, advise that feelings are normal; refrain from display of distaste or alarm at surgical site	E. Reduces embarrassment caused by exposure of surgical procedure(s)
F. Diversional activities such as relaxation exercises, TV, radio, music, reading, tapes, guided imagery; encourage to continue usual interests	F. Reduces anxiety and promotes comfort
G. Allow to participate in planning of care to maintain usual activities when possible	G. Allows for some control over situations

INTERVENTION	RATIONALE
H. Support grieving for loss of life-style and restrictions in activities, changes in physical appearance and use of alternative speech methods	H. Provides assistance in adaptation to changes imposed by surgical procedure

NURSING DIAGNOSES

Risk for infection related to inadequate primary defenses (surgical incision, stasis of pulmonary secretions), invasive procedures (trachesotomy tube, wound tubes and drainage)

Risk for impaired skin integrity related to mechanical external factor of pressure of tubes, internal factor of secretions or fluid accumulation in neck dissection wound

Altered oral mucous membrane related to mechanical trauma resulting from placement of nasogastric tube, surgery involving oral cavity, ineffective oral hygiene

EXPECTED OUTCOMES

Adequate defenses and wound healing with complications prevented evidenced by temperature, respirations, WBC within normal range, oral and nasopharyngeal mucosa clean and free of irritation and breakdown, absence of redness, swelling, purulent drainage at wound site(s)

INTERVENTION	RATIONALE
I. Assess for:	
A. Oral cavity for dryness, decreased secretions, dry sore lips	A. Results from NPO status and mouth dryness
B. Stoma and/or incision for redness, swelling, irritation, odor, lesions, crusts	B. Indicates inflammation/infection or dried secretions that predispose to skin breakdown
C. Nasal mucosa for pain, redness, breaks, facial irritation from tape	C. Indicates irritation from pressure and securing of nasogastric tube

INTERVENTION	RATIONALE
D. Tracheal ischemia and possible necrosis	D. Results from excess pressure on tracheal mucosa
E. Wound skin flap elevation	E. Indicates infection of neck dissection wound
F. Respiratory rate and breath sounds and bloody secretions	F. Symptoms of respiratory infection associated with artificial airway
II. Monitor, describe, record: A. Temperature q4h and PRN	A. Elevations indicate infection
B. WBC	B. Increases indicate infection
C. Wound drain and drainage for color, consistency, and if amount is increasing or decreasing q4h for 24 to 48 hours	C. Indicates patency of tubing and time that drainage tube and suction device can be removed
III. Administer: A. Antibiotic PO, IV, TOP at wound sites	A. Acts to prevent cell wall synthesis to destroy microorganisms in the prevention or treatment of infection
B. Corticosteroid PO, IV	B. Acts as an anti-inflammatory agent to reduce inflammation and increase body defenses in acute infection
C. Antipyretic PO	C. Acts to reduce temperature

INTERVENTION	RATIONALE
IV. Perform/provide:	
A. Environment with optimal temperature, humidity, and ventilation, free of smoking or other irritants	A. Promotes comfort and respiratory ease
B. Avoid exposure to visitors or staff with upper respiratory infection	B. Prevents transmission of infectious agents
C. Elevate head and support with pillows to maintain alignment	C. Reduces stress on incisional area
D. Use sterile technique and all sterile equipment and supplies for treatments, tracheostomy and wound care, dressings of lint-free material around stoma, pressure dressing on neck dissection surgical site	D. Prevents contamination by pathogens
E. Cleansing of stoma, tracheostomy tube, change tubes and tape when wet or soiled, humidification and oxygen tubing change as indicated by policy	E. Prevents accumulation of secretions, promotes cleanliness and prevents infection
F. Tape nasogastric tube to avoid pressure on mucosa, avoid moving tube and secure to avoid pull on tube, change position of tube taping daily	F. Prevents irritation and breakdown of mucosa

INTERVENTION	RATIONALE
G. Offer anesthetic gargle or deodorizing mouthwash or irrigation with water, saline, hydrogen peroxide solution	G. Provides cleansing of mouth to prevent infection and odors
H. Use tooth brush or small washcloth to brush tongue and sides of mouth	H. Cleanses and moisturizes mouth
I. Vaseline to lips	I. Provides moisture to dry lips to prevent cracking

NURSING DIAGNOSES

Altered nutrition, less than body requirements related to inability to ingest food because of biologic factors (dysphagia, impaired olfactory and gustatory perception, presence of tracheostomy tube) causing inadequate nutritional status

Impaired swallowing related to mechanical obstruction (tracheostomy tube, gastrostomy tube), dry oral cavity and pain, and neuromuscular impairment resulting from removal of structures needed for swallowing during neck surgery

EXPECTED OUTCOMES

Nutritional status maintained evidenced by weight range within baseline determinations, removal of nasogastric tube and feedings with progressive increase in oral intake of nutrients as appetite and swallowing improve

INTERVENTION	RATIONALE
I. Assess for: A. Presence of nasogastric tube and initiation of liquid formula feedings	A. Usually present immediately postoperative to remove gastric secretions and later for tube feedings if oral intake is not tolerated (can continue for up to 2 weeks)

INTERVENTION	RATIONALE
B. Weight loss, skinfold thickness, anorexia, intake of food groups and calories for 24 hours	B. Signs and symptoms of possible malnutrition state
C. Effect of coughing, swallowing on appetite and amount of food intake	C. Coughing, dysphagia cause decreased food intake
II. Monitor, describe, record:	
A. Weight on same scale, same time of day, same clothing q2days or as appropriate	A. Indicates weight changes that can reveal malnutrition
B. Transferrin, albumin, Hb	B. Indicates nutritional status
III. Administer:	
A. Vitamin/minerals PO	A. Supplements diet to ensure adequate intake of these requirements when oral intake has been established
IV. Perform/provide:	
A. Nasogastric feedings as bowel sounds return by bolus, gravity or pump regulated drip as tolerated	A. Method of feeding until swallowing and appetite returns, or in some cases until tube has been removed and stoma healed to allow for coughing and to prevent aspiration
B. Place in high Fowler's or sitting position during meals	B. Enhances passage of food by gravity

INTERVENTION	RATIONALE
C. Small, frequent feedings beginning with a thickened pureed diet, refrain from offering liquids	C. Reduces risk of aspiration of liquids until swallowing ability returns
D. Graduated diet to foods that are easy to swallow such as inclusions of foods with smooth texture, moist foods while avoiding sticky foods, milk and filling mouth with food	D. Improves ability to swallow and ingestion of nutrients
E. Allow time needed to eat slowly and not feel rushed, privacy if embarrassed by eating difficulty	E. Preserves self-esteem while adjusting to effects of the surgery
F. Suggest holding lips closed and tilt head to nonsurgical side when foods are in the mouth prior to swallowing	F. Assists to swallow foods
G. Oral care and rest period prior to meals, hard candy to suck before mealtime	G. Promotes comfort of mucous membranes and appetite
H. Consult with nutritionist for meal planning	H. Provides assistance for dietary intake according to personal preferences

NURSING DIAGNOSES

Impaired verbal communication related to surgical procedure (laryngectomy), physical barrier of tracheostomy, and psychological barrier (depression) causing inability to speak and interact with others

Impaired social interaction related to communication barriers (inability to speak) resulting from laryngectomy causing isolation, depression

EXPECTED OUTCOMES

Adequate communication established and improved interactions with others evidenced by use of alternate temporary methods of communications initially and progressing to mastery of techniques to restore speech

INTERVENTION	RATIONALE
I. Assess for:	
A. Ability to write, interest and prospects for speech and relearning to speak	A. Provides data regarding alternate methods of communication
B. Usual pattern of interacting, social relationships and activities	B. Provides a baseline to compare with progress in resocialization and communication based on realistic goals
IV. Perform/provide:	
A. Calm approach with time and patience for communication	A. Facilitates communications and reduces fear and anxiety
B. Pencil-and-paper, magic slate; allow time to write questions and answers	B. Method to ask questions and make requests when needed for the first few days postoperatively
C. Explanations of all procedures and answer all questions, be as anticipatory as possible in providing information and care	C. Reduces anxiety when not able to communicate needs
D. Allow to answer with a nod of the head, blink of eyes, or hand motions	D. Nonverbal responses to questions that can avoid frustrations associated with voice loss

INTERVENTION	RATIONALE
E. Place call light nearby within reach and assure that it will be answered promptly and that help is near	E. Facilitates communication in presence of voice loss and allays anxiety
F. Use touch in communication	F. Provides calm and caring attitude
G. Inform that speech might be possible when tracheostomy cuff is deflated	G. Possible with some types of tubes
H. Encourage slow gradual resumption of vocal sounds beginning with a whisper and progressing to more substantial sounds while occluding the stoma, or to take in a bolus of air and compress lips to simulate sounds by "plosive speech," or esophageal speech by swallowing and retaining air in the esophagus and speaking before reswallowing the air, if any are appropriate to produce vocal sounds	H. Surgical procedure can preserve some or all of vocal cords, alternate methods of making vocal sounds can be learned
I. Assist to use an artificial larynx if appropriate, 3 to 4 days following surgery	I. An electronic device causing vibrations that produce speech
J. Assist to use and reinforce instructions by speech pathologist for voice prosthesis, 5 to 6 days following surgery	J. Device inserted into a tracheoesophageal puncture to form a fistula to hold a voice prosthesis that produces speech

INTERVENTION	RATIONALE
K. Positive encouragement and praise any attempts at socialization with family/ friends	K. Promotes and reinforces social interaction
L. Apply a sign to the bed indicating that patient is unable to speak	L. Notifies personnel that patient requires special communication method
M. Reassurance that speech rehabilitation can be very successful and various methods can be provided to regain speech ability	M. Provides encouragement and support
N. Suggest visit from one who has had the same surgery and arrange visits with a speech pathologist	N. Provides information and support from those with knowledge, understanding and can provide needed reassurance and therapy

NURSING DIAGNOSIS

Knowledge deficit related to disease process, life-style changes and follow-up care (tracheostomy/stoma care, exercise program, nutritional regimen and method, use and care of artificial larynx/voice prosthesis, reduction of safety hazards, signs and symptoms to report to physician)

EXPECTED OUTCOMES

Knowledge and understanding of disease and ongoing care with life-style modified evidenced by performance of planned care and treatment regimen for wound and stoma healing, daily nutritional and exercise routine, pain control, and use and care of alternate voice device

INTERVENTION	RATIONALE
I. Assess for:	
A. Readiness, willingness, and motivation to learn, discharge care and lifestyle changes	A. Learning can best take place if client is receptive and compliance is more likely to occur
B. Health practices, health beliefs, ethnic identity (religion, diet, language), value orientations, family interactions and cooperation	B. Factors to incorporate into teaching plan to facilitate learning and compliance with long-term care
IV. Perform/provide:	
A. Acknowledgment of perceptions with a nonjudgmental attitude	A. Establishes nurse–patient relationship in an accepting environment
B. Explanations that are clear, accurate in understandable terms, small amount of information over time	B. Prevents misconceptions, erroneous attitudes and beliefs about disease
C. Demonstrations of all procedures with supervised return demonstrations with time for questions	C. Method that allows for visualization and practice of all care measures
D. Environment conducive to learning with space, lighting, and proper equipment and supplies	D. Distractions or discomfort will interfere with learning
E. As much control over lifestyle change decisions as possible, include in discharge planning	E. Allows power to be given or retained by patient

INTERVENTION	RATIONALE
F. Teaching aids (pamphlets, video tapes, pictures, written instructions)	F. Reinforces learning
G. Team of resource personnel/professionals	G. Nutritionist, social worker, counselor, speech pathologist, and others can assist in teaching specific care and providing support for desired changes

V. Teach patient/family:

INTERVENTION	RATIONALE
A. Disease process and pathophysiology, surgical procedure performed, and general follow-up care, stages of grieving process and that expressions of grief are allowed and accepted	A. Promotes understanding of disease that facilitates compliance and provides a caring attitude
B. Grooming and dressing options when in public (scarf, ascot, loose shirt, turtleneck top)	B. Preserves self-image by some masking of stoma and scarring
C. Inform family of their influences on patient's perception of self by their responses to appearance	C. Prevents negative feedback by significant others
D. Dietary modification with instruction in administration of tube feedings and care of equipment, formula, and nasogastric tube	D. Provides nutritional requirements for general health and to promote wound healing

INTERVENTION	RATIONALE
E. Administration and rationale of all prescribed medications with written schedule of times and dosages, side effects to expect and to report	E. Promotes compliance of complete medication regimen
F. Oral care with irrigation or cleansing with soft brush or cloth	F. Maintains oral hygiene and comfort
G. Cleansing of stoma, tracheostomy tube, changing tube and ties as needed, suctioning procedure (oral and tracheal)	G. Maintains patent artificial airway
H. Dressing change at stoma and incisional sites	H. Maintains skin integrity
I. Insertion and removal of tube and to have an outer cannula and obturator on hand if needed	I. Precaution for emergency situation such as tube dislodgement
J. Care and use of artificial larynx or voice prosthesis as appropriate to include cleansing, insertion, maintaining puncture site opening, replacement if needed	J. Reinforces instruction of speech pathologist and physician
K. Range of motion, muscle strength exercises, application of heat to shoulder if painful	K. Restores full movement of shoulder following neck dissection surgery

INTERVENTION	RATIONALE
L. Environment free of smoking, avoid hot foods/drinks that can burn mucosa, constrictive clothing around neck, water from entering stoma, use of aerosols or powders	L. Precautions necessary to prevent injury or complications with tracheostomy or nerve damage
M. Humidification of air by placing pans of water in all rooms	M. Assists to liquefy and loosen secretions for easier removal
N. Cover stoma with light shield when using shower or having a haircut; wear a protective shield at all times to cover stoma	N. Prevents entry of foreign material
O. Inform that ability to hold breath, blow nose, sense of smell and taste is lost or impaired	O. Protective mechanism removed when tracheostomy performed
P. Progressive activity routine allowing for restriction of lifting heavy objects with arm on the surgical side	P. Supports life-style change to maintain self-care and independence
Q. Suggest home modifications to support energy and endurance level	Q. Conserves energy while maintaining control of self-care
R. Report hemoptysis, coughing, nausea or vomiting with tube feedings, changes in wound appearance, painful shoulder	R. Indicates possible complications of surgery or postoperative care procedures

INTERVENTION	RATIONALE
S. Inform to wear emergency alert bracelet or identification card in wallet or purse	S. Informs of presence of stoma and voice prosthesis
T. Contact support groups such as Lost Chord Club, Speech and Hearing Association, American Cancer Association for information/educational materials, home care assistance	T. Provides assistance and support for adaptation to voice loss

pleuritis/pleural effusion

DEFINITION
Pleuritis is the inflammation of the parietal pleura of the lungs associated with pulmonary disorders such as pneumonia, pneumothorax, or pleural effusion. Pleural effusion is the accumulation of fluid in the pleural space caused by conditions such as congestive heart failure, pleuritis, tumor, trauma, or any disorder that interferes with the secretion or drainage of the pleural fluid. If the fluid becomes thick and purulent, it is termed empyema. If surgical procedures are planned to treat fibrothorax or recurrent pleural effusion this plan can be used in association with the PREOPERATIVE CARE and POSTOPERATIVE CARE plans

NURSING DIAGNOSES
Pain related to physical injuring agent of pressure resulting from inflammatory process and increasing buildup in pleural space

Ineffective breathing pattern related to restricted lung expansion and respiratory effort resulting from pain with inspiration, inflammatory response of fluid accumulation in pleural spaces

EXPECTED OUTCOMES
Pain managed and controlled and breathing effort achieved evidenced by respiration rate, depth, ease within baseline levels without dyspnea, verbalization that pain relief achieved with analgesia allowing breathing to improve

INTERVENTION	RATIONALE
I. Assess for:	
A. Respiratory rate, ease, depth, chest movement, use of accessory muscles, dyspnea and rapid, shallow breathing, decreased chest wall movement, cough for severity and frequency, decreased breath sounds, tactile fremitus, dullness on percussion	A. Provides data base of respiratory function that changes with inflammation/fluid accumulation that increase pain and distress
B. Pleural pain severity, onset, side affected, type of pain (stabbing, sharp)	B. Verbal descriptors of pain caused by pressure on nerve endings in the parietal pleura
C. Restlessness, holding the chest, moaning, crying, reduced respiratory effort and lung expansion, exertional dyspnea	C. Nonverbal descriptors of pain if not able to communicate pleural pain and symptoms of pleural fluid accumulation
II. Monitor, describe, record:	
A. VS and temperature q4h	A. Indicates respiratory dysfunction and potential infection
B. ABGs, pulmonary function tests	B. Diagnostic test and/or procedure to determine lung ventilation and function
C. Chest x ray	C. Reveals presence of fluid or air in pleural space
III. Administer:	
A. Analgesic PO	A. Acts to reduce pain depending on severity and respiratory rate

INTERVENTION	RATIONALE
B. Antibiotic PO	B. Acts to destroy infectious agents as a preventive measure or therapy
C. Antitussive PO	C. Acts to reduce cough or treat unproductive cough
D. Oxygen via nasal cannula	D. Corrects hypoxia if present

IV. Perform/provide:

INTERVENTION	RATIONALE
A. Elevate head of bed to position of comfort, support chest with pillow when moving, coughing, and on inspiration	A. Facilitates breathing and reduces chest movement when coughing or deep breathing
B. Periods of rest in a quiet, calm, dimmed environment; minimize visitors and procedures	B. Reduces stimuli that increases pain
C. Humidity to environment by cool-air vaporizer	C. Provides moisture to the air to ease breathing and coughing and facilitate removal of secretions
D. Assistance to physician in performing intercostal nerve block	D. Controls pain when pharmacological interventions are ineffective
E. Deep-breathing exercises, incentive spirometry q1–2h	E. Inflates and expands the lungs and mobilizes secretions for removal
F. Prepare for and assist in thoracentesis if appropriate	F. Removes excess fluid from pleural space to ease breathing and for laboratory analysis of the fluid

NURSING DIAGNOSIS
Knowledge deficit related to information regarding follow-up care (medications, activity) and prevention of recurrence of disorders

EXPECTED OUTCOMES
Knowledge and understanding of care requirements following discharge evidenced by progressive resolution of pain and respiratory effort as inflammation and fluid accumulation subside

INTERVENTION	RATIONALE
V. Teach patient/family:	
A. Plan rest periods and activities within defined limitations	A. Prevents fatigue and allays pain
B. Avoid smoking and exposure to those with upper respiratory infections	B. Prevents transmission of infectious agents to already compromised respiratory system
C. Continued administration of prescribed medications with action, dose, frequency, times, side effects with antibiotics taken until complete prescription is administered	C. Ensures ongoing treatment of disorder(s) to prevent recurrence
D. Report pain in chest, changes in breathing, fever, chills, diaphoresis	D. Signs and symptoms of possible infection or pleural effusion
E. Comply with physician follow-up appointments and chest x rays	E. Monitors respiratory status for needed changes or to discontinue therapy

pneumonia

DEFINITION
Pneumonia is an inflammation of the lung involving a segment or lobes of the lung in response to the invasion by micro-organisms (bacteria, fungi, viruses, protozoa, mycoplasmas), inhalation of toxic materials (gases, chemicals, dusts), or aspiration of substances (foods, fluids, vomitus, secretions). Depending on the areas affected, pneumonia can be referred to as bronchial (bronchioles and alveoli), interstitial (air and vascular structures), alveolar (air spaces), or necrotic (death of an area of lung). Risk factors include smoking, environmental pollution, chronic pulmonary disorders or infections, immunosuppression, postoperative states, and older adults

NURSING DIAGNOSES
Ineffective airway clearance related to tracheobronchial secretion resulting from inflammation and mucus accumulation in airways, and decreased energy and fatigue resulting in decreased ability to cough and causing stasis of secretions

Ineffective breathing pattern related to decreased lung expansion, energy and fatigue resulting from pain and inflammatory process causing anxiety, inadequate ventilation

EXPECTED OUTCOMES
Improved and adequate respiratory and ventilation function evidenced by respiratory rate, ease, depth, breath sounds within baseline parameters, effective removal of secretions causing airway clearance and patency

INTERVENTION	RATIONALE
I. Assess for:	
A. Respiratory rate, depth, ease, noting dyspnea, shallow or irregular breathing, use of accessory muscles, cough and sputum production and removal, crackles or bronchial breath sounds on auscultation, increased tactile fremitus, dull percussion in identified areas	A. Provides data baselines and changes indicating inflammatory process
B. Changes in mental status (restlessness, confusion, lethargy), especially in the older adult, cyanosis, pleuritic pain, fever, chills, diaphoresis, fatigue	B. Indicates possible decreases in oxygenation or as a result of infection
C. Quality of cough, ability to raise secetions including consistency and characteristics of sputum	C. Removes secretions that prevent obstruction of airways and stasis leading to further infection and consolidation and clearing airways facilitates breathing
II. Monitor, describe, record:	
A. VS with R and breath sounds q2–4h or as needed	A. Indicates airway movement, resistance, changes indicating increasing severity of disease
B. ABGs, pulse oximetry	B. Indicates need for supplemental oxygen if hypoxemia present, or presence of hypercapnia

INTERVENTION	RATIONALE
C. Chest x ray	C. Provides extent and location of pneumonia such as scattered with patchy shadows in bronchopneumonia, fluffy shadows in alveolar pneumonia, fibrosis in interstitial pneumonia, cavity formation in necrotic pneumonia
D. Sputum culture and sensitivities	D. Identifies infectious agent and effective antibiotic agent
III. Administer:	
A. Antibiotic PO, IV	A. Acts by binding to cell wall of micro-organism preventing synthesis and destroying pathogens
B. Antitussive/expectorant PO	B. Acts on bronchial cells to increase fluid production and promote expectoration, reduces surface tension of secretions, both to relieve nonproductive cough
C. Bronchodilator PO, IV	C. Acts to dilate bronchi in reversible airway obstruction
D. Mucolytic INH	D. Decreases viscosity of mucus for easier removal
E. Oxygen via nasal cannula	E. Supplement oxygen to maintain optimal level for tissue oxygenation

INTERVENTION	RATIONALE
IV. Perform/provide:	
A. Place in semi-Fowler's position on bed rest with restricted activities	A. Provides needed rest and reduce need for oxygenation, facilitates comfort and ease of breathing
B. Assist to change sidelying position q2h	B. Prevents aspiration, especially in those whose mentation is affected
C. Assist in deep breathing, coughing, incentive spirometer q2h, pillow to splint chest when coughing	C. Improves ventilation and respiratory status and comfort during coughing
D. Increased fluid intake to 2L/day if permitted and if cough dry and hacking	D. Liquefies secretions for easier removal
E. Humidified air via cool-mist vaporizer, postural drainage if condition warrants this procedure	E. Facilitates the removal of secretions, moistens mucous membranes
F. Orotracheal suctioning as appropriate and if ordered	F. Removes secretions when other methods have failed
G. Oral care after expectoration and provide tissues and bag for proper disposal	G. Promotes comfort and prevents transmission of organisms

NURSING DIAGNOSES

Pain related to physical injuring agent of microbial invasion and inflammation of lung tissue causing discomfort with breathing, coughing, and positioning

Hyperthermia related to illness of inflammation/infectious process causing stimulation to the regulating center in the hypothalamus

EXPECTED OUTCOMES
Relief or control of pain and temperature reduced and within baseline parameters evidenced by verbalizations that pain absent and comfort increased following analgesic, temperature in range of 98.6°F (37°C) maintained

INTERVENTION	RATIONALE
I. Assess for: A. Pleuritic pain, type, severity, frequency or continuous, presence of headache with temperature	A. Reveals pain descriptors associated with chest pain caused by inflammation
B. Elevated temperature, chills, malaise, sweats, diaphoresis, hot/flushed skin	B. Indicates signs and symptoms of infectious process of lung
II. Monitor, describe, record: A. VS and temperature q4h	A. Increased BP, P, R associated with pain and temperature elevation
B. WBC, differential	B. Elevation of WBC indicates presence of infectious process (pulmonary or spread to other sites)
C. Sputum culture	C. Identifies causative agent to determine antibiotic regimen
III. Administer: A. Antipyretic PO	A. Acts to reduce temperature and promote comfort
B. Analgesic PO while noting effect on respirations	B. Acts to reduce chest pain according to severity

C. Antimicrobial PO, IV

C. Acts to interfere with cell wall synthesis and cause death of pathogens

IV. Perform/provide:
   A. Calm, restful environment with optimal warm temperature and ventilation, warm blankets and change of damp linens or clothing

   A. Prevents stimuli that increases pain and chilling associated with fever

   B. Bed rest if pain present or rest periods before and after activity

   B. Exertion and fatigue increase pain perception

   C. Semi-Fowler's, sidelying position, pillow to splint chest during coughing

   C. Reduces pain and promotes comfort by reducing strain on affected side

   D. Backrub, sponge bath, relaxation techniques

   D. Cooling measures to decrease temperature and promote comfort

   E. Fluid intake of 2 to 3 L/day as permitted, warm fluids if chilled

   E. Replaces fluid lost from diaphoresis as temperature increases or persists

NURSING DIAGNOSES

Activity intolerance related to imbalance between oxygen supply and demand (inflammatory process) causing tissue hypoxia, weakness, fatigue, and increased energy requirements to perform ADL

Sleep pattern disturbance related to internal factors of illness (nocturnal dyspnea, coughing, pleuritic pain) and psychological stress (anxiety) causing disruption of sleep, fatigue

EXPECTED OUTCOMES

Progressive increase in activity tolerance and return to sleep and rest pattern with reduction in fatigue level evidenced by increased performance of ADL with decreased dyspnea, increased energy and endurance, VS stable before, during, and after activity, uninterrupted sleep with verbalizations that feeling more rested and less anxious

INTERVENTION	RATIONALE
I. Assess for: A. Level of fatigue, weakness, and potential for activity progression, effect on respirations, dyspnea with activities	A. Provides baseline and allows for planning activities and need for assistance
B. Interest and ability in performing ADL with or without assistance	B. Readiness and increased energy level necessary for successful program
C. Sleep/rest pattern, wakefulness during night, irritability, lethargy	C. Optimal rest and sleep necessary to reduce fatigue and perform activities
D. R >20/minute, P >120/bpm and not returning to pre-activity level within 3 minutes, palpitations, dyspnea, dizziness, chest pain, weakness, and stopping activity if symptoms appear	D. Signs and symptoms of activity intolerance leading to fatigue
III. Administer: A. Sedative PO, unless respirations <12/minute	A. Acts on limbic and subcortical levels of CNS and increases sleep time
B. Oxygen via nasal cannula	B. Supplements oxygen during daily activities or sleep as needed

INTERVENTION	RATIONALE
IV. Perform/provide:	
A. Bed rest during acute state in a position of comfort with body parts supported with pillows	A. Conserves energy and provides needed rest
B. Perform or assist in ADL and other activities as needed, place all articles and call light within reach to use as desired	B. Conserves energy while preserving as much control and independence as possible
C. Increase activities gradually from sitting up in bed, in chair, walking in room, to bathroom, and in hall with daily increase in distance and ADL activities	C. Progressive change in activities increases with endurance and energy level and prevents symptoms of activity intolerance
D. Place bed in low position and clear pathways if ambulating independently with a walker or cane, inform to get out of bed slowly and take time needed for slow progress in ambulation	D. Prevents falls if weak until endurance returns
E. Organize activities around rest periods in a quiet, calm, dimly lit, environment free of stimuli and respiratory irritants	E. Permits rest without interruptions
F. Assist to assume preferred position for sleep, offer backrub, oral care, extra pillows, other activities based on sleep pattern	F. Provides for usual bedtime rituals to ensure comfort and sleep

INTERVENTION	RATIONALE
G. Restrict visitors and limit time of visit	G. Prevents additional stimuli that interferes with rest and causes fatigue

NURSING DIAGNOSIS

Knowledge deficit related to disease process, medications, life-style changes, and follow-up care (dietary for weight control, exercise program, respiratory health practices, reduction of risk factors such as stress, smoking)

EXPECTED OUTCOMES

Knowledge and understanding of disease, and ongoing care with life-style modified to reduce risk factors associated with respiratory disease evidenced by verbalizations of and understanding and compliance with medication, immunization, and dietary regimen, activity routine and restrictions with participation in pulmonary rehabilitation, signs of symptoms to report and ongoing physician monitoring of respiratory status

INTERVENTION	RATIONALE
I. Assess for: A. Readiness, willingness, and motivation to learn, discharge care and life-style changes	A. Learning can best take place if client is receptive and compliance is more likely to occur
B. Health practices, health beliefs, ethnic identity (religion, diet, language), value orientations, family interactions and cooperation	B. Factors to incorporate into teaching plan to facilitate learning and compliance
IV. Perform/provide: A. Acknowledgment of perceptions with a nonjudgmental attitude	A. Establishes nurse–patient relationship in an accepting environment

INTERVENTION	RATIONALE
B. Explanations that are clear, accurate in understandable terms, small amount of information over time	B. Prevents misconceptions, erroneous attitudes and beliefs about disease
C. Environment conducive to learning with space, lighting, and proper equipment and supplies	C. Distractions or discomfort will interfere with learning
D. As much control over lifestyle change decisions as possible	D. Allows power to be given or retained by patient
E. Teaching aids (pamphlets, videotapes, pictures, written instructions)	E. Reinforces learning
F. Team of resource personnel/professionals	F. Nutritionist, social worker, counselor, pulmonary rehabilitation therapist, and others can assist in teaching specific care and providing support for desired changes
V. Teach patient/family:	
A. Anatomy, function of the lungs, pathophysiology, and the convalescence process that takes about 6 to 8 weeks following discharge, longer for the older adult and those with chronic lung disease	A. Promotes understanding of disease that facilitates compliance

INTERVENTION	RATIONALE
B. Risk factors such as overweight, stress, smoking, exercise deficit, alcohol intake, chronic pulmonary disease	B. Contributes to information about factors that can be modified with life-style changes
C. Dietary modification with sample menus for restricted calories, list of foods to include and restrict and caloric content, tips on purchasing and preparing foods, amount of alcohol intake to allow/day	C. Reduces risk factor associated with overweight
D. Administration and rationale of all prescribed medications (antibiotics, bronchodilators), written schedule of times and dosages, side effects to expect and to report, demonstrate use of handheld inhalers and allow to return demonstration	D. Promotes compliance of complete medication regimen
E. Fluid intake of 10 to 12 glasses/day or amount allowed	E. Maintains daily fluid needs
F. Continue coughing and deep-breathing exercises, inform of resources to obtain small-volume nebulizer, incentive spirometer if needed	F. Maintains respiratory health status

INTERVENTION	RATIONALE
G. Progressive activity routine allowing for restrictions, rest periods when needed during activity, to cease activity if dizzy, dyspneic or has pain; take steps to arrange for pulmonary rehabilitation program if ordered	G. Supports life-style change to maintain respiratory status
H. Avoid stressful situations, consider counseling or stress-reduction program to assist in development of coping and problem-solving skills	H. Prevents risk factor associated with respiratory dysfunction
I. Encourage to avoid groups or persons with upper respiratory disease or during flu season	I. Prevents transmission of infectious agents
J. Report temperature elevation, chills, dyspnea, pulse irregularity, activity intolerance, continued fatigue, chest pain, change in cough and sputum characteristics (yellow, rust colored), irritability, restlessness to physician	J. Indicates possible recurrence or complication of pneumonia (pleural effusion, atelectasis)
K. Importance of having pneumovax immunization, keeping appointments as scheduled, notify physician prior to using any other medications	K. Protects against bacterial pneumonia

INTERVENTION	RATIONALE
L. Contact support groups to stop smoking, for weight reduction, alcoholism, American Lung Association for information/educational materials	L. Provides assistance to reduce risk factors

pneumothorax/hemothorax

DEFINITION

Pneumothorax is the collection of air in the pleural space between the parietal and visceral pleurae causing a loss of negative intrathoracic pressure resulting in partial or complete lung collapse. It can be simple or closed (puncture or tear in bronchi or alveoli, spontaneous rupture of a bleb) or open (traumatic puncture into the chest wall), or tension (a combination of both usually associated with chest injury). Hemothorax is the accumulation of blood and fluid in the pleural space that results from an injury associated wtih laceration of the lungs, heart, great vessels, intercostal arteries or veins in the chest wall or diaphragm causing total or partial lung collapse. Situations that can predispose to these conditions are trauma (rib fracture, flail chest, renal biopsy, resuscitation) and diseases (chronic obstructive pulmonary disease, pulmonary tumor)

NURSING DIAGNOSES

Ineffective breathing pattern related to pain and decreased lung expansion causing anxiety (fear of suffocation), inadequate ventilation

Impaired gas exchange related to altered oxygen/carbon dioxide exchange resulting from reduced surface area of lungs caused by partial or total collapse

Anxiety related to change in health status (impaired ventilation), threat of death (complication of tension pneumothorax, hypovolemia caused by hemothorax)

EXPECTED OUTCOMES

Improved chest expansion with adequate ventilation and oxygenation as pain is reduced and lung reinflated evidenced by respiratory rate and ease returned to normal parameters, ABGs within normal levels; anxiety within manageable levels evidenced by verbalization of decreased fear and apprehension, more relaxed expression and appearance

INTERVENTION	RATIONALE
I. Assess for: A. Respiratory rate, ease, depth, tachypnea, dyspnea, use of accessory muscles, unequal chest movements, coughing, diminished breath sounds, hyperresonance on percussion	A. Provides data base of respiratory function affected by air, fluid, blood accumulation in pleural space
B. Restlessness, irritability, confusion, tachycardia, changes in mentation, cyanosis	B. Indicates decreased oxygenation leading to hypoxia
C. Level of anxiety, tremors, restlessness, feelings of uncertainty and apprehension	C. Anxiety commonly associated with dyspnea and other symptoms of respiratory distress
II. Monitor, describe, record: A. VS q4h, R q30 minutes	A. Indicates change caused by respiratory function
B. ABGs, pulse oximetry	B. Reveals hyper- or hypoventilation, oxygenation with decreased PaO_2 and increased $PaCO_2$ levels, oxygen saturation with oximetry
C. Chest x ray, pulmonary function	C. Diagnostic procedures that reveal vital capacity and fluid or air in pleural space, degree of collapse, presence of mediastinal shift, lower diaphragm

INTERVENTION	RATIONALE
III. Administer:	
A. Antibiotic PO, IM	A. Acts to prevent infection if collapse is caused by open wound
B. Tetanus toxoid, immune globulin IM	B. Acts as prophylaxis following injury
C. Oxygen via nasal cannula	C. Provides supplemental oxygen based on ABG, pulse oximetry results
IV. Perform/provide:	
A. Calm, quiet environment	A. Prevents stimuli that increase fear and anxiety
B. Place in semi- or high Fowler's position and avoid any pressure on chest	B. Promotes ease of breathing and chest expansion
C. Change position q2h	C. Improves breathing and gas exchange
D. Allow or restrict activity as tolerated with rest periods as needed	D. Prevents change in breathing patterns caused by exertion
E. Remain during periods of dyspnea, tachypnea, request to mimic own slower respirations	E. Provides support and assists to reduce anxiety and moderate respiratory pattern
F. Deep breathing exercises or incentive spirometry q2–4h	F. Assists in ventilation and fluid removal
G. Prepare for and assist with large-bore needle and valve attachment insertion procedure	G. Provides temporary decompression via aspiration of air, fluid, or blood

INTERVENTION	RATIONALE
H. Prepare for and assist with chest tube insertion and suction/drainage with monitoring patency of tube and collection system	H. Removes fluid, air, blood and promotes lung reexpansion by reestablishing negative pressure in chest

NURSING DIAGNOSES

Pain related to physical injury of trauma causing pressure or air in pleural space, chest tube causing irritation of skin at insertion site

   Risk for impaired skin integrity related to pressure or instability of chest tube

EXPECTED OUTCOMES

Pain relieved or controlled evidenced by verbalization that pain minimized, chest tube stable, and insertion site free of redness and excoriation

INTERVENTION	RATIONALE
I. Assess for:	
A. Pain on affected side with chest movement, breathing, coughing, severity (tightness, bubbling sensation in chest)	A. Pain descriptors determine need for analgesia and severity or extent of lung collapse, possible bleeding or accumulation of fluid
B. Pain, soreness at tube insertion site, irritation or breakdown of skin at the site	B. Movement of chest tube can cause pain, irritation of skin leading to breakdown and infection
III. Administer:	
A. Analgesic IM if R >12/minute	A. Acts to interfere with CNS pain pathways and given while evaluating effect on respirations

INTERVENTION	RATIONALE
IV. Perform/provide:	
A. Restful, quiet environment	A. Reduces stimuli that can increase pain
B. Analgesic 30 minutes prior to coughing and breathing exercises, other painful activities	B. Allows for more effective breathing when pain is relieved
C. Splint chest with a pillow when coughing and deep-breathing	C. Supports and reduces movements that cause pain
D. Change position with smooth, gentle movements, taking time to allow patient to assist	D. Prevents unnecessary pain
E. Position on affected side for limited periods of time	E. Facilitates drainage and chest expansion
F. If chest tube present, position on side without tubing and use pillow to support tubing, secure tubing, and use extra length of tubing if needed	F. Prevents tension, movement, or pulling on tube that causes pain and irritation

NURSING DIAGNOSIS

Knowledge deficit related to follow-up care following removal of chest tube (wound care, activity restrictions, breathing exercises, appointments with physician), prevention of recurrence of pneumothorax (spontaneous), and signs and symptoms to report

EXPECTED OUTCOMES

Knowledge and understanding of care requirements following tube removal and discharge evidenced by compliance with measures and appointments to prevent complications or recurrence of condition

INTERVENTION	RATIONALE
V. Teach patient/family:	
A. Inform that spontaneous pneumothorax can recur and to report chest pain or breathing difficulty immediately	A. Possible in as many as 50% of those experiencing lung collapse
B. Demonstrate wound care, removal and application of pressure dressing, allow to return demonstration, inform to report redness, swelling, purulent drainage, temperature elevation and chills	B. Promotes appropriate care of tube insertion site until healing is complete
C. Avoid lifting heavy objects, strenuous exercise or activity, exposure to changes in barometric pressure or possibly altitude	C. Activity restrictions to prevent recurrence of spontaneous pneumothorax
D. Encourage to stop smoking, suggest assistance from program to stop smoking	D. Reduces risk for recurrence of pneumothorax
E. Antibiotic therapy to continue for prescribed time	E. Prevents pulmonary or insertion site infection
F. Inform to practice deep breathing exercises as advised by physician	F. Strengthens chest muscles and promotes ventilation
G. Written reminder of appointment date and time for follow-up visit to physician	G. Promotes compliance with follow-up monitoring of health status

pulmonary embolism

DEFINITION

A condition characterized by blockage of the pulmonary vasculature by some foreign matter such as blood clot, air, tumor tissue, bone, fat, or a tip or piece of an IV catheter/cannula. It is most commonly caused by thrombus of the veins of the extremities or pelvis. Risk factors associated with this condition include trauma or surgery on the legs or pelvis, immobility, obesity, and clotting disorders. The most serious complication is the obstruction of blood flow and perfusion of a portion of the lung leading to hypoxemia, and in cases of embolism of the larger pulmonary vessel, leading to atelectasis and possible reduced cardiac output. This plan can be used in association with ACUTE VENOUS INSUFFICIENCY (THROMBOPHLEBITIS/THROMBOSIS)

NURSING DIAGNOSES

Pain related to physical injuring agent of inflammatory process of the lung, pulmonary ischemia resulting from occlusion of blood flow by emboli

Ineffective breathing pattern related to inflammatory process, pain, and anxiety causing restricted lung expansion and respiratory effort

Impaired gas exchange related to altered blood flow and decreased perfusion (occlusion by emboli), and altered oxygen supply (atelectasis) causing hypoxemia

EXPECTED OUTCOMES

Pain, anxiety managed and controlled, and breathing effort improved, tissue oxygenation achieved evidenced by respiration rate, depth, ease within baseline levels without dyspnea, ABGs within normal levels, verbalization that pain relief achieved with analgesia allowing anxiety to subside

INTERVENTION	RATIONALE
I. Assess for:	
A. Pleuritic pain including severity, location, onset, associated nonverbal manifestations such as restlessness, diaphoresis, tachycardia, increased BP, facial expressions	A. Common symptom of pulmonary embolism usually with an abrupt onset and affected by breathing pattern
B. Respiratory rate, ease, depth, chest movement, use of accessory muscles, dyspnea, shallow breathing, cough for severity, frequency, and hemoptysis, decreased breath sounds, crackles on auscultation	B. Provides data base of respiratory function that changes with inflammation/pulmonary emboli that increase pain and distress; changes indicate size of emboli and possible alveolar damage caused by atelectasis
C. Irritability, confusion, lethargy with dyspnea and tachypnea	C. Signs and symptoms of hypoxemia
D. Anxiety level during pain and dyspnea	D. Inability to breathe causes fear and apprehension
II. Monitor, describe, record:	
A. VS with emphsis on R q15 min or as appropriate	A. Indicates respiratory dysfunction and possible hemodynamic abnormalities caused by vasoconstriction of arterioles resulting from histamine, serotonin, protoglandin, and catecholamine release by the clot

INTERVENTION	RATIONALE
B. ABGs, pulse oximetry	B. Diagnostic test and/or procedure to determine arterial oxygen or oxygen saturation to determine hypoxemia and need for supplemental oxygen
C. Chest x ray	C. Reveals density of infarction, pulmonary effusion, or consolidation
D. Perfusion and ventilation nuclear scan	D. Reflects pulmonary circulation and gas movement through lungs to determine obstructed blood flow, size of clot
E. Pulmonary angiography	E. Determines emboli in pulmonary vascular system, filling defect in pulmonary vessel
F. ECG	F. Reflects pattern indicating pulmonary emboli
III. Administer: A. Analgesic IV	A. Acts to reduce pain depending on severity and respiratory rate, usually morphine is drug of choice, as it also allays anxiety
B. Oxygen via nasal cannula or face mask	B. Corrects hypoxia if present

INTERVENTION	RATIONALE
IV. Perform/provide:	
A. Place in semi- or high Fowler's position, support chest with pillow when moving, coughing, and on inspiration, change position q2h for comfort and to ease breathing	A. Facilitates breathing and reduces chest movement and pain when coughing or deep-breathing
B. Periods of rest in a quiet, calm, dimmed environment, maintain bed rest and minimize visitors and procedures	B. Reduces stimuli that increases pain, anxiety
C. Relaxation exercises, back-rub, position of comfort with supportive aids, quiet diversional activities	C. Nonpharmacological interventions to reduce pain
D. Deep-breathing exercises, incentive spirometry q1–2h	D. Inflates and expands the lungs and prevents atelectasis
E. Remain during dyspneic and painful episodes, suggest patient mimic nurse's slowing of breathing pattern	E. Provides support and reassurance to reduce pain and anxiety

NURSING DIAGNOSES

Risk for injury related to complications of pulmonary embolism and treatment regimen causing bleeding, heart failure, recurrent or extension of embolism

Altered protection related to drug therapy (anticoagulant) causing altered clotting of blood and risk for excessive bleeding

EXPECTED OUTCOMES
Risk of complications minimized or eliminated evidenced by absence of signs and symptoms of right heart failure, spontaneous active bleeding, continued or extended pumonary embolism

INTERVENTION	RATIONALE
I. Assess for:	
A. Increased P, peripheral edema, distended neck veins, extra heart sounds or murmurs auscultated, enlarged liver, restlessness, anxiety	A. Signs and symptoms of right-sided heart failure
B. Ecchymosis, petechiae, bleeding from gums and mucous membranes, joints for pain and swelling, blood in urine or feces, hemoptysis, epitaxis	B. Indicates bleeding caused by anticoagulant therapy
C. Persistent chest pain, increasing respiratory changes with cough and hemoptysis, hypoxemia	C. Indicates recurrence or extension of pulmonary embolism
II. Monitor, describe, record:	
A. VS, CVP q4h	A. Complications can cause hypotension, tachycardia, tachypnea, dyspnea
B. Hct, Hb, platelet count	B. Decreases with excessive bleeding
C. PT, PTT for prolonged time	C. Acts to monitor and regulate heparin dosage with PTT maintained at 2 to $2\frac{1}{2}$ times control, warfarin dosage with PT maintained at $1\frac{1}{2}$ to 2 times control

INTERVENTION	RATIONALE
III. Administer:	
A. Anticoagulant IV initially followed by PO	A. Acts to potentiate the effect of antithrombin III to prevent thrombus formation or extension of thrombi (heparin) or interfere with synthesis of clotting factors to prevent thrombo-embolism
B. Vitamin K, protamine sulfate on hand	B. Enhances clotting should bleeding become profuse, protamine for heparin and vitamin K for warfarin therapy
IV. Perform/provide:	
A. Bed rest in semi- to high Fowler's position, restrict activities involving Valsalva maneuver (straining or holding breath)	A. Improves comfort and prevents recurrence or extension of embolism
B. Use smallest-gauge needle for injections and apply pressure to site until bleeding stops	B. Prevents trauma that causes bleeding
C. Avoid overinflation of BP cuff, use of rectal thermometer, dental floss, hard toothbrush, straight razor for shaving	C. Traumatizes skin or mucous membranes that causes bleeding
D. Pad bed rails and assist to move in bed if restless	D. Prevents trauma

INTERVENTION	RATIONALE
E. Remain and support patient if complication occurs, prepare for surgical procedure if appropriate (embolectomy)	E. Provides caring and reduces fear and anxiety

NURSING DIAGNOSIS

Knowledge deficit related to follow-up discharge care, including medications and side effects, measures to avoid thrombus formation, signs and symptoms to report, and compliance with laboratory and physician appointments

EXPECTED OUTCOMES

Knowledge of medication regimen and implications, restrictions in activities, and necessary physician and laboratory appointmens needed evidenced by compliance with precautions to avoid complications of bleeding and recurrence of embolism

INTERVENTION	RATIONALE
V. Teach patient/family:	
A. Course of anticoagulant therapy (usually up to 6 months)	A. Provides information needed to ensure compliance with long-term medication regimen
B. Medication administration with dose, side effects, take same time each day, not to skip or change dose	B. Promotes compliance and prevents recurring thrombi
C. Avoid taking aspirin or other OTC drugs or alcohol without notifying physician	C. Enhances action of anticoagulant
D. Importance of having laboratory testing done as scheduled	D. Determines correct dosage of anticoagulant or need for adjustment

INTERVENTION	RATIONALE
E. Use safety razor, soft toothbrush, avoid straining at defecation or blowing nose hard, activities that can traumatize the skin such as walking barefoot, sports, or games	E. Prevents trauma and bleeding episode
F. Apply prolonged pressure on an area that is bleeding	F. Assists to stop the bleeding
G. Avoid sitting or standing for prolonged periods, crossing legs when sitting, wearing restrictive clothing such as garters, girdles	G. Promotes blood flow and prevents recurrence of thrombosis
H. Report excessive bleeding from any site, chest pain, dyspnea, redness and swelling in an extremity, extreme anxiety, restlessness	H. Permits early interventions to treat complication of bleeding or recurring pulmonary embolism

pulmonary resection
(lobectomy/segmental/pneumonectomy)

DEFINITION

Pulmonary resection is the surgery (also known as thoracotomy) of the lung involving procedures to remove a portion of or a total lung depending on the type and area affected by disease. It can be performed to remove a wedge (small, diseased area near the surface of the lung for biopsy or to resect a small lesion), segmental (limited area of diseased tissue such as tumor, blebs that includes bronchiole and alveoli), lobectomy (entire lobe of the lung to remove tumor), or pneumonectomy (entire lung for cancer, bronchiectasis, abscesses, or tuberculosis). Closed chest drainage is usually used following the surgery to allow for the drainage of air and fluid from the pleural space, reestablish negative pressure to reexpand the lung, and equalize the pressure on both sides to prevent lung collapse. The drainage consists of closed systems that operate by gravity, water seal, and suction. This plan, which includes interventions specific to these procedures, can be used in association with the NEOPLASM (CHEMOTHERAPY/EXTERNAL AND INTERNAL RADIATION), PNEUMOTHORAX/HEMOTHORAX, PREOPERATIVE CARE, and POSTOPERATIVE CARE plans

NURSING DIAGNOSES

Ineffective airway clearance related to tracheobronchial secretion increases resulting from inflammation and mucus accumulation in airways, and weakness and trauma of surgery with decreased ability to cough causing stasis of secretions

Ineffective breathing pattern related to decreased lung expansion, resulting from pain, fear of dislodging chest tube causing anxiety, inadequate removal of secretions and ventilation

Impaired gas exchange related to altered oxygen supply resulting from a reduction in surface for gas exchange with removal of portion or complete lung

EXPECTED OUTCOMES

Improved and adequate respiratory function, ventilation, and tissue oxygenation evidenced by respiratory rate, ease, depth, and breath sounds within baseline parameters, effective removal of secretions with airway clearance and patency, ABGs within normal range

INTERVENTION	RATIONALE
I. Assess for:	
A. Respiratory rate, depth, ease, noting dyspnea, orthopnea, tachypnea, use of accessory muscles	A. Provides data baselines and changes indicating respiratory dysfunction postoperatively
B. Decreased breath sounds on auscultation before and after coughing	B. Results from ineffective air movement and can result in stasis of secretions
C. Amount of chest drainage, patency of drainage tubes and system	C. Reveals if bleeding present and if negative pressure and lung inflation is maintained, all of which affect breathing pattern
D. Changes in mental status (restlessness, confusion, lethargy) cyanosis, fatigue	D. Indicates decreases in oxygenation and hypoxemia
II. Monitor, describe, record:	
A. VS with R and breath sounds q2–4h or as needed until stable	A. Indicates airway movement, changes related to chest drainage and pressures, possible respiratory failure
B. ABGs, pulse oximetry	B. Indicates need for supplemental oxygen if hypoxemia (hypoventilation) present, or presence of hypercapnia (chronic respiratory acidosis)

INTERVENTION	RATIONALE
C. Chest x ray	C. Reveals pulmonary infection or atelectasis
III. Administer:	
A. Bronchodilator IV	A. Acts to dilate airways and prevent obstruction
B. Oxygen via nasal cannula	B. Supplements oxygen to maintain optimal level for tissue oxygenation
IV. Perform/provide:	
A. Place in semi-Fowler's position on bed rest, or on back or operative side as ordered based on removal of a portion of complete lung	A. Provides for lung expansion and drainage of fluid and air by chest tubes, and allows for lung reexpansion following surgery
B. Assist in deep-breathing, coughing exercises q1–2h for 24 to 48 hours, arrange for these exercises when analgesia is at an optimal level	B. Improves ventilation and coughing to remove secretions, clears and dilates the airways to promote full lung expansion
C. Assist to splint chest during coughing and breathing exercises and inform that this will not dislodge the drainage tube(s)	C. Promotes comfort and support to the incisional area
D. Increased sips of fluid if permitted	D. Liquefies secretions for easier coughing and removal
E. Humidified air via cool-mist vaporizer	E. Facilitates the removal of secretions, moistens mucous membranes

INTERVENTION	RATIONALE
F. Orotracheal suctioning as appropriate and if ordered	F. Removes secretions when other methods have failed
G. Maintain patency and function of drainage tubes and system, including drainage amount and characteristics, patency of tubes and apparatus functioning, appropriate bubbling in water-seal compartment, correct pressure and suction, placement of the drainage system and tubing (these are system type dependent)	G. Promotes lung reexpansion and drainage of fluid and air
H. Oral care after expectoration and provide tissues and bag for proper disposal	H. Promotes comfort and prevents transmission of organisms

NURSING DIAGNOSES

Pain related to physical injury of intercostal nerves during surgery and presence of chest tubes

Impaired physical mobility related to pain and discomfort resulting from surgical affect on muscles on operative side

EXPECTED OUTCOMES

Pain reduced or controlled evidenced by verbalization that comfort increased and less analgesia required, improvement in arm and shoulder mobility and function evidenced by prevention of adhesions and progressive use of affected side

INTERVENTION	RATIONALE
I. Assess for:	
A. Chest pain at incisional and tube sites, feeling of numbness or heaviness, severity and effect on movement and breathing	A. Surgical trauma causes severe pain because of large incision, severance of nerves, and presence of chest tubes
B. Ability to move arm and shoulder on operative side, difficulty in positioning, effect of pain on ability to use the affected side	B. Surgery can involve muscle incision and immobility
III. Administer:	
A. Analgesic IV, patient-controlled device	A. Acts on CNS to interfere with pain pathways for consistent pain relief
IV. Perform/provide:	
A. Pain relief before too severe and prior to required breathing activities without depressing respirations and coughing	A. Provides adequate pain relief and promotes comfort at consistent level
B. Calm, restful environment with optimal temperature, ventilation, and noise free	B. Prevents stimuli that increases pain
C. Bed rest if pain present or rest periods before and after activity	C. Exertion and fatigue increase pain perception
D. Semi-Fowler's, sidelying position, pillow to splint chest during coughing	D. Reduces pain and promotes comfort by reducing strain on affected side and enhances lung expansion

INTERVENTION	RATIONALE
E. Avoid sidelying position on operative side with wedge or segmental procedure performed, and lateral position following pneumonectomy	E. Reduces expansion of remaining portion of lung, lung tissue can become compressed with mediastinal shift if a complete lung is removed
F. Position change q2h with support of tubing	F. Improves circulation and drainage via the chest tube without dislodgment or change in intrapleural pressure
G. Range of motion (passive) to the arm and shoulder of the operative side q4–6h for 24 hours postoperatively, progress to active ROM and self-care activities as tolerated using the affected arm and shoulder	G. Prevents adhesions in the operative area caused by surgery on the muscles
H. Backrub, relaxation exercises, music, other diversional activities	H. Nonpharmacological measures to promote comfort
I. Rest periods between activities as needed and based on respiratory status	I. Prevents fatigue and discomfort

NURSING DIAGNOSES

Risk for infection related to inadequate primary defenses (surgical incisions), invasive procedures (chest tubes and drainage system)

Risk for impaired skin integrity related to mechanical external factor of pressure of chest tube at insertion site

EXPECTED OUTCOMES

Adequate defenses and wound healing with complications prevented evidenced by temperature, WBC within normal range, area around tube insertion pink, dry, with absence of irritation or drainage, secure connections of drainage apparatus

INTERVENTION	RATIONALE
I. Assess for:	
A. Area around tube insertion, patency in removing fluids, color of drainage and if increasing or decreasing q4h for 24 to 48 hours	A. Infectious agents can be introduced into chest cavity or risk for infection resulting from stasis of fluid
B. Incision for redness, swelling, drainage, irritation of skin at tube site, healing of site following removal of tube	B. Indicates inflammation/infection or excoriation of skin caused by chest tube pressure and movement
C. Respiratory rate and breath sounds changes	C. Symptoms of pulmonary infection associated with contamination of or ineffective drainage system
II. Monitor, describe, record:	
A. Temperature q4h and PRN	A. Elevations indicate infection
B. WBC	B. Increases indicate infection
III. Administer:	
A. Antibiotic PO, IV, TOP at tube insertion site	A. Acts to prevent cell wall synthesis to destroy microorganisms in the prevention or treatment of infection

INTERVENTION	RATIONALE
IV. Perform/provide:	
A. Environment with optimal temperature, humidity, and ventilation, free of smoking or other irritants	A. Promotes comfort and respiratory ease
B. Avoid exposure to visitors or staff with upper respiratory infection	B. Prevents transmission of infectious agents
C. Elevate head and support with pillows to maintain alignment	C. Reduces stress on incisional area
D. Use sterile technique and all equipment and supplies for treatments, wound care and dressings, maintenance of chest drainage	D. Prevents contamination by pathogens
E. Secure chest tube to avoid pressure and pull on tube, avoid moving tube with position change	E. Prevents irritation and breakdown of skin

NURSING DIAGNOSIS

Risk for injury related to complications of pulmonary edema or pneumothorax/hemothorax and malfunction of chest tube and drainage system causing air, fluid, or blood accumulation in pleural space

EXPECTED OUTCOMES

Risk of complications minimized or eliminated evidenced by lung reexpansion and maintenance of respiratory baseline parameters

INTERVENTION	RATIONALE
I. Assess for:	
A. Respiratory rate, ease, depth, tachypnea, dyspnea, use of accessory muscles, unequal chest movements, diminished or absent breath sounds, dullness on percussion, blood in drainage system and on dressings	A. Provides data base of respiratory function affected by blood accumulation in pleural space
B. Restlessness, irritability, confusion, tachycardia, changes in mentation	B. Indicates expended pneumothorax
C. Level of anxiety, tremors, restlessness, feelings of uncertainty and apprehension	C. Anxiety commonly associated with dyspnea and other symptoms of respiratory distress
D. Increased P, dyspnea, orthopnea, cough with frothy sputum, adventitious sounds auscultated, cyanosis	D. Signs and symptoms of pulmonary edema
E. Absent drainage, bubbling of water in system, tidaling of water levels, kinking or compression of tubing or other obstruction, air leaks with loose connections, pump or power source problems, placement of drainage bottles at lower level than chest	E. Indicates malfunction of chest drainage system preventing reexpansion of lungs
II. Monitor, describe, record:	
A. VS q4h or as appropriate	A. Reveals changes indicating postoperative complication

INTERVENTION	RATIONALE
B. ABGs, pulse oximetry	B. Reveals need for supplemental oxygen
C. Chest x ray	C. Reveals reexpansion status or possible collapse
III. Administer: A. Oxygen via nasal cannula or face mask	A. Provides supplemental oxygen to treat hypoxemia
IV. Perform/provide: A. Bed rest in semi- to high Fowler's position, restrict activities as ordered depending on procedure	A. Improves comfort and prevents risks for complications
B. Maintain drainage system and suction levels, tape all connections securely, ensure patency of tubing, avoid allowing drainage system to be raised higher than the chest	B. Promotes lung reexpansion
C. Maintain pressure dressing at tube insertion site	C. Prevents complications associated with chest tube drainage
D. Assist with tube clearing, insertion of new tube(s), or thoracentesis	D. Interventions to correct mediastinal shift or chest tube malfunction
E. Change or maintain positions depending on type of surgery performed	E. Positioning important to proper drainage and prevention of drainage into areas that cause complications or prevent reexpansion

NURSING DIAGNOSES

Knowledge deficit related to disease process, medications, life-style changes and follow-up care (dietary requirements, exercise program, respiratory health practices, reduction of risk factors such as stress, smoking), measures to prevent infection, signs, and symptoms to report to physician

Noncompliance related to health beliefs, cultural values evidenced by inability to implement proposed therapeutic regimen and failure to maintain health status

EXPECTED OUTCOMES

Knowledge and understanding of disease, and ongoing care with life-style modified to enhance wellness associated with lung surgery evidenced by verbalizations of and understanding and compliance with medication, immunization, and dietary regimen, activity routine and restrictions with participation in pulmonary rehabilitation, signs and symptoms to report and ongoing physician monitoring of respiratory status

INTERVENTION	RATIONALE
I. Assess for: A. Readiness, willingness, and motivation to learn, discharge care and life-style changes	A. Learning can best take place if client is receptive and compliance is more likely to occur
B. Health practices, health beliefs, ethnic identity (religion, diet, language), value orientations, family interactions and cooperation	B. Factors to incorporate into teaching plan to facilitate learning and compliance with long-term care
IV. Perform/provide: A. Acknowledgment of perceptions with a nonjudgmental attitude	A. Establishes nurse–patient relationship in an accepting environment

INTERVENTION	RATIONALE
B. Explanations that are clear, accurate in understandable terms, small amount of information over time	B. Prevents misconceptions, erroneous attitudes and beliefs about disease and surgical procedure
C. Environment conducive to learning with space, lighting, and proper equipment and supplies	C. Distractions or discomfort will interfere with learning
D. As much control over lifestyle change decisions as possible, include in discharge planning	D. Allows power to be given or retained by patient
E. Teaching aids (pamphlets, videotapes, pictures, written instructions)	E. Reinforces learning
F. Team of resource personnel/professionals	F. Nutritionist, social worker, counselor, pulmonary rehabilitation therapist, and others can assist in teaching specific care and providing support for desired changes
V. Teach patient/family: A. Anatomy, function of the lungs, pathophysiology, and effects of surgery	A. Promotes understanding of disease that faciliates compliance
B. Risk factors such as malnutrition, stress, smoking, exercises	B. Contributes to information about life-style changes that can be modified
C. Dietary modification and daily fluid intake of 10 to 12 glasses/day if allowed	C. Reduces risk factor associated with malnutrition or fluid deficit

INTERVENTION	RATIONALE
D. Administration and rationale of all prescribed medications (antibiotics, bronchodilators, anti-inflammatory), written schedule of times and dosages, side effects to expect and to report, demonstrate administration of oxygen, and allow to practice the procedures involved with this treatment	D. Promotes compliance of complete medication regimen
E. Wound care and reporting of any changes such as redness, swelling, drainage	E. Provides for early treatment and interventions to prevent serious complications
F. Environment free of smoking, pollutants, change filters monthly, remove offensive odors	F. Provides air free of irritants that provoke coughing and changes in compromised respiratory system
G. Continue coughing and deep-breathing exercises, inform of oxygen and equipment administration safety measures to follow in use of oxygen	G. Maintains respiratory health status and prevents complications or safety hazards
H. Progressive activity routine allowing for restrictions, rest periods when needed during activity, to cease activity if dizzy, dyspneic, continue arm and shoulder exercises on operative side and avoid lifting heavy objects, take steps to arrange for pulmonary rehabilitation program if ordered	H. Supports life-style change to maintaining respiratory status

INTERVENTION	RATIONALE
I. Suggest home modifications to support energy and endurance level	I. Conserves energy while maintaining control of self-care
J. Avoid stressful situations, consider counseling or stress-reduction program to assist in development of coping and problem-solving skills	J. Prevents risk factor associated with chronic pulmonary disease
K. Encourage to avoid groups or persons with upper respiratory disease or during flu season	K. Prevents transmission of infectious agents
L. Report temperature elevation, chills, dyspnea, pulse irregularity, activity intolerance, continued fatigue, chest pain, change in cough and sputum characteristics (yellow, rust colored), irritability, restlessness to physician	L. Indicates possible recurrence or complication of pneumonia (pleural effusion, atelectasis)
M. Contact support groups to stop smoking, for financial counseling, American Lung and Cancer Associations for information/educational materials	M. Provides assistance to reduce risk factors

rhinoplasty/septoplasty

....

DEFINITION
Rhinoplasty is the surgical reconstruction of the nose usually done to correct a deformity or for cosmetic reasons. Septoplasty is the surgical correction of the nose resulting from septal deviation or trauma that requires realignment or removal of bone and cartilage. Both procedures are usually performed with the use of a local anesthetic by injection and/or topical application

NURSING DIAGNOSES
Ineffective breathing pattern related to nasal obstruction resulting from surgical packing, splints, dressing postoperatively

    Altered oral mucous membrane related to mouth breathing resulting from nasal packing and edema postoperatively

    Pain related to physical injury of trauma resulting from surgery causing pressure of edema and ecchymosis

EXPECTED OUTCOMES
Ventilation by alternate breathing pattern temporarily attained evidenced by mouth breathing with moist, intact oral membranes maintained; pain controlled evidenced by verbalization that comfort achieved with analgesia

INTERVENTION	RATIONALE
I. Assess for: A. Respiratory rate, ease, depth, any distress caused by adapting to mouth breathing	A. Provides data regarding ability to maintain adequate ventilation

INTERVENTION	RATIONALE
B. Oral mucosa for dryness, irritation, breaks, complaints of thirst	B. Indicates risk for damage caused by mouth breathing
C. Pain severity, type of dressing, internal or external nose splint, nose mold, amount of edema	C. Provides information for analgesia administration, dressing displacement
D. Posterior throat, nasal packing for blood	D. Indicates amount of bleeding and risk for hemorrhage

III. Administer:

A. Mild analgesic PO	A. Acts to reduce pain by interfering with CNS pathways

IV. Perform/provide:

A. Place in semi- to high Fowler's position	A. Promotes comfort and breathing, reduces edema
B. Assist to breathe deeply through the mouth four times/hour, avoid coughing if possible	B. Ensures adequate ventilation
C. Ice pack q4h	C. Reduces edema and pain by vasoconstriction of vessels
D. Humidification continuously via cool-air vaporizer	D. Provides moisture in the air breathed to prevent oral dryness
E. Increase fluid intake to 2 L/day if permitted	E. Provides hydration and prevents dry oral mucous membrane

INTERVENTION	RATIONALE
F. Apply water-soluble jelly to lips and oral cavity using cotton swab	F. Provides lubrication and prevents dryness and cracking
G. Allow to rinse mouth frequently and gently brush teeth twice/day	G. Reduces discomfort of mouth dryness
H. Avoid disturbing dressings, splint, or packing when giving care	H. Prevents accidental displacement
I. Change dressing under the nose PRN using sterile technique	I. Promotes comfort and prevents transmission of microorganisms
J. Assist to remove packing in 24 to 48 hours postoperatively	J. Allows for nose breathing and promotes comfort
K. Cleanse mouth with half-strength hydrogen peroxide following packing removal	K. Promotes cleanliness by removing postoperative debris

NURSING DIAGNOSES

Body image disturbance related to physical factor of facial discoloration, presence of dressing or splint; psychological factor of fear of unsatisfactory outcome of cosmetic surgery

Knowledge deficit related to postoperative care (medications, follow-up appointments, activities to avoid), possible complication of bleeding, healing process and when to expect results

EXPECTED OUTCOMES

Knowledge and compliance with follow-up care evidenced by successful outcome of surgery within 3 months without discomfort or complications

INTERVENTION	RATIONALE
V. Teach patient/family:	
A. Inform that surgery is usually successful, and allow several weeks before judging resuls	A. Reduces apprehension about outcome of surgery and allows time for complete healing
B. Inform that nose will remain edematous and face discolored following removal of packing and splint	B. Promotes positive self-image as swelling subsides
C. Avoid blowing nose, and sneeze with mouth open after removal of packing, avoid Valsalva movement until healing is complete	C. Prevents bleeding
D. Avoid touching splint or packing if still in place	D. Prevents displacement
E. Sleep with head of bed elevated	E. Enhances breathing and comfort
F. Continue soft dietary and fluid inclusion for up to 1 week	F. Provides necessary fluid and nutritional intake
G. Report fresh bleeding or oozing of blood to physician	G. Indicates presence of bleeding and intervention for control

tonsillitis/tonsillectomy

DEFINITION
The tonsils are lymphoid masses of tissue located on the posterior walls of the oropharynx. Infections of this tissue can be chronic or acute most commonly caused by the *Streptococcus* and complicated by pneumonia, nephritis, rheumatic fever as well as otitis media and abscess in acute episodes. Surgical removal (tonsillectomy) is performed to relieve chronic enlargement of this tissue that obstructs the passage of air in and out of the respiratory tract or to treat chronic infections. The adenoids can be removed at the same time (adenoidectomy). In the adult, a local anesthetic is usually used to perform a tonsillectomy. This plan can be used in association with the PREOPERATIVE CARE and POSTOPERATIVE CARE plans

NURSING DIAGNOSES
Pain in throat related to physical injuring agent of bacterial infection preoperatively or trauma of surgery postoperatively

Risk for physical injury related to complication of surgical procedure causing hemorrhage

EXPECTED OUTCOMES
Pain relieved or controlled and expected minimal amount of bleeding postoperatively evidenced by verbalization that pain has subsided and progressively able to swallow without discomfort, absence of excessive immediate or delayed bleeding

INTERVENTION	RATIONALE
I. Assess for:	
A. Throat pain, difficulty in swallowing, elevated temperature, malaise, redness and swelling of tonsils	A. Signs and symptoms of tonsillitis
B. Throat pain, referred ear pain	B. Pain can be expected for 7 to 10 days postoperatively
C. Excessive bleeding at back of throat, bright red bleeding on expectoration or vomitus	C. Indicates risk for hemorrhage during first 12 to 24 hours postoperatively or in delayed hemorrhage 7 to 10 days postoperatively before healing is complete
II. Monitor, describe, record:	
A. VS q15 min initially, then q4h, axillary temperature q4h	A. Tachycardia, hypotension indicates hemorrhage, elevated temperature associated with tonsillitis
III. Administer:	
A. Mild analgesic, antipyretic PO (avoid aspirin)	A. Acts to control pain by interference with CNS pathways and reduce temperature; aspirin increases bleeding tendency
B. Antibiotic PO, IM	B. Acts to reduce pain by treating the infectious process
IV. Perform/provide:	
A. Bed rest during the acute stage of tonsillitis	A. Promotes comfort during curative phase of infection
B. Place in sidelying position following surgery	B. Allows drainage of secretions via the mouth to prevent aspiration

INTERVENTION	RATIONALE
C. Throat gargle with saline solution two to four times/day	C. Promotes comfort and relieves throat pain in tonsillitis
D. Ice pack to throat q4h	D. Promotes comfort and vasoconstriction to control edema and bleeding postoperatively
E. Clear cool fluids, ice chips, gelatin, ice cream, custard	E. Provides needed fluid intake and foods of smooth consistency for easier swallowing and minimal irritation to throat

NURSING DIAGNOSIS

Knowledge deficit related to treatment for tonsillitis, preoperative and postoperative follow-up care, healing process, signs and symptoms to report

EXPECTED OUTCOMES

Knowledge and understanding of treatments and care associated with tonsillitis/postoperative tonsillectomy evidenced by compliance with medication administration, dietary and fluid requirements, activities to avoid, and verbalization of symptoms to report to physician

INTERVENTION	RATIONALE
V. Teach patient/family:	
A. Course of disease or postoperative care and healing process that is completed in 2 to 3 weeks	A. Provides information needed for compliance with treatments and when to resume normal activities and diet
B. Rest periods with activities increased as tolerated	B. Allows for convalescence without complications

INTERVENTION	RATIONALE
C. Administration of medications (analgesic, antipyretic, antibiotic regimen) with action, times, dosage, frequency, side effects, and to take all of the prescribed antibiotic	C. Promotes compliance with therapy to reduce pain, fever, and ensures destruction of infectious organism
D. Use throat spray, gum, or lozenge for throat soreness	D. Provides anesthesia to reduce pain
E. Encourage liquid intake and soft foods, avoid spicy, hot, rough consistency foods, citrus juices for 1 to 2 weeks	E. Provides adequate fluid and food intake without irritating sore throat
F. Avoid use of straw, coughing, clearing throat, blowing nose, or sneezing postoperatively	F. Irritates throat and disturbs clotting process caused by suction or pressure
G. Inform that ear pain can occur and this is not unusual	G. Referred pain is common as nerve pathways are disturbed
H. Report bleeding that occurs 5 to 10 days postoperatively	H. Delayed bleeding can occur as tough fibrous membrane begins to break away from operative site

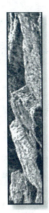

Renal/Urinary Systems Standards

renal/urinary systems data base

chronic renal failure

nephrectomy/nephrostomy

renal/urinary tract calculi/litholapaxy

renal/urinary tract infections
(cystitis/glomerulonephritis/pyelonephritis)

urinary diversion/cystectomy (continent vesicostomy/cutaneous
ureterostomy/ileal conduit)

renal/urinary systems data base

HISTORICAL DATA REVIEW
Past Events:
1. Acute and/or chronic renal and urinary disease or disorders, presence of other diseases that affect the renal/urinary systems (diabetes, neuromuscular disorders, gastrointestinal disorders, sexually transmitted diseases, vascular disorders)
2. Signs and symptoms related to renal or urinary tract disorders (pain, edema, elevated blood pressure, weight gain, mentation changes, fatigue, skin and mucous membrane dryness, pruritis, and turgor changes, altered urinary pattern, fever, chills, tingling in extremities)
3. Renal/bladder disorders, hypertension, diabetes of family members
4. Tobacco/alcohol/caffeine use, exposure to environmental nephrotoxic substances, dietary restrictions, treatments
5. Medications (prescription and over-the-counter) for renal/urinary conditions and nephrotoxic drugs
6. Anxiety, stressors, depression, presence of urinary diversion, rehabilitation associated with incontinence, dietary restrictions and inclusions (acid-ash or low-purine diet, protein, sodium, potassium, calcium)
7. Hospitalizations and feelings about care, surgery associated with kidneys, ureters, or urinary bladder

Present Events:
1. Medical diagnoses associated with or affecting renal and urinary organ structure and function, patency of urinary tract
2. Urine amount and characteristics (color, odor, clarity, sedimentation, hematuria, mucus, pus), need for increases or restrictions of fluids
3. Urinary incontinence, retention, bladder distention
4. Abnormal urinary pattern, anuria, oliguria, polyuria, nocturia, frequency
5. Flank pain, dysuria, burning on urination

6. Fluid intake and output (I&O) amounts and types for a specific time interval
7. Electrolyte profile and balance
8. Dehydration (skin turgor, itching, dryness of lips, skin, mucous membranes)
9. Edema of face, extremities, and sacral area, weight gain, blood pressure elevation
10. Behavior such as alertness, cognitive ability, level of consciousness
11. Activities of daily living and effect on continence (toileting), self-esteem, mentation changes, restlessness, insomnia
12. Preferences in toileting, treatments for renal function (dialysis), urinary function (indwelling catheter, intermittent catheterization)

PHYSICAL ASSESSMENT DATA REVIEW

1. Kidney size and movement, masses in flank area palpated
2. Abdominal or bladder distention
3. Dullness over bladder if distended percussed
4. Possible bruit with stenosis of renal artery

NURSING DIAGNOSES CONSIDERATIONS

1. Altered urinary elimination
2. Fluid excess
3. Functional incontinence
4. Risk for fluid volume deficit
5. Risk for infection
6. Knowledge deficit
7. Reflex incontinence
8. Self-care deficit (toileting)
9. Stress incontinence
10. Total incontinence
11. Urge incontinence
12. Urinary retention

GERIATRIC CONSIDERATIONS

Renal/urinary changes in geriatric patients occur over long periods as a result of renal diseases, urinary tract infections, organ atrophy, or trauma. Renal function involves excretion, secretion, and regulation, and aging diminishes these processes and their effect on urination. The most

common disorders affecting these systems in the older adult are incontinence, retention, and urinary tract infection. Changes associated with aging that should be considered when assessing the geriatric patient include:

1. Reduced renal tissue growth resulting in decreased organ size and
   decreased number and increased size of nephrons resulting in a reduction in renal function and efficiency
2. Glomeruli sclerosis and afferent arteriole atrophy resulting in degeneration of glomeruli and glomerular filtration rate (GFR)
3. Decreased renal blood flow, GFR, and tubular function resulting in reduced concentration of urine and drug clearance
4. Increased blood urea nitrogen (BUN) and decreased muscle mass
   causing decreased creatinine production and clearance resulting in
   need for age adjustments when noting laboratory values
5. Decreased reabsorption of glucose and sodium resulting in longer
   time for acid–base problems to be resolved
6. Decreased cell mass resulting in reduced intracellular body water
   with extracellular fluid remaining the same, decreased water content
   of tissues resulting in a reduced total body water content
7. Bladder becomes more funnel shaped with decreased capacity resulting in urinary frequency and possibly nocturia
8. Increased bladder and perineal muscle weakness resulting in retention and stress incontinence in women; enlarged prostate in men resulting in urgency and frequency, dribbling of urine
9. Decreased bladder muscle tone and sphincter relaxation resulting in
   frequency
10. Decreased ability to empty bladder completely resulting in urinary
    stasis and urinary tract infection
11. Decreased inhibitory neural impulses to bladder resulting in loss of
    bladder contractions and the control of bladder function that cause
    incontinence

DIAGNOSTIC LABORATORY TESTS AND PROCEDURES

1. Abdominal flat plate (KUB), intravenous pyelogram (IVP), retrograde
   pyelogram, cystoscopy, renal angiography, computerized tomography
   (CT), cystourethrography, manometric bladder/urethra studies, ultrasonography, nuclear scan, electromyography of perineal muscles
   and sphincters, renal biopsy and cytology
2. Urinalysis (routine, serial, culture), creatinine clearance, concentra-

tion and dilution tests, blood urea nitrogen (BUN), serum creatinine, complete blood count (CBC), electrolyte panel

MEDICATIONS

1. Analgesics; phenazopyridine
2. Anticholinergics: propantheline bromide, imipramine hydrochloride
3. Antimicrobials: sulfisoxazole, trimethoprim combined with sulfamethoxazole, cephalexin monohydrate, ciprofloxacin, penicillin
4. Antispasmodics: flavoxate hydrochloride
5. Cholinergics: bethanechol chloride, dicyclomine hydrochloride
6. Diuretics: furosemide (loop), mannitol (osmotic), chlorothiazide (thiazide)
7. Incontinence agents: oxybutynin chloride, verapamil hydrochloride, propanolamine hydrochloride
8. Urinary antiseptics: nitrofurantoin, methenamine mandelate, nalidixic acid

chronic renal failure

DEFINITION

Chronic renal failure (CRF) is a progressive, irreversible impairment in renal function causing the loss of the ability to excrete water and non-metabolized solutes. This eventually leads to a gradual accumulation of uremic toxins (uremia). The most common causes or risk factors involved in development of the disease are acute renal failure, diabetes mellitus, chronic glomerulonephritis or pyelonephritis as well as hypertension, renal obstructions, and lupus erythematosus. Functioning nephrons decrease as the disease progresses resulting in reduced glomerular filtration rate (GFR). Uremia becomes evident when the GFR level is <10 to 20 mL/minute. Medical intervention includes renal dialysis (peritoneal or hemodialysis), and surgical care involves kidney transplant if available. This plan includes care of the major manifestations of CRF and, if kidney transplant is planned, can be used in association with PREOPERATIVE CARE and POSTOPERATIVE CARE plans

NURSING DIAGNOSES

Anxiety related to threat to or change in health status (long-term progression of disease), threat of death (poor prognosis and early death), threat to self-concept (change in life-style and roles associated with illness and dialysis therapy) causing inability to manage feelings of uncertainty about outcome of the illness and apprehension regarding availability of kidney for transplantation

Ineffective individual coping related to inability to cope with illness (poor prognosis, long-term dialysis), personal vulnerability (inadequate family support system), and life-style and role changes (difficulty in adjustment to treatment plan resulting in chronic anxiety, depression and worry, inability to problem-solve and meet basic needs)

Powerlessness related to hospitalization and treatments, lack of control over illness or self-care resulting in increased apprehension and tension, feelings of helplessness and hopelessness as condition deteriorates, dependence on others for care

EXPECTED OUTCOMES

Anxiety and fear within manageable levels, development of coping and problem-solving skills, verbalizations that anxiety is decreasing, optimal participation and receptive attitude in planning for ongoing care and life-style changes needed to manage disease and chronic anxiety

INTERVENTION	RATIONALE
I. Assess for:	
A. Level of anxiety, use of coping mechanisms, stated fears of disease outcome, life-style changes, feelings of hopelessness	A. Anxiety can range from mild to severe, verbalizations assist to identify feelings and inappropriate use of coping skills
B. Restlessness, complaining, joking, withdrawal, depression, agitation, demanding behaviors	B. Nonverbal expressions of anxiety and personality changes when not able to communicate feelings and realization that dialysis is a permanent part of life
C. Personal resources to cope with stress, anxiety, and interest in learning to problem-solve	C. Support systems and personal strengths assist to develop coping skills and plan their life realistically
D. Feelings and response to change in life-style, declining ability to carry out role and participate in activities, changes in appearance and treatments as disease progresses	D. Changes in roles and self-concept common problems associated with CRF
E. Expressed feelings of anger, fear, hostility, apathy, hopelessness	E. Results from feelings of powerlessness as disease progresses leading to increased debilitation and finally death

INTERVENTION	RATIONALE
III. Administer: A. Anti-anxiety agent PO	A. Acts to reduce anxiety level and provides calming effect and rest, depresses subcortical levels of CNS, limbic system
IV. Perform/provide: A. Environment conducive to rest, and expressions of fear and anxiety, avoid anxiety-producing situations	A. Decreases stimuli that cause stress/anxiety, venting of feelings decreases anxiety
B. Orient to hospital room, staff, equipment, routines, and policies regarding visiting hours, others	B. Reduces anxiety and provides comfort and adjustment to a new situation
C. Suggest new methods to enhance coping skills and problem solving, allow to externalize and identify those that help	C. Offers alternative coping strategies that allow for release of anxiety and fear
D. Positive feedback regarding progress made, focus on abilities rather than inabilities	D. Provides support for adaptive behavior, promotes self-worth and responsibility
E. Diversional activities such as relaxation exercises, TV, radio, music, reading, tapes, guided imagery	E. Reduces anxiety and promotes comfort
F. Allow visitors according to desire and condition, avoid stressful situations	F. Promotes support from significant others/family to decrease anxiety

INTERVENTION	RATIONALE
G. Allow to participate in planning of care to maintain usual activities when possible, include family as appropriate	G. Allows for some control over situations
H. Support grieving for loss of life-style and restrictions in activities, changes role and independence	H. Provides assistance in adaptation to changes imposed by disease such as permanent dialysis
I. Information about economic/legal/social resources, recent research and treatments available, government assistance, psychological counseling, support group if advised	I. Provides information and promotes control over present and future life-style changes, assists with finances, medical and surgical care, reducing anxiety

NURSING DIAGNOSES

Altered nutrition: Less than body requirements related to inability to ingest food because of biologic factors (anorexia, accumulation of nitrogen waste in renal dysfunction) resulting in dietary restrictions of protein, reduced intake of nutrients

Altered oral mucous membrane related to restriction in fluid intake resulting in xerostomia, discomfort, stomatitis

Constipation related to less than adequate dietary bulk, fluid intake, and physical activity, medication administered to control increases in electrolytes

EXPECTED OUTCOMES

Adequate nutritional intake within protein restriction and constipation prevented or resolved evidenced by dietary intake of 2000 calories/day with return of appetite, and soft, formed feces eliminated daily or q2 days, maintenance or improvement in energy, activity level and endurance within limitations evidenced by participation in ADL, absence of circulatory complications with RBC, platelets within normal range and no bleeding from mucous membranes or gastrointestinal tract

INTERVENTION	RATIONALE
I. Assess for:	
A. Dietary pattern and intake, including calories, basic four food groups, vitamins and minerals, acceptance of special diet	A. Provides baseline data for possible nutritional deficiencies; dietary restrictions of protein reduces levels of nitrogenous wastes
B. Stomatitis, oral pain, periodontitis, oral pain, state of oral care, dryness of oral mucosa, effect on eating	B. Indicates changes in oral mucosa caused by inflammatory process and fluid intake, formation of ammonia from salivary urea
C. Anorexia, nausea, vomiting, salty bitter taste in mouth, fishy, ammonia odor to breath	C. Results from dislike of diet, manifestations of renal failure
D. Bowel pattern and characteristics with presence of constipation, abdominal distention or fecal impaction, decrease in activities	D. Provides data to normalize adequate bowel elimination, constipation can result from administration of phosphate-binding agents
II. Monitor, describe, record:	
A. Weight on same scale, same time and same clothing daily/weekly	A. Monitors gains and losses indicating nutritional deficiencies as disease progresses
III. Administer:	
A. Bulk laxative PO	A. Acts to provide bulk to feces for easier passage and prevent constipation to avoid using agents containing sodium or calcium

INTERVENTION	RATIONALE
B. Antiemetic IV, PO	B. Acts to reduce vomiting by enhancing gastric empty-ing to block stasis
C. Multivitamin PO	C. Acts to provide supplemen-tary support for dietary re-strictions
IV. Perform/provide: A. Environment conducive to eating (quiet, relaxed, pleasant, odor free)	A. Anorexia is a common problem that worsens as disease progresses
B. Special diet consisting of appropriate protein, carbo-hydrate, and fats with a usual intake of 20 to 50 g/day of protein and 100 g/day of carbohydrate and total intake of 2000 calo-ries/day	B. Provides diet with maxi-mum protein allowances with foods that include complete amino acids, pro-tein content depends on renal impairment deter-mined by BUN level, carbo-hydrates prevent fat break-down and tissue catabolism
C. Dietary supplements and food inclusions (high caloric) but based on defi-ciency	C. Provides foods to treat de-ficiencies, prevents hy-poproteinemia, hyperlipi-demia, minimize uremic toxicity
D. Small, frequent meals of soft foods spread over 24 hours, avoid hot, spicy, foods, caffeine-containing beverages	D. Provides optimal nutri-tional intake while pre-venting discomfort of oral mucous membranes

INTERVENTION	RATIONALE
E. Inclusions of high-fiber foods in restricted diet if possible, encourage as much activity as allowed	E. Provides bulk to feces to prevent constipation
F. Oral care with soft brush, mouth rinses prior to and after meals with saline or hydrogen peroxide solution, position dentures in place if needed for meals	F. Prevents irritation of oral mucosa and promotes comfort
G. Fluid intake allowed, hard candy, chewing gum	G. Provides fluids to alleviate dry mouth and constipation
H. Referral to nutritionist	H. Assists to modify diet to include and exclude foods

NURSING DIAGNOSES

Fluid volume excess related to compromised regulatory mechanism (renal dysfunction) resulting in progressive failure causing sodium and water retention and possible cardiovascular changes (hypertension, heart failure)

Fluid volume deficit related to failure of regulatory mechanisms (renal dysfunction), and reduced fluid intake resulting in electrolyte imbalance (hypernatremia, hyperkalemia, hypocalcemia, hyperphosphatemia, hypermagnesemia) as intake is increased beyond restrictions or disease progresses and kidneys fail to excrete these electrolytes

EXPECTED OUTCOMES

Fluid volume excess or deficit reduced or resolved evidenced by P, BP, R, peripheral pulses, capillary refill time, and breath sounds within normal baseline determination and absence of cardiac complications, I&O ratio in balance, weight and edema reduced, Na, K, Ca, Mg, P levels within normal ranges

INTERVENTION	RATIONALE
I. Assess for:	
A. P rate and rhythm (irregular of <60 or >100/bpm), reduced or increased BP, rapid and labored respirations (>20), apical pulse (<60/bpm)	A. Identifies changes associated with decreased CO caused by heart failure in the presence of fluid retention or overload
B. Lung sounds for crackles, abnormal heart sounds, dyspnea, jugular vein distention, cyanosis, decreased mental alertness or thought processes, peripheral edema, urinary output of <30 mL/hour, coolness and pallor to extremities with decreased pulses, capillary refill of <3 seconds	B. Identifies changes associated with fluid volume excess and perfusion problems in other system functions that result in organ dysfunction
C. Fluid daily intake, preferred fluids, calculated daily fluid restrictions	C. Determines if adjustment in fluid intake is needed and/or restrictions in intake are followed
D. Dry skin and mucous membrane, thirst, poor skin turgor, decreased urinary output	D. Indicates risk for dehydration
E. Muscle weakness, flaccidity, twitching, cramping, increased bowel sounds, diarrhea, irregular P, and abnormal ECG readings	E. Signs and symptoms of hyperkalemia resulting from decreased renal tubular function as medications and dietary intake late in the disease contribute to K excesses

INTERVENTION	RATIONALE
F. Muscle cramps, numbness or tingling in fingers or toes, changes in mentation, possible seizures	F. Signs and symptoms of hypocalcemia resulting from reduced intestinal absorption of Ca or possibly a secretion of the parathyroid gland
G. Weakness, lethargy, restlessness, mentation changes, thirst, vomiting, diarrhea	G. Signs and symptoms of hypernatremia resulting from inability of nephrons to filter out Na; gastrointestinal symptoms result from hyponatremia
H. Muscle cramps, paresthesia, seizure activity	H. Signs and symptoms of hyperphosphatemia as kidneys fail to excrete P
I. Nausea, vomiting, hypotension, bradycardia, reduced deep-tendon reflexes, confusion	I. Signs and symptoms of hypermagnesemia as kidneys fail to excrete Mg
II. Monitor, describe, record: A. VS, q1–4h as appropriate	A. Indicates hemodynamic stability to determine cardiac function status and potential for failure, increases in BP and P associated with increasing levels of electrolytes
B. I&O q1h for output of <30 mL/hr or as appropriate for greater intake than output with fluid excess, and increased output with diuretic therapy	B. Indicates kidney perfusion and function, effect of diuretic therapy

INTERVENTION	RATIONALE
C. Weight daily at same time, on same scale, wearing same clothing	C. Monitors degree of fluid excess and effectiveness of therapy
D. ABGs, electrolytes, BUN, creatinine, glucose, uric acid	D. Indicates impact of condition on organ and system functions; evaluates K of >5.0 mEq/L, Na of >150 mEq/L, Ca of <6.0 mEq/L, P of >2.0 mEq/L, and Mg of >3.0 mEq/L
E. Urinalysis for hematuria, Sp.Gr., electrolyte, creatinine clearance	E. Determines kidney ability to concentrate urine, excrete electrolytes, and kidney damage

III. Administer:

A. Diuretic PO, IV while monitoring electrolyte imbalance, with potassium replacement if needed	A. Acts to increase water in hyponatremia (loop diuretic) or hypernatremia (thiazide diuretic) and potassium excretion depending on the type administered
B. Vasodilator PO	B. Acts to increase renal blood flow to prevent fluid and Na retention that leads to hypertension
C. Antihypertensive PO	C. Acts to treat hypertension in Na and water retention to reduce and control BP by action on peripheral vasculature, inhibits angiotensin-converting enzyme

INTERVENTION	RATIONALE
D. Anticonvulsive PO	D. Acts to prevent seizure activity by reducing electrical discharges in the motor cotex in electrolyte imbalance
E. Calcium, Vitamin D IV, PO	E. Acts to prevent or maintain calcium level or counteract high K levels
F. Cation exchange resin REC	F. Acts to exchange Na for K in treatment of hyperkalemia if K is >7 mEq/L
G. Phosphate binder PO	G. Acts to bind with dietary phosphates in hyperphosphatemia

IV. Perform/provide

A. Bed rest with activity restrictions if appropriate	A. Provides rest without excessive activity that promotes catabolism
B. Place in semi-Fowler's position with periodic changes for comfort	B. Promotes breathing with less effort, venous return in presence of edema
C. Fluid restrictions of 400 to 1000 mL/24 hours plus amount of fluid loss or as ordered, spread over 24 hours ($\frac{1}{2}$ during day, $\frac{1}{3}$ during evening, $\frac{1}{6}$ during night)	C. Amount of restriction depends on kidney's ability to secrete water

INTERVENTION	RATIONALE
D. Na intake of 500 to 2300 mg/day and K intake of 1500 to 2500 mg/day restrictions	D. Impaired kidney function reduces ability to excrete Na and K, Na increases water retention in extracellular compartments causing fluid excess and fluid overload potential
E. Mouth care q4h, offer hard candy, ice chips, popsicle, add to intake record	E. Promotes comfort and moisture to allay dry mouth
F. Cautious administration of IV solutions avoiding Na if fluids are retained, close monitoring of rate of infusion	F. Improves fluid intake if advised without causing fluid retention
G. Dietary restrictions as follows:	G. Prevents electrolyte imbalances
a. Avoid table salt, snack foods, MSG in foods, bacon, luncheon meats, beverages and juices containing Na	a. High in Na and disallowed on limited diet
b. Avoid bananas, tomatoes, fruit juices, potatoes	b. Foods high in K
c. Avoid peanuts, peas, corn, and poultry, organ meats, milk, eggs	c. Foods high in P
d. Avoid legumes, whole-grain bread, and cereals	d. Foods high in Mg
e. Include dairy foods	e. Provides Ca replacement
H. Referral to nutritionist	H. Assists in meal planning to adhere to restrictions and inclusions

NURSING DIAGNOSES

Risk for infection related to chronic disease and inadequate secondary defenses resulting from buildup of nitrogenous wastes, immunosuppression from medication regimen, inadequate primary defenses of broken skin resulting from peritoneal dialysis catheter insertion site and dialysis procedure

Risk for impaired skin integrity related to external factor of immobility (activity intolerance) resulting in pressure to skin, bony prominences and edematous parts, internal factor of progressive illness resulting in pruritus, edema, dryness causing scratching and irritation or disruption to skin

Risk for injury related to physical factor of broken skin associated with hemodialysis venous access patency and infection

EXPECTED OUTCOMES

Infection free and intact skin evidenced by absence of redness at pressure points, breaks, or scratches, signs and symptoms of respiratory, urinary, or oral infections evidenced by WBC, temperature, urine and sputum cultures, respirations and urinary pattern within normal determinations

INTERVENTION	RATIONALE
I. Assess for:	
A. Elevated temperature, chills, adventitious breath sounds, sputum color changing to yellow or greenish, positive sputum culture	A. Indicates pulmonary infection caused by stasis of secretions in the presence of change in mobility status (immobility)
B. Cloudy, foul-smelling urine, positive urine culture, burning, urgency, and frequency	B. Indicates urinary infection caused by stasis of urine
C. Pain, redness, swelling of oral cavity mucous membranes, ammonia breath, positive culture	C. Indicates infection of mucous membranes, increased urea and ammonia from bacterial breakdown of urea results in odor to breath

INTERVENTION	RATIONALE
D. Skin dryness, itching, redness at pressure points	D. Results from pruritis and dry skin, urea crystallization on skin (uremic frost), constant pressure on skin leads to decreased circulation and breakdown
E. Dry, brittle hair and nails, sallow yellowish color of skin	E. Results of retention of urinary chromogens and decreased oil gland activity
F. Skin around catheter insertion site for peritoneal dialysis for redness, swelling, drainage, color of peritoneal dialysis dialysate	F. Indicates infection associated with peritoneal dialysis

II. Monitor, describe, record:

INTERVENTION	RATIONALE
A. Temperature q4h	A. Indicates elevations in presence of infection
B. Culture of urine, sputum, blood, skin	B. Indicates presence of and identifies pathogens
C. WBC, differential	C. Increases in presence of infection to WBC of >12,000/mm^3

III. Administer:

INTERVENTION	RATIONALE
A. Antibiotic PO	A. Acts to destroy pathogens by inhibiting cell wall synthesis
B. Antipyretic PO	B. Acts to reduce temperature
C. Antipruritic PO, TOP	C. Acts to relieve itching

INTERVENTION	RATIONALE
IV. Perform/provide:	
A. Change positions q2h, protect susceptible body parts	A. Reduces prolonged pressure on bony prominences
B. Careful handwash technique prior to performing any care or treatment	B. Prevents transmission of microorganisms
C. Comply with sterile technique standards for all invasive procedures, use gloves and masks when performing peritoneal dialysis	C. Prevents introduction of pathogens to susceptible areas
D. Oral care, including brushing with soft brush, flossing of teeth	D. Promotes cleanliness of oral mucous membranes
E. Ensure fluid intake according to calculated restrictions	E. Dilutes urine and prevents stasis of urine in the bladder
F. Deep breathing and coughing exercises as appropriate	F. Promotes ventilation, removal of secretions to prevent stasis
G. Cool room temperature with cool compresses to pruritic areas	G. Promotes comfort and allays itching
H. Soothing emollients such as baking soda or cornstarch in bath water, use mild soap and warm water and gently pat dry	H. Removes uremic frost and allays itching

INTERVENTION	RATIONALE
I. Apply pressure to affected areas, discourage scratching (diversional activities)	I. Decreases tendency to scratch
J. Adequate fluid and nutritional intake according to restrictions	J. Provides proper nourishment to body cells to protect from infection
K. Change dressing on cannula if in place, avoid BP or blood withdrawal on arm with access	K. Protects access site from infection and clotting

NURSING DIAGNOSES

Risk for activity intolerance related to presence of renal dysfunction (weakness, peripheral neuropathy), inadequate nutritional intake, presence of circulatory problem (kidney's inability to produce erythropoietin resulting in anemia)

Sexual dysfunction related to disease process resulting in impotence, libido problems, reduced sperm mobility, menstrual irregularities, testicular changes

EXPECTED OUTCOMES

Optimal activity level and endurance within limitations evidenced by participation in ADL, absence of weakness, pain in feet and legs; sexual pattern enhanced evidenced by verbalization of sexual activity resumed with more satisfying level of satisfaction compatible with functional changes

INTERVENTION	RATIONALE
I. Assess for: A. Level of fatigue, weakness, and potential for activity progression, bed rest status	A. Provides baseline and allows for planning activities and need for assistance

INTERVENTION	RATIONALE
B. Interest and ability in performing ADL with or without assistance, factors that precipitate fatigue	B. Readiness and increased energy level necessary for successful program for self-care
C. Sleep/rest pattern, wakefulness during night	C. Optimal rest and sleep necessary to reduce fatigue and perform activities
D. R > 20/minute, P > 120/bpm and not returning to pre-activity level within 3 minutes, palpitations, dyspnea, dizziness, chest pain, weakness, and stopping activity if symptoms appear	D. Signs and symptoms of activity intolerance leading to fatigue
E. Amenorrhea, infertility, testicular atrophy, psychophysiological factors associated with libido changes; expression of feelings regarding sexual performance and satisfaction	E. Signs and symptoms of reproductive changes associated with CRF

III. Administer:

A. Androgens PO	A. Acts to correct sexual dysfunction
B. Hematopoietic agent PO	B. Acts to stimulate RBC production

IV. Perform/provide:

A. Enforced bed rest and activity restrictions if needed	A. Provides needed rest to prevent fatigue and improve activity tolerance

INTERVENTION	RATIONALE
B. Perform or assist in ADL and other activities as needed, place all articles and call light within reach to use as desired	B. Conserves energy while preserving as much control and independence as possible
C. Increase activities gradually from sitting up in bed, in chair, walking in room, to bathroom, and in hall with daily increase in distance and ADL activities	C. Progressive change in activities increases with endurance and energy level
D. Organize activities around rest periods in a quiet, calm, dimly lit, stimuli-free environment	D. Permits rest without interruptions
E. Assist to assume preferred position for sleep, offer backrub, oral care, extra pillows, other activities based on sleep pattern	E. Provides for usual bedtime rituals to ensure comfort and sleep
F. Referral to sex therapist, counseling	F. Provides needed support to overcome concerns and gain information needed to improve sexual function

NURSING DIAGNOSES

Sensory/perceptual alterations (visual, auditory) related to neurological deficit resulting from cranial nerve involvement causing hearing deterioration (high-frequency deficit), eye irritation, and uremic amaurosis (possible sudden temporary blindness)

Altered thought processes related to physiological factor of CNS involvement resulting from high level of nitrogenous wastes causing inaccurate interpretation of the environment or inappropriate thinking abilities

EXPECTED OUTCOMES

Optimal neurological function evidenced by management or control of sensory and mental changes resulting from renal functional deterioration, orientation to time, place, person, event

INTERVENTION	RATIONALE
I. Assess for: A. Attention span, confusion, impaired memory, judgment, reasoning, concentration, ability to identify specific areas of deficit, irritability	A. Provides information about mental state
B. Hearing threshold level, irritated appearance of eyes	B. Results of cranial nerve involvement, calcium deposits in the eyes
IV. Perform/provide: A. Interaction for brief periods and allow time for responses, speak slowly and clearly, and use name	A. Provides stimulation and reality orientation
B. Place calendar, radio, TV, newspaper, and encourage visitors	B. Provides stimulation and reminders in the environment
C. Maintain a structured routine as much as possible	C. Allows for successful thinking when knows what to expect
D. Include family members to assist in planning, problem-solving with patient	D. Provides support and interest by significant others

NURSING DIAGNOSES

Knowledge deficit related to information regarding the disease and life-style changes, treatment regimens (fluids/dietary/activities/dialysis), measures to prevent complications, medical monitoring of disease

Anticipatory grieving related to loss of physiopsychosocial well-being, loss of renal function, independence, roles, and potential for premature death

EXPECTED OUTCOMES

Adequate knowledge of ongoing regimens evidenced by compliance with preventive information, absence of infections, verbalization of signs and symptoms to report and adaptation to life-style that support optimal wellness, ability to express grief and initiate grieving process

INTERVENTION	RATIONALE
I. Assess for:	
A. Readiness, willingness, and motivation to learn, discharge care, and life-style changes	A. Learning can best take place if client is receptive and compliance is more likely to occur
B. Health practices, health beliefs, ethnic identity, value orientations, family interactions and cooperation	B. Factors to incorporate into teaching to facilitate learning and compliance with long-term care
C. Expression of anger, withdrawal and denial, inability to concentrate, insomnia, sadness, hostility	C. Initial stage of grieving
D. Home for kitchen, bathroom, and bedroom provisions needed for peritoneal dialysis if applicable	D. Provides information about safety precautions and sanitary practices

INTERVENTION	RATIONALE
IV. Perform/provide:	
A. Acknowledgment of perceptions with a nonjudgmental attitude	A. Establishes nurse–patient relationship in an accepting manner
B. Explanations that are clear, accurate in understandable terms, small amount of information over time	B. Prevents erroneous information, allows for patience, time, and understanding of new procedures to learn for regulation of the disease
C. Environment conducive to learning with space, lighting, and proper equipment and supplies	C. Distractions or discomfort will interfere with learning
D. As much control over lifestyle change decisions as possible, including family in discharge planning	D. Allows power to be given or retained by patient
E. Teaching aids (pamphlets, videotapes, pictures, written instructions)	E. Reinforces learning
F. Demonstration of procedures and time for return demonstration and practices with encouragement	F. Hands-on experience enhances and reinforces learning

INTERVENTION	RATIONALE
V. Teach patient/family:	
A. Pathophysiology of the disease, changes in the systems, risks for deterioration of renal function, the chronic, progressive nature of the disease, prognosis and control of symptoms with treatment, effect on life-style	A. Promotes understanding of disease and risk factors for complications and progressive failure of renal function
B. Explain grieving process, and allow to express feelings in an accepting environment	B. Facilitates grieving process
C. Reasons for fluid and food restrictions, amounts allowed each day and how to divide over 24-hour period	C. Information increases compliance
D. Foods and fluids to allow and restrict, list of these and sample menus that include complete proteins (fish, poultry, meats) and carbohydrates (jellies, marshmallows, sugar, candies)	D. Promotes adequate intake without adverse effects on kidney function, encourages inclusion of all amino acids and concentrated carbohydrates
E. How to measure and record I&O on a daily basis, weight q2days	E. Provides information regarding fluid balance
F. How to take BP, allow to return demonstration and practice	F. Monitors BP for increases indicating progressive renal failure

INTERVENTION	RATIONALE
G. Administration of medications including amount, time, frequency, side effects, how to take and expected results, signs, and symptoms to report	G. Ensures compliance with optimal effect with safe administration
H. How to plan to limit, modify, or increase activity according to level of tolerance and realistic goals	H. Allows for control while achieving progress and avoiding fatigue
I. Inform that mental and sensory changes subside with treatment	I. Changes are caused by accumulation of toxic substances that kidneys are unable to excrete
J. Report changes in breathing, nausea, temperature, sputum, urinary output, edema, change in urine characteristics, other persistent complaints	J. Indicates possible infection and other fluid balance complications
K. Report skin changes or breaks, color or integrity, mouth soreness	K. Predisposes or indicates presence of infection
L. Report muscle cramps, tremors, weakness, vomiting, lethargy, confusion, diarrhea	L. Signs and symptoms of electrolyte imbalance
M. Avoid exposure to those with infections and smoking, review other measures to prevent infection	M. Prevents transmission of pathogens to patients

INTERVENTION	RATIONALE
N. Community resources such as economic, social, psychological counseling, American Kidney Association	N. Provides information, support, and supplies
O. Remind to keep appointments with physician as scheduled	O. Provides monitoring of disease and treatments

nephrectomy/nephrostomy

DEFINITION

Nephrectomy is the surgical removal of a kidney to treat malignancy, polycystic kidney, and extensive trauma to the organ. It can also be removed from a donor for transplantation into a donee. The procedure can range from removal of a kidney and upper portion of the ureter to radical surgery that includes the kidney, adrenal gland, and retroperineal lymphatics depending on the underlying disorder. The procedure can be preceded by radiation therapy to reduce the size of a tumor and is usually followed by radiation and chemotherapy. Nephrostomy is the surgical incision into the kidney to remove calculi (lithotomy) or tube insertion for drainage of the kidney in hydronephrosis. This plan involves the care of these procedures and can be used in association with NEOPLASM, RENAL/URINARY CALCULI, PREOPERATIVE CARE and POSTOPERATIVE CARE plans

NURSING DIAGNOSES

Risk for impaired skin integrity related to external factor of excretions (urine) resulting from wound drainage tubes (nephrostomy) postoperatively

Risk for infection related to inadequate primary defenses of surgical incision to drain kidney and invasive procedure of urinary catheterization

EXPECTED OUTCOMES

Skin intact and free from excoriation at incisional site, and urinary drainage and output clear and odorless evidenced by absence of redness, irritation, and breaks at drainage site around nephrostomy tube and swelling, pain, and exudate at incisional site, absence of dysuria, cloudy, foul-smelling urine

INTERVENTION	RATIONALE
I. Assess for:	
A. Irritation, excoriation, or redness at drainage site or incisional site	A. Constant leakage of drainage around tube irritates the skin
B. Urinary drainage on dressings and frequency of changes	B. Wet, soiled dressings are irritating to skin and wound
C. Nephrostomy tube and urinary catheter for patency, presence of kinks or dislodgement	C. Prevents backup or stasis of urine in kidney pelvis or urinary bladder
D. Urine and drainage characteristics (cloudiness, foul odor)	D. Signs of infection
II. Monitor, describe, record:	
A. I&O q1–4h to include nephrostomy drainage in output total	A. Dressings saturated with urine drainage are weighed and output considered
B. WBC, urine and wound culture	B. Increased WBC and positive urine or wound cultures indicate infection and identifies the microorganism
III. Administer:	
A. Antibiotic IV, PO	A. Acts to prevent or treat infection by inhibiting cell wall synthesis
B. Fluid IV	B. Ensures excretion of waste products via urine preoperatively and replaces excessive fluid losses postoperatively

IV. Perform/provide:

A. Change dressings PRN using sterile technique, cleanse and redress incisional site	A. Initially the dressings are saturated with urine, and then drainage is gradually reduced
B. Careful handling of nephrostomy tube and catheter, tape securely to flank and position to prevent kinking or obstruction to flow	B. Tube can become dislodged or flow obstructed, secure tubing ensures that fear of dislodging tube during deep breathing or movement is reduced
C. Nephrostomy tube clamping and eventual removal	C. Preparation for removal of tube if urinary flow via normal route is reinstituted
D. Fluid intake to 2 to 3 L/day if allowed	D. Promotes urine output, dilutes urine, prevents urinary stasis and infection

NURSING DIAGNOSES
Knowledge deficit related to general preoperative care information, follow-up care, including wound care, medications, health of remaining kidney, measures to treat underlying condition leading to renal complications

Dysfunctional grieving related to actual loss of body part (kidney) resulting in expression of distress, sadness, and denial

EXPECTED OUTCOMES
Adequate information and teaching about follow-up care for renal surgery and initial resolution of grief evidenced by verbalization and performance of care required to protect remaining kidney (activity/fluid/diet/medications), and expression of feelings about loss and beginning interest and participation in care

INTERVENTION	RATIONALE
V. Teach patient/family:	
A. Stages of grieving and assist to identify and adapt to grief and responses to expect	A. Facilitates resolution of grief resulting in acceptance of loss
B. Dressing change and wound protection during bathing	B. Maintains clean dry wound
C. Measures to prevent urinary infection or renal calculi as follows: a. Fluid intake of 2 to 3 L/day b. Acid-ash diet c. Void when urge is felt d. Wipe from front to back and maintain clean perineum	C. Ensures appropriate follow-up care to prevent complications
D. Medication administration to include dose, frequency, time, how to take drug(s), condition being treated, expected effects, side effects, and what to do if they occur	D. Protects remaining kidney by treating underlying condition
E. Avoid excessive exercises or lifting heavy objects, contact sports, or any trauma to the remaining kidney, plan for rest periods during convalescence	E. Activity restrictions following surgery to allow for healing and prevent trauma

INTERVENTION	RATIONALE
F. Report any redness, swelling, or pain at wound site, change in urinary pattern, output, characteristics, weight gain, flank pain, temperature	F. Signs and symptoms of possible infection or calculi/pathology in remaining kidney
G. Inform of planned chemotherapy or radiation therapy	G. Postoperative therapy for renal malignancy
H. Suggest counseling if appropriate	H. Provides support for grief resolution

renal/urinary tract calculi/litholapaxy

DEFINITION

Calculi are stones of varied sizes formed in the kidney (nephrolithiasis) or in the urinary bladder (urolithiasis). They are formed from insoluble substances that are normally excreted by the kidneys and remain there or lodge in the ureters as they move down into and remain in the urinary bladder. The types of stones include calcium, struvite, uric acid, and cystine. Their development can be associated with infection/inflammation, urinary pH, urinary stasis, hypercalciuria, hypercalcemia, some medications, and genetic factors. Risk factors include immobility, neurogenic bladder, dehydration, and the long-term use of an indwelling catheter. Litholapaxy is a procedure performed to remove calculi from the bladder via a cystoscope by crushing the stone and irrigating the bladder to wash out the fragments. A cystolithotomy can also be performed via a superpubic surgical incision into the bladder to remove the stones. Another procedure to remove calculi is percutaneous lithotripsy in which tubes are inserted into a small incision at the site, a contrast medium injected, and forceps used to remove the stones. If a procedure to remove the calculi is performed, this plan can be used with NEPHRECTOMY/NEPHROSTOMY, PREOPERATIVE CARE, and POSTOPERATIVE CARE plans.

NURSING DIAGNOSIS

Pain related to physical injury agents of pressure of calculi or obstruction from calculi lodged in the tract resulting in inflammation/irritation and/or obstruction of urine flow

EXPECTED OUTCOMES

Pain reduced or controlled evidenced by decrease in request of analgesic, absence of restlessness, moaning, anxiety

INTERVENTION	RATIONALE
I. Assess for:	
A. Pain severity and characteristics, sharp, dull, or aching, colic type, duration and if constant or intermittent, factors that aggravate or relieve pain	A. Source of pain can be ureteral or renal and radiate downward to the thigh and genitalia (ureteral) or from the lumbar region to the testicle/bladder (renal), characteristics depend on the site, size, and movement of the calculi
B. Nausea, vomiting, diaphoresis, urinary frequency	B. Symptoms associated with severe pain
C. Restlessness, grimacing, crying, moaning	C. Nonverbal expressions of pain
II. Monitor, describe, record:	
A. Abdominal flat plate x ray (KUB)	A. Reveals presence of calculi, and obstruction responsible for pain
B. VS q2–4h	B. Responses to severe pain
III. Administer:	
A. Analgesic (narcotic) IM	A. Acts to control pain before becoming severe and control gate closing
B. Antispasmodic PO	B. Acts to relax muscle spasms caused by calculi and reduce pain
IV. Perform/provide:	
A. Evaluation of effect of analgesic 30 minutes, $1\frac{1}{2}$, and 3 hours after administration	A. Determines response and need to repeat, increase, or change medication if pain is extremely severe

INTERVENTION	RATIONALE
B. Moist heat to flank area PRN	B. Relieves pain by vasodilation to increase circulation to the site
C. Remain until severe pain subsides, maintain calm attitude	C. Provides support and reassurance to decrease anxiety that increases pain
D. Encourage and assist in activities according to ability and pain episodes (10 minutes, q2h), and schedule ambulation 30 minutes following analgesic or between attacks of pain	D. Provides activity at optimal times to prevent or reduce pain while encouraging passage of the stone
E. Positive remarks regarding the effectiveness of pain relief measures	E. Confidence expressed by staff improves effect of medication
F. Quiet environment with opportunity for relaxation/breathing techniques, guided imagery	F. Reduces stimuli and pain perception, provides distraction

NURSING DIAGNOSES

Altered urinary elimination related to mechanical trauma resulting from calculi in the tract, irritation and obstruction causing hematuria, retention preoperatively

Risk for fluid volume deficit related to altered intake, losses through normal routes (vomiting, hemorrhage) postoperatively

EXPECTED OUTCOMES

Optimal fluid intake and output evidenced by resumption of normal urinary flow and characteristics following stone passage or removal, fluid intake increased with I&O balanced and absence of excessive losses postoperatively

INTERVENTION	RATIONALE
I. Assess for:	
A. Pattern of urinary elimination including amount, frequency, urgency, dysuria, incontinence, retention, odor, color, sedimentation, blood, pus, mucus	A. Provides data to identify abnormal variations and/or constituents
B. Bladder distention by palpation, flank pain radiating downward	B. Indicates obstruction affecting the urinary flow
C. NPO status, vomiting preoperatively	C. Affects fluid intake and loss that can affect fluid balance
D. Nausea, emesis, dry hot skin, poor skin turgor, dry mucous membranes, thirst, lethargy, weight loss (5%), possible temperature elevation	D. Identifies postoperative causes of fluid loss leading to dehydration
II. Monitor, describe, record:	
A. I&O q4–8h preoperatively, q1–2h postoperatively, include urinary drainage from catheter/nephrostomy or other tubes	A. Determines fluid balance and need for fluid/electrolyte replacement, fluid intake should equal urinary output plus 800 mL
B. Urinalysis (RBC, WBC, pH, Sp.Gr.), electrolytes	B. Presence of RBC, WBC indicates irritation of mucosa by calculi, K decreases indicate depletion with fluid loss
C. Urinalysis, 24-hour specimen	C. Reveals output of crystals in urine predisposing to calculi

INTERVENTION	RATIONALE
D. KUB, IVP, retrograde pyelography	D. Reveals calculi (calcium and cystine) and obstruction if present
III. Administer:	
A. Anti-emetic IM	A. Acts to reduce nausea and vomiting by blocking chemoreceptor acting on vomiting center
B. Fluids, electrolytes IV	B. Replacement therapy if fluids lost pre- or postoperatively
C. Antibiotic PO	C. Acts to prevent or treat urinary tract infection
IV. Perform/provide:	
A. Environment free from odors, quiet and restful, avoid stressful situations	A. Reduces stimulation of vomiting center
B. Straining of all urine through layers of gauze, advise not to discard urine without pouring through the strainer provided	B. Determines if stones have been passed
C. Urinary catheterization or assist with ureteral catheter placement	C. Relieves distention caused by retention or obstruction
D. Fluid intake of 3 to 4 L/day if permitted, one glass/hour throughout the day and two glasses at bedtime and if awake at night	D. Ensures urinary output of 2 to 3 L/day (30 mL/hr or 200 to 400 mL/voiding) to remove concentrates and prevent urinary stasis

INTERVENTION	RATIONALE
E. Clear liquid, bland, soft foods, dry foods if nauseated, allow time, advise to eat and drink slowly, and offer small feedings six times/day	E. Progressive diet as tolerated to prevent fullness and nausea

NURSING DIAGNOSIS
Knowledge deficit related to follow-up care, including fluid, nutritional, medication requirements to prevent recurrence

EXPECTED OUTCOMES
Adequate knowledge and understanding of preventive care evidenced by compliance with daily fluid intake, nutritional inclusions and restrictions, and medication regimen

INTERVENTION	RATIONALE
V. Teach patient/family:	
A. Prepare a schedule to drink fluids q1h and void q2h, increase if ill with diarrhea, vomiting, temperature	A. Dilutes urine and encourages flow with an intake of 2 to 3 L/day
B. Continue straining urine and report any noted	B. Assists to recognize passage of stones
C. Dietary changes as follows:	C. Dietary inclusions and restrictions vary with type of stones
a. Avoid tea, coffee, colas, beer, chocolate, citrus fruits, peanuts, beans, cabbage, apples, others	a. Advised for those with oxalate stones
b. Avoid cheeses, organ meats, wine (low-purine diet)	b. Advised for those with uric acid stones

INTERVENTION	RATIONALE
c. Avoid milk and dairy products	c. Advised for those with calcium stones
D. Medications as follows:	D. Medication inclusion and restriction vary with type of stones
a. Avoid calcium-containing antacids, phosphates, diuretics, allopurinol	a. Advised for those with calcium stones
b. Allopurinol, magnesium oxide, cholestyramine, pyridoxine	b. Advised to prevent oxalate and uric acid stones
c. Citrate, sodium bicarbonate	c. Advised to alkanize urine and prevent uric acid stones
d. Ammonium salts, methionine	d. Advised to acidify urine to prevent calcium and struvite stones
E. Report pain, changes in urinary pattern, hematuria	E. Allows for early intervention in recurrence of calculi

renal/urinary tract infections
(cystitis/glomerulonephritis/pyelonephritis)

DEFINITION

Urinary tract infection (UTI) includes cystitis (bladder and urethra), pyelonephritis (renal pelvis, interstitial tissue, renal tubules), and glomerulonephritis (renal glomeruli, tubular, interstitial, and vascular areas). Most common site of infection is the urinary bladder usually caused by *Escherichia coli, Pseudomonas, Enterobacter,* and *Candida.* The highest risk for the condition is in women because of the close proximity of a short urethra to the anus, and of the hormonal changes associated with pregnancy and aging. Catheterization and an indwelling catheter are the other major causes of urinary tract infection. Pyelonephritis is often the extension of bladder infection via the ureter or occurs as a result of calculi, hydronephrosis, or trauma and can be an acute or chronic condition. Those with chronic calculi and cystitis, as well as diabetes are at risk for this condition. Glomerulonephritis, considered to be an immunologic disorder, most often follows (within 2–3 weeks) a bacterial or viral infection in other parts of the body (infectious glomerulonephritis). Other conditions, infectious and systemic, also can cause this disease. This plan includes the care associated with infections of the kidneys or urinary bladder.

NURSING DIAGNOSES

Pain related to physical injuring agents of bacterial invasion of areas of the renal/urinary organs resulting in inflammation/infection, damage to renal function

Hyperthermia related to illness (infectious process) resulting in discomfort and risk for fluid imbalance

EXPECTED OUTCOMES

Pain and hyperthermia reduced or controlled evidenced by verbalization that pain relieved during urination, rest, or activity and reduced requests for analgesic, VS, and temperature within baseline levels

INTERVENTION	RATIONALE
I. Assess for:	
A. Low back or suprapubic pain, malaise, dysuria	A. Indicates urinary bladder infection caused by irritation to the bladder wall and urethral mucosa
B. Pain in the abdomen or flank area (unilateral or bilateral), radiating pain down a ureter, headache, nausea, vomiting, generalized edema	B. Indicates infection of the kidney(s)
C. Urine for cloudiness, foul odor, hematuria	C. Indicates infection in the tract
D. Temperature for persistent low-grade elevation, sudden onset of a high fever, chills, diaphoresis	D. Indicates infection in the tract
II. Monitor, describe, record:	
A. VS and temperature q4h	A. Determines increases caused by infectious process
B. I&O q4–8h with attention to output of <250 mL/8 hours	B. Correlates fluids to determine imbalance
C. Urine culture, urinalysis	C. Bacterial count of >100,000/mL in culture results indicate infection, RBC, WBC, increased pH indicate infection, RBC, casts, proteinuria, increased Sp. Gr., decreased pH indicate glomerulonephritis

INTERVENTION	RATIONALE
III. Administer: A. Antipyretic PO	A. Acts to reduce temperature by inhibiting heat-regulating center
B. Antimicrobial PO	B. Acts to inhibit cell wall synthesis or interfere with biosynthesis of proteins to eliminate infection depending on medication administered
C. Analgesic, and evaluate effect 30 minutes, $1\frac{1}{2}$, and 3 hours to determine response, urinary analgesic for pain caused by irritation, antispasmodic for bladder muscle spasms	C. Controls pain and need to repeat before pain becomes severe in renal pain
IV. Perform/provide: A. Warm sitz bath or heat to perineum three times/day	A. Promotes comfort in presence of dysuria
B. Blankets, additional warmth if needed	B. Allays chilling and increases comfort
C. Fluids at least two to three L/day if allowed (cystitis, pyelonephritis)	C. Replaces fluid loss as result of temperature and diaphoresis
D. Quiet, restful environment, schedule activities around rest periods	D. Stimuli increases discomfort

NURSING DIAGNOSES

Altered urinary elimination related to trauma of infectious process

Risk for fluid volume deficit related to excessive losses through normal routes (diaphoresis, vomiting, diarrhea) resulting from temperature, responses to infectious process causing possible dehydration

Fluid excess related to compromised regulatory mechanism resulting from glomerular damage with reduction in glomerular filtration rate (GFR) causing increased fluid retention

EXPECTED OUTCOMES

Resumption of baseline urinary pattern and fluids in balance evidenced by absence of dysuria, urgency, frequency (cystitis and pyelonephritis), and signs and symptoms of dehydration with resolution of infection, fluid volume excess progressively resolved evidenced by absence of edema, oliguria, abnormal breath sounds, neck vein distention, and VS, I&O, and weight within baseline parameters

INTERVENTION	RATIONALE
I. Assess for:	
A. Dysuria, frequency, urgency, nocturia, foul odor, hematuria, pyuria, mucus	A. Indicates presence of infection that causes irritation of bladder, reveals by-products of bacterial action
B. Oliguria, edema, respiratory changes and crackles, neck vein distention, change in mentation, hematuria or smoky appearance, lethargy, increased BP and P	B. Indicates renal impairment, reduced GFR, damaged glomeruli causing fluid retention in body tissues as kidneys are unable to excrete urine and the fluid is returned to tissues via circulation
C. Skin for temperature, color, dryness or moistness, turgor, thirst	C. Indicates possible dehydration associated with fluid depletion resulting from losses associated with elevated temperature, vomiting

INTERVENTION	RATIONALE
II. Monitor, describe, record:	
A. I&O q1–4h as appropriate with attention to output below 30 mL/hr	A. Determines if imbalance is present and fluid lost or retained
B. BUN, creatinine	B. BUN of >25 mg/mL, creatinine of >1.5 mg/dL indicates renal impairment
C. Creatinine clearance, urinalysis	C. Decreased in renal impairment, urinalysis reveals hematuria, proteinuria and decreased pH
D. Cystoscopy, intravenous pyelogram (IVP), flat plate (KUB)	D. Reveals abnormalities of renal/urinary system that can lead to infection
E. VS q4h in presence of edema	E. BP increases and tachycardia associated with fluid overload potential
F. Weight daily or as appropriate on same scale, at same time, wearing same clothing	F. Monitors gains and losses to determine fluid retention or dehydration
III. Administer:	
A. Diuretic IV, PO	A. Acts on tubules, loop of Henle to facilitate excretion of urine and Na, Cl, and water
B. Potassium chloride IV, PO	B. Replaces K lost with diuretic therapy
C. Anti-inflammatory agent PO	C. Acts to support body defenses in glomerulonephritis

INTERVENTION	RATIONALE

IV. Perform/provide:

A. Fluid intake of 2 to 3 L/day for fluid deficit, limit fluid intake to 500 to 1000 mL/day, offer ice, popsicle for thirst

A. Achieves and maintains fluid balance if deficit or retention is present

B. Limit protein and Na intake

B. Adjusted to level of renal impairment (proteinuria), Na reduction to prevent fluid retention

C. Commode or close proximity to bathroom

C. Urgency can cause incontinence and embarrassment

NURSING DIAGNOSIS

Knowledge deficit related to follow-up care including fluid/dietary/medication regimen and measures to prevent infection recurrence, care/precautions (fluids, activity, nutrition, infection) needed to prevent complications depending on renal damage, signs and symptoms to report

EXPECTED OUTCOMES

Adequate information to control and/or prevent infections of the urinary/renal system and their complications or recurrence evidenced by compliance with self-administration of medications, restriction/promotion of fluid/diet/activity regimens, verbalization of signs and symptoms to report

INTERVENTION	RATIONALE

V. Teach patient/family:

A. Anatomy and physiology of the urinary/renal systems, pathology and effect on body systems

A. Information regarding the condition as a basis for rationale for treatment regimen enhance understanding

INTERVENTION	RATIONALE
B. Medication administration to include, dose, time, frequency, and side effects, special attention to antimicrobial therapy and their effects	B. Prevents errors in administration of drug(s) and possible complications if fluid intake is not adequate
C. Fluid intake of vitamin C, acid-ash diet that includes meats, eggs, cranberries, whole grains, cheese, avoid vegetables except legumes, and foods containing baking soda	C. Manages fluid/dietary regimen for urinary infection to acidify the urine
D. Increase fluid intake to 2 to 3 L/day or limit fluids to 1000 mL/day, offer a written schedule to follow	D. Ensures an adequate urinary output or prevents fluid retention
E. Low protein and Na, high-calorie diet, offer sample menus and list of foods to include and exclude	E. Allows the kidneys to rest by avoiding need for protein catabolism, prevents fluid retention with Na intake
F. Activity schedule adjusted to renal impairment, rest periods and diversional activities	F. Activity can be limited for weeks in glomerulonephritis as this can increase catabolic activity
G. Collection of clean-catch urine specimen, allow to demonstrate	G. Provides specimen for culture to determine bacterial count
H. Empty bladder completely and frequently (q4h), wear cotton underwear, and avoid tight-fitting pants	H. Prevents urinary stasis and medium for bacteria and irritation of genitalia

INTERVENTION	RATIONALE
I. Women to wipe from front to back, and wash genital and rectal areas after urination, defecation, intercourse	I. Prevents contamination from genitalia with passage of bacteria into the urethra
J. Report persistent or recurring symptoms, any change in temperature, weight loss or gain, fatigue, weakness, restlessness, edema, nausea, vomiting, as well as increased P, BP, changes in urinary pattern, amount, gross urine characteristics	J. Indicates that treatment is ineffective or infection has recurred
K. Maintain regular physician visits as scheduled	K. Monitors conditions and need to adjust therapy

urinary diversion/cystectomy
(continent vesicostomy/cutaneous ureterostomy/ileal conduit)

DEFINITION

Urinary diversion is a surgical procedure associated with the removal of the total urinary bladder performed to treat bladder malignancy. A segmental or partial cystectomy can also be performed if the prognosis is a more favorable one. The total cystectomy generally includes removal of the bladder and urethra in women and the bladder, urethra, seminal vesicles, and prostate in men. A more radical procedure includes removal of pelvic lymph nodes and reproductive organs. It can also be done to establish urinary drainage in those with spinal cord injury (neurogenic bladder), congenital anomalies (meningomyelocele), obstructive conditions, severe and persistent cystitis with hemorrhage, or trauma of the lower tract preventing normal function. Types of diversion include a cutaneous ureterostomy in which the end(s) or a section of the ureter(s) are brought to the surface of the abdominal wall with one or two stomas, or a vesicostomy in which the end of the ureter is brought to the surface of the abdomen at the bladder site and formation of a stoma. Drainage of urine from these procedures can be accomplished by intermittent catheterization. Another procedure is the ileal conduit (most common procedure) in which a portion of the terminal ileum is brought to the skin surface and stoma formed with implantation of the ureters into this segment of the intestine. This allows the urine to flow into the conduit developed by the bowel with elimination by intestinal peristalsis and collection provided via an appliance and collecting system. This plan includes care of the urinary diversion procedure and can be used in association with SPINAL CORD INJURY, NEOPLASM, PREOPERATIVE CARE, and POSTOPERATIVE CARE plans

NURSING DIAGNOSES

Anxiety related to threat to or change in health status causing inability to manage feelings of uncertainty and apprehension regarding uncertain prognosis, disfigurement caused by the ostomy, and ability to manage permanent urinary diversion

Ineffective individual coping related to inability to cope with change in control of urinary elimination, change in appearance (body image), and future life-style changes

Body image disturbance related to biophysical factor of change in structure and function of body part (change in urinary pattern with urinary diversion), and change in appearance (permanent ostomy on surface of abdomen), embarrassment of ostomy presence, impotency affecting sexual function/pattern resulting from surgical diversion procedure

EXPECTED OUTCOMES

Anxiety and fear within manageable levels, development of coping and problem-solving skills, body image improved evidenced by verbalizations that anxiety is decreasing, fear reduced, participation in care activities and receptivity to planning for ongoing ostomy care, change in urinary elimination and sexual pattern, and management of chronic anxiety

INTERVENTION	RATIONALE
I. Assess for:	
A. Level of anxiety, use of coping mechanisms, stated fears of uncertainty of disease outcome, life-style changes	A. Anxiety can range from mild to severe and high level associated with urinary diversion, assists in identifying inappropriate use of coping skills
B. Restlessness, diaphoresis, complaining, joking, withdrawal, talkativeness, increased P and R	B. Nonverbal expressions of anxiety when not able to communicate feelings
C. Personal resources to cope with stress, anxiety, and interest in learning to problem-solve, use of defense mechanisms	C. Support systems and personal strengths assist to develop coping skills

INTERVENTION	RATIONALE
D. Feelings and response to change in appearance, permanent stoma, ability to carry out role and participate in care/social activities, fear of sexual inadequacy, sterility	D. Changes in body image and self-concept a common and serious problem with changes in structure and function of a body organ
E. Looking or touching stoma, hiding stoma, feeling or preoccupation with the change, negative expressions about changes in life-style	E. Responses to presence of stoma, negative or positive

III. Administer:

A. Anti-anxiety agent PO	A. Acts to reduce anxiety level and provides calming effect and rest, depresses subcortical levels of CNS, limbic system

IV. Perform/provide:

A. Environment conducive to rest, time to express fears and anxiety, avoid anxiety-producing situations	A. Decreases stimuli that cause stress/anxiety, venting of feelings decreases anxiety
B. Suggest new methods to enhance coping skills and problem solving, allow to externalize and identify those that help	B. Offers alternative coping strategies that allow for release of anxiety and fear
C. Positive feedback regarding progress made, focus on abilities rather than inabilities	C. Provides support for adaptive behavior, promotes self-worth and responsibility

INTERVENTION	RATIONALE
D. Avoid verbal or nonverbal reactions to stoma care or other procedures, display of distaste or alarm of surgical site	D. Promotes comfort with nurse–patient relationship
E. Privacy when dressings or appliance are changed, advise that feelings about the ostomy are normal	E. Reduces embarrassment caused by exposure of surgical procedure
F. Diversional activities such as relaxation exercises, TV, radio, music, reading, tapes, guided imagery, encourage to continue usual interests	F. Reduces anxiety and promotes comfort
G. Allow to participate in planning of care to maintain usual activities when possible, allow to participate in ostomy care as soon as possible	G. Allows for some control over situations
H. Support grieving for loss of life-style and restrictions in activities, changes in physical appearance and alternative urinary elimination	H. Provides assistance in adaptation to changes imposed by disease
I. Suggest visit from one who has had urinary diversion surgery and has made a successful recovery	I. Provides support and information from a reliable source

NURSING DIAGNOSES

Risk for infection related to inadequate primary defenses (surgical incision) resulting in wound infection, invasive procedures (wound tubes, intermittent catheterization) resulting in urinary tract infection

Risk for impaired skin integrity related to mechanical external factor of presence of collection appliance resulting in peristomal skin irritation, internal factor of secretions or wound drainage at wound site resulting in irritation and breakdown

EXPECTED OUTCOMES

Skin intact, healing, and free from breakdown at peristomal and wound site, urinary drainage in collecting system or via catheterization clear and odorless evidenced by absence of redness, irritation, excoriation at peristomal skin site, and swelling, pain, and exudate at incisional site, and absence of dysuria, cloudy, foul-smelling urine, temperature, culture, and WBC within normal levels

INTERVENTION	RATIONALE
I. Assess for:	
A. Irritation, excoriation, or redness at peristomal skin site, itching or burning under appliance, drainage from stoma	A. Constant changing of temporary pouch, prolonged use of more permanent appliances, or urine seepage around bag not properly applied can irritate skin
B. Drainage on dressings with redness and swelling at incisional site	B. Indicates wound infection
C. Color of stoma changing from pink or red to bluish or purple	C. Indicates poor blood supply to stoma
D. Position of collection pouch and tubing for patency, presence of kinks or dislodgement	D. Prevents backup or stasis of urine in conduit

INTERVENTION	RATIONALE
E. Urine and drainage characteristics (cloudiness, foul odor) from catheter, ureteral stents, or collection pouch	E. Signs of urinary infection
F. Patency of stoma, ureteral catheters, suprapubic catheter, presence bladder distention if partial cystectomy	F. Indicates possible obstruction of urine flow caused by edema, stenosis, or clogging of catheter with mucus
II. Monitor, describe, record: A. VS and temperature q4h	A. Temperature elevation indicates infection
B. I&O q1–4h to include ostomy drainage and intermittent amounts in output total, q2h following removal of stents if used	B. Provides a ratio to determine fluid imbalance, a decrease in output can indicate obstruction
C. WBC, urine and wound culture	C. Increased WBC of >10,000/mm^3 and positive urine or wound cultures indicate infection and identify the microorganism
D. Routine urinalysis	D. RBC, WBC, casts, hematuria indicates infection, pH for alkaline urine that irritates skin
III. Administer: A. Antibiotic PO, TOP	A. Acts to prevent or treat infection by inhibiting cell wall synthesis

INTERVENTION	RATIONALE
B. Antipyretic PO	B. Acts to reduce temperature

IV. Perform/provide:

A. Proper handwash prior to any care or contact	A. Prevents transmission of pathogens
B. Use sterile technique and all sterile equipment, supplies, and dressings for wound and stoma care	B. Prevents contamination by pathogens
C. Dressing change of q4–8h for 24 hours postoperatively or as needed if wet	C. Prevents contact of secretions with skin and promotes cleanliness, prevents infection
D. Fluid intake to 2 to 3 L/day if allowed	D. Promotes urine output, dilutes urine, prevents urinary stasis and infection
E. Empty pouch when $\frac{1}{3}$ full, place pouch and drainage collection bag below level of bladder or away from stoma	E. Prevents reflux of urine
F. Check for residual urine after catheter removed, if one is in place post-operatively	F. Identifies stasis of urine and potential for infection
G. Intermittent catheterization beginning when appropriate healing achieved	G. Prevents urinary stasis and potential for infection

INTERVENTION	RATIONALE
H. Cleanse peristomal area with mild soap and warm water, gently pat dry	H. Cleanses secretions or debris from peristomal skin
I. Apply light to stoma covered with light dressing q4h, avoid use of soap, skin barrier, adhesive if skin irritated	I. Treatment for peristomal irritation
J. Apply skin barrier or skin sealant and then adhesive material when changing appliance, perform patch test prior to application (United Skin Prep and Hollister Skin Gel as sealants, Karaya and Stomahesive as skin barriers), antibiotic powder or ointment if ordered to peristomal skin if yeast infection present	J. Protects skin from contact with irritating substances and possible allergic reaction
K. Use a two-piece appliance if possible, change only when needed or ordered	K. Allows for changing of pouch without removing the skin adhesive plate, changes are more frequent early in postoperative period

INTERVENTION	RATIONALE
L. Remove and apply appliance and pouch as follows:	L. Ensures proper use of urinary collection system
a. Change appliance before morning meal or at night q4–5 days or longer if more permanent type used	a. Ostomy less likely to be active
b. Measure stoma for proper fit of appliance (opening should not extend more than $\frac{1}{4}$ inch from stoma)	b. Ensures proper fit to prevent leakage around stoma
c. Gently remove appliance in direction of hair growth and any substances with solvent prior to washing	c. Prevents skin damage when cleansing and changing appliance
d. Cover stoma with tampon or tissue when changing appliance	d. Absorbs urine when changing appliance and prevents contact with peristomal skin
e. Fill in any irregular spaces around stoma with ostomy paste	e. Ensures seal to prevent leakage
f. Remove air pockets when applying pouch, empty q2–3h or when $\frac{1}{3}$ full	f. Prevents pull from skin due to heavy bag
g. Allow space of two fingers between skin and belt attached to appliance	g. Prevents pressure of belt or fasteners on belt to skin
M. Referral to enterostomal therapist if needed	M. Provides problem-solving assistance to prevent complications

NURSING DIAGNOSES

Knowledge deficit related to general postoperative care information, follow-up care including wound/ostomy procedures, intermittent self-catheterization, measures to prevent complications

EXPECTED OUTCOMES

Adequate information and teaching about follow-up care evidenced by performance of care required for proper ostomy function and prevention of complications associated with urinary diversion surgical procedure, expression of feelings about participation in care of ostomy

INTERVENTION	RATIONALE
V. Teach patient/family:	
A. Dressing change and wound/stoma protection during bathing	A. Maintains clean dry wound and stoma
B. Removal and application of appliance, pouch application and emptying, leg bag as appropriate with associated skin care, allow to demonstrate and practice	B. Ensures proper and safe care and use of ostomy supplies
C. Proper cleansing of pouches, use of deodorant tablets in pouch	C. Minimizes embarrassing odors from long-term use or reused pouch
D. Intermittent self-catheterization of vesicostomy q3–4h, care and preparation of catheters for future use	D. Ensures removal of urine at appropriate times from pouch created to hold urine
E. Inform that stoma size will reach permanent status by 4 months	E. Prevents anxiety caused by changes in stoma
F. Medication administration to include dose, frequency, time, how to take drug(s), condition being treated, expected effects, side effects, and what to do if they occur	F. Protects or treats infection or skin irritation

INTERVENTION	RATIONALE
G. Avoid excessive exercises or lifting heavy objects, contact sports, or any trauma to the abdomen, plan for rest periods during convalescence	G. Activity restrictions following surgery to allow for healing and prevent trauma
H. Fluid intake of 2 to 3 L/day spread over 24 hours to include acidic liquids and foods that form acid ash such as meat, poultry, fish, eggs, whole grains	H. Ensures adequate fluid intake to dilute urine, encourage output, and lower pH to prevent infection
I. Suggest wearing loose or full clothing, use pads to cover stoma	I. Covers appliance, prevents soiling of clothing and revealing presence of bag
J. Suggest alternative sexual activities, covering stoma during sexual activity, possibility of penile implant or sexuality counseling	J. Assistive aids can enhance sexual satisfaction
K. Report any redness, swelling, or pain at wound site, change in urinary pattern, output, characteristics, temperature elevation, stoma changes	K. Signs and symptoms of possible complications of urinary diversion
L. Inform of planned chemotherapy or radiation therapy if appropriate	L. Postoperative therapy for bladder malignancy
M. Suggest counseling if appropriate, community agencies such as American Cancer Society, Ostomy Club	M. Provides support and information

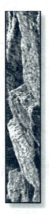

Neurological System Standards

neurological system data base

cerebrovascular accident

intracranial/spinal infections (brain abscess/encephalitis/meningitis)

intracranial trauma (contusion/laceration)

seizure disorders

spinal cord trauma

transient ischemic attack/carotid endarterectomy

neurological system data base

....

HISTORICAL DATA REVIEW
Past events:
1. Acute and/or chronic motor or sensory disease or disorders, presence of other disorders that affect the neurological system (trauma, diabetes, hypertension, anemia, infectious diseases, fluid and electrolyte imbalances, congenital disorders)
2. Chronic signs and symptoms related to neurological disorders (behavioral changes, syncope, vertigo, motor changes [weakness, tremor, mobility difficulty], seizures, changes in thought processes, sensory changes [pain, visual, auditory, tactile, olfactory, gustatory])
3. Neurological disease, hypertension, epilepsy, Alzheimer's or dementia or mental retardation of family members
4. Childhood diseases (measles, meningitis, poliomyelitis, neuromuscular disorders) and immunizations for influenza, poliomyelitis, measles
5. Anxiety, tobacco/alcohol/drug use, exposure to environmental toxic agents, sleep pattern, exercise routine
6. Treatments, rehabilitation associated with speech, mental, or neuromuscular deficits
7. Medications (prescription and over-the-counter) for neurological and other conditions, use of mind-altering drugs
8. Hospitalizations and feelings about care, surgery associated with or affecting the brain or spinal cord

Present events:
1. Medical diagnoses associated with or affecting organ structure or function of the neurological system
2. Motor deficits for gait, coordination, balance, paralysis, posture, muscle weakness/tone/spacticity/flaccidity, range of motion
3. Sensory deficits for numbness, paresthesia, visual, hearing or other sensory perceptual loss

4. Mental deficits for memory, consciousness, orientation, speech, concentration
5. Behavior for combativeness, aggression, agitation, lability, euphoria, depression
6. Activities of daily living and effect of neurological status on self-care, body image, self-esteem, and personal appearance

PHYSICAL ASSESSMENT DATA REVIEW

1. General appearance for affect, posture, personal care
2. Vital signs and temperature, pulse at carotid and temporal sites, nystagmus, pupil shape, position, size, and reaction to light
3. Bruits at carotid, eye, temporal, and mastoid sites
4. Symmetry, size, shape of head, neck, back; masses, depressions of head and muscles, shape, tone, atrophy of muscles palpated
5. Superficial reflexes for abdominal, plantar, corneal, anal, and gag; deep reflexes for biceps, triceps, patellar, and Achilles
6. Cranial nerves including 1 through 12; spinal nerves including cervical 4–8, thoracic 1–12, lumbar 1–5, and sacral 1–5

NURSING DIAGNOSES CONSIDERATIONS

1. Altered thought processes
2. Altered tissue perfusion (cerebral)
3. Body image disturbance
4. Bowel incontinence
5. Dysreflexia
6. Risk for disuse syndrome
7. Risk for infection
8. Risk for injury
9. Impaired physical mobility
10. Impaired verbal communication
11. Ineffective thermoregulation
12. Knowledge deficit
13. Reflex incontinence
14. Self-care deficits
15. Sensory/perceptual alterations
16. Sexual dysfunction
17. Sleep pattern disturbance
18. Total incontinence
19. Unilateral neglect

GERIATRIC CONSIDERATIONS

Nervous system changes in geriatric patients depend on the integrative abilities associated with the aging process. These changes vary with individuals and the degree of deficit experienced results from the amount and rapidity of functional and structural alterations in the nervous and other systems. There is a decline in sensory/motor flexibility but intellectual, communicative, and comprehension abilities are usually maintained. Changes in circulation affect oxygen supply to the brain and can cause mentation, sensory perception, and movement deficits. Neurological changes associated with aging that should be considered when assessing the geriatric patient include:

1. Decreased weight of brain resulting in reduced number of neurons, atrophy of convolutions and widening of sulci and gyri, ventricle dilatation
2. Increased accumulation of lipofuscin pigment resulting in abnormal position of cell nuclei, senile plaque, or lesion development
3. Decreased oxygen consumption resulting in reduced glucose utilization and intracellular energy; changes in circulation and blood flow to the brain that affect mental acuity, movement, sensory perception, and capacity to cope with events
4. Decreased neurons resulting in reduced strength of transmission from the brain to body areas and change in threshold for arousal of organ/system; decreased dendrites in nerve, synapses, lesions on axons resulting in reduced peripheral nerve conduction and slowed reaction time
5. Decreased norephinephrine, increased serotonin and monoamine oxidase resulting in neurotransmitter functional change and depression; decreased dopamine resulting in Parkinson's disease
6. Synaptic metabolic changes resulting in sleep disturbance, temperature control, and depression; extrapyramidal changes resulting in reduced movement and blinking, and changes in affect
7. Decreased deep-reflex intensity in arms, absence of ankle reflexes, plantar reflex absence with foot problems
8. Increased recovery time of autonomic nervous system resulting in increased time in returning to baselines following stimulation with anxiety following overstimulation
9. Electroencephalography (EEG) changes of one cycle lower than in other adult stages
10. Changes in stages in sleep such as longer time spent in stages I and II, reduced or eliminated stage IV resulting in need for more time to

fall asleep, frequent wakenings, decreased intensity of sleep, feeling of fatigue or not getting enough sleep and tension; reduced REM resulting in less dreaming, irritability, lethargy; increased napping, sleep apnea, and insomnia

DIAGNOSTIC LABORATORY TESTS AND PROCEDURES

1. X-ray of skull and spinal column, computerized tomography (CT), magnetic resonance imaging (MRI), positron emission tomography (PET), single photon-emission computerized tomography (SPECT), ultrasonography, Doppler scan (carotid), evoked potential tests (EP), electroencephalography (EEG), myelography, electromyography (EMG), perfusion tests, vestibular tests, cortical function tests, angiography, lumbar puncture and cerebrospinal fluid (CSF) cytology/culture, muscle biopsy
2. Complete blood count (CBC), electrolyte panel, drug level and toxicity tests, tissue culture of blood, skin, wound, or bone marrow

MEDICATIONS

1. Analgesics: aspirin, acetaminophen, codeine sulfate, indomethacin
2. Anti-anxiety agents: diazepam, oxazepam
3. Anticoagulants/antiplatelets: warfarin, heparin, aspirin, dipyridamole
4. Anticonvulsants: phenytoin, valproic acid, phenobarbital, carbamazepine
5. Antidepressants: amitriptyline hydrochloride, noriptyline hydrochloride, fluoxetine hydrochloride, nortriptyline hydrochloride
6. Antihypertensives: see Cardiovascular System Data Base (Medications)
7. Antimicrobials: acyclovir, amphotericin B, penicillins, tetracyclines, erythromycin, cephalosporins, chloramphenicol
8. Antiparkinson's agents: levodopa with carbidopa, amantadine hydrochloride, benztropine mesylate, procyclidine hydrochloride, bromocriptine mesylate, selegiline hydrochloride
9. Antipsychotics: halperidol, thiothixine, chlorpromazine
10. Cholinergic-acetylcholinesterases: neostigmine bromide, pyridostigmine bromide
11. Corticosteroids: dexamethasone, prednisone
12. Diuretics: furosemide (loop), mannitol (osmotic), chlorothiazide (thiazide)

cerebrovascular accident

DEFINITION

A cerebrovascular accident (CVA), also known as a stroke, is the interruption in the blood supply to a localized portion of the brain. It can result when cerebral blood vessels are narrowed or occluded (ischemic type) caused by thrombosis associated with atherosclerosis, or embolism associated with tumor, fat, blood clot, or bacteria. It can also result when atherosclerotic and hypertensive cerebral vessels rupture causing bleeding into the tissues (hemorrhagic type). Less common causes are spasm of cerebral arteries or compression of cerebral vessels resulting from disorders of the brain. Risk factors include age, obesity, smoking, stress, and presence of atherosclerosis, diabetes, heart disease, hypertension, transient ischemic attacks, and a family history of CVA. This plan includes care specific to this condition and can be used in association with the HYPERTENSION and TRANSIENT ISCHEMIC ATTACKS/CAROTID ENDARTERECTOMY care plans

NURSING DIAGNOSES

Ineffective individual coping related to situational crises of risk for or actual disabilities and psychophysiological changes (sensory, motor, and communication), and inability to manage stress, cope with change in appearance and future life-style changes caused by illness (possible transfer to long-term facility and/or rehabilitation)

Self-esteem disturbance related to neurological damage/deficits causing a loss in function and capabilities and feelings of helplessness, depression

Body image disturbance related to biophysical, psychosocial, and cognitive-perceptual factors causing changes in physical/mental/sensory/motor functions

EXPECTED OUTCOMES

Progressive acknowledgment and adaptation to changes in body functions and ability to cope evidenced by verbalizing positive statements about body changes and feeling less helpless and hopeless, development and utilization of coping skills, personal aids and assistance, return of interest in appearance and social participation

INTERVENTION	RATIONALE
I. Assess for: A. Use of coping mechanisms, stated fears of uncertainty of disease outcome, lifestyle changes, reactions to loss of motion, speech, vision, sensation	A. Assist to identify inappropriate use of coping skills, feelings of grief over losses associated with stroke
B. Negative expressions about body appearance, feelings of helplessness and uselessness, withdrawal behavior	B. Indicates difficulty in coping and decrease in self-esteem and body image
C. Personal resources to cope with stress of illness, and interest in learning to problem-solve	C. Support systems and personal strengths assist to develop coping skills
D. Feelings about inability to carry out role, participate in activities and need to modify life-style	D. Decline in self-esteem common in those left with neurological deficits
IV. Perform/provide: A. Environment conducive to rest, expression of fears and concerns, avoid anxiety-producing situations	A. Decreases stimuli that cause stress, venting of feelings assists to cope with changes and reduces anxiety

INTERVENTION	RATIONALE
B. Listen and clarify perceptions and information given, correct misconceptions, and assist to understand condition	B. Promotes successful resolution of crisis and establishes positive coping mechanisms
C. Allow time to verbalize feelings of denial, anger, or resentment, comments about appearance and possible loss of abilities in a nonjudgmental environment	C. Promotes temporary use of defense mechanisms to assist in reducing negative feelings
D. Discuss strengths and abilities with honesty, discuss realistic expectations of what can be accomplished with specialized therapy	D. Promotes self-esteem and develops trust in the nurse–patient relationship
E. Suggest new methods to enhance coping skills and problem solving, allow to externalize and identify those that help	E. Offers alternative coping strategies that allow for release of anxiety and promote hope for optimal outcome
F. Encouragement and positive feedback regarding progress made, focus on abilities rather than disabilities	F. Provides support for adaptive behavior, promotes self-worth and responsibility for independence
G. Allow to participate in planning of care and to maintain usual routine activities when possible	G. Allows for some control over situations
H. Support grieving for loss of life-style and restrictions in activities, changes in physical appearance	H. Provides assistance in adaptation to changes imposed by condition

INTERVENTION	RATIONALE
I. Explain that inappropriate behavioral responses are caused by the brain damage and usually improve with time and physical care	I. Prevents feelings of guilt and shame regarding feelings and behaviors that are unfamiliar to the patient
J. Include family in information regarding condition and support participation in care when possible	J. Provides opportunity for involvement and understanding of care

NURSING DIAGNOSES

Altered cerebral tissue perfusion related to interruption of arterial or venous flow resulting from obstruction or rupture of vessels in an area of the brain causing possible increase in intracranial pressure (ICP) and neurological deficits

Altered thought processes related to physiological change resulting from reduced cerebral blood flow causing impaired sensations and inaccurate interpretation of the environment

Pain related to biologic and physical factors of pressure or irritation to pain-sensitive areas resulting from hemorrhagic stroke, cerebral infarction, or carotid artery occlusive stroke

EXPECTED OUTCOMES

Pain controlled or relieved and progressive improvement in tissue perfusion and mental function evidenced by absence of increased ICP, stability of Glasgow Coma Scale, decreasing signs and symptoms of motor/sensory/mental dysfunction, and ability to cooperative and participate in activities

INTERVENTION	RATIONALE
I. Assess for: 　A. Headache, onset and severity, site such as frontal, temporal, neck or occipital areas	A. Results from pressure on cerebral structures with severity depending on whether ischemic or hemorrhagic CVA

INTERVENTION	RATIONALE
B. Level of consciousness, dizziness, visual and pupillary changes, perceptual deficits, aphasia or speech impairment, motor deficit such as paralysis, parasthesia, restlessness, delirium, lethargy, reflex activity	B. Neurological manifestations of reduced cerebral perfusion or increased intracranial pressure (ICP) caused by hemorrhage or hematoma (see specific nursing diagnosis for sensory/motor or other deficits)
C. Respiratory hyperventilation, bounding and slow pulse, increased BP, vomiting, seizures, agitation, confusion, lethargy	C. Signs and symptoms of increasing ICP or intracranial hypertension resulting from brain tissue compression or cerebral ischemia
II. Monitor, described, record: A. Glasgow Coma Scale	A. Provides measurement of level of consciousness, pupil reaction and motor activity to determine deficits, stability, or improvement
B. VS q2–4h or as appropriate	B. Indicates rise in ICP, possible rise in BP
C. Cerebral angiography	C. Identifies arterial obstruction or hemorrhagic causes of CVA and areas of the brain involved
D. Brain scan, computed tomography (CT) scan	D. Identifies hematoma, infarct, or arteriovenous malformation
E. CSF analysis	E. Bloody fluid indicates hemorrhage as the cause of CVA

INTERVENTION	RATIONALE
F. PT, PPT	F. Reveals blood coagulation that can lead to embolic CVA if time prolonged, also monitors anticoagulant therapy if given for adjustments if needed

III. Administer:

INTERVENTION	RATIONALE
A. Anticoagulant PO, IV, antiplatelet agent PO	A. Acts to prevent clot formation and improve cerebral perfusion
B. Hemostatic agent IV	B. Acts to prevent rebleeding after a clot has formed at the site
C. Osmotic diuretic IV	C. Acts to reduce cerebral edema that predisposes to ICP
D. Sedative PO, IV	D. Acts to control restlessness, anxiety, or delirium

IV. Perform/provide:

INTERVENTION	RATIONALE
A. Elevate head of bed to semi-Fowler's position if allowed, maintain head and neck in midline, and avoid turning or flexing the head	A. Promotes cerebral drainage to prevent ICP
B. Restrict fluid intake as ordered	B. Prevents ICP
C. Schedule care and activities to avoid excessive movement, anxiety, muscle tension, distended bladder or bowel impaction	C. Prevents increased BP and ICP

INTERVENTION	RATIONALE
D. Environment that is understanding and nonjudgmental as attempts are made to regain normalcy	D. Provides support and empathy for those experiencing behavior changes and promotes cooperation
E. Reorient as consciousness improves, especially if confused or aphasic or with memory loss	E. Prevents disorientation and regression
F. Place familiar articles within reach and view, face patient and speak slowly and clearly, repeat words when needed	F. Promotes return of memory, attention span and orientation
G. Gentle handling and use of safety measures such as soft toothbrush, electric razor, avoiding injections and sharp objects if possible	G. Prevents bleeding if anticoagulant therapy is administered
H. Prepare for surgical procedure if appropriate	H. Possible vessel ligation for bleeding, or removal of enlarging hematoma

NURSING DIAGNOSES

Altered nutrition: less than body requirements related to inability to ingest food resulting from anorexia, impaired chewing and swallowing (paralysis of tongue, one side of face), inability to feed self causing risk for aspiration and malnutrition

Risk for fluid volume deficit related to deviations affecting access to and intake of fluids resulting from physical immobility and impaired swallowing reflex (paralysis)

Risk for aspiration related to impaired swallowing, depressed gag reflex resulting from neuromuscular paralysis or deficits causing choking, coughing, and possible aspiration pneumonia

Feeding self-care deficit related to inability to use eating utensils to bring foods or fluids from dish or cup to mouth, resulting from upper extremity paralysis

EXPECTED OUTCOMES
Adequate oral fluid and nutritional intake, absence of aspiration evidenced by stable weight with dietary and fluid intake ingested for age, height, frame with absence of choking and coughing during meals as swallowing ability improves, and breath sounds and respiratory status within baseline parameters

INTERVENTION	RATIONALE
I. Assess for:	
A. Total daily amount of oral intake of food and fluid, anorexia, ability to feed self	A. Provides data about nutritional and fluid status and need for alternate route or assistance in oral feedings to avoid frustration caused by eating difficulties
B. Ability to swallow, cough, and clear airway, presence of gag reflex	B. Prevents choking or aspiration
C. Dyspnea, confusion, crackles on auscultation, elevated temperature	C. Indicates possible aspiration pneumonia
II. Monitor, describe, record:	
A. Weight daily or as needed at same time, on same scale, wearing same clothing	A. Reveals losses that can result from inadequate intake of food and fluid
B. I&O ratio q8h	B. Determines fluid balance and need for increased intake

INTERVENTION	RATIONALE
IV. Perform/provide:	
A. Quiet, clean environment during meals, allow time to eat, chew, and swallow slowly	A. Promotes appetite and prevents choking caused by rushing
B. Place in sitting or upright position in bed for meals or drinking and maintain position for 30 minutes after meal	B. Permits gravity flow of food and fluid to prevent aspiration
C. Support the head if voluntary control is limited by placing hand on forehead to maintain upright position	C. Prevents hyperextension that can lead to aspiration while eating
D. Feed slowly with small bites and sips placed into unaffected side of mouth, alternate solid and liquid intake	D. Allows to feel more in control of food and prevents food left in mouth on affected side
E. Touch lips with utensil, stroke under the chin, or apply pressure to the chin to open mouth or pressure above upper lip to close mouth	E. Assists to open and close mouth if patient is unable to do this without assistance
F. Foods and liquids that are thick in texture and will not stick to mouth and that are warm rather than hot or cold, allow to suck the food from the utensil or use straw	F. Easier to control and swallow without chewing or running out of the mouth, perception deficit can prevent identification of hot or cold

INTERVENTION	RATIONALE
G. Use of tongue blade to correct tongue protrusion and movement	G. Promotes tongue movement to enhance eating if partially paralyzed
H. Ice, popsicle prior to meals, fluids in sips q2h up to 1 to 2 L/day if allowed	H. Stimulates secretion of saliva and ensures appropriate fluid intake
I. If choking, allow to remove food without assistance unless breathing affected requiring suctioning	I. Prevents aspiration of food if choking
J. Check mouth after meals for food left on affected side, oral care following meals to remove all food	J. May not be aware of food and choke on remains
K. Assist to use one hand to eat and use assistive aids/utensils	K. Promotes self-feeding and independence
L. Arrange food and utensils on tray within view, avoiding side affected by hemianopsia, remove items that are not needed from tray	L. Prevents spilling and promotes self-feeding
M. Initiate tube feedings and care procedures if oral intake is not effective	M. Supplies nutritional intake and prevents aspiration
N. Secure nutritionist consult if advised	N. Assists in providing an adequate nutritional program

NURSING DIAGNOSES

Impaired physical mobility related to neuromuscular and perceptual or cognitive impairments resulting in paralysis and immobility and causing motor activity deficits, loss of muscle strength and mass, altered sexuality patterns

Risk for trauma related to internal factor of weakness, balancing difficulty, reduced muscle coordination, reduced sensory perceptions (visual, tactile) resulting in falls, burns, or other injury

Bathing/Hygiene, Dressing/Grooming self-care deficit related to impaired physical mobility (paralysis), unilateral neglect, and sensory/perceptual alterations (visual, tactile, kinesthetic) resulting from neurological deficit and narrowed perceptual fields

EXPECTED OUTCOMES

Progressive adequate physical activity evidenced by optimal mobility, transfer, ambulation with use of aids, absence of muscular atrophy, weakness, contractures, performance of ADL with improvement leading to independence in self-care, and no evidence of physical trauma during independent activities

INTERVENTION	RATIONALE
I. Assess for:	
A. Type and severity of mobility impairment, muscle flaccidity, spasticity, and coordination, reflexes, ability to walk, sit, move in bed, presence of paralysis including side or limbs affected	A. Provides data regarding mobility and ability to perform activities within limitations without injury or frustration
B. Sensory deficits affecting mobility such as visual, tactile perception	B. Affects ability to protect self from injury by falling, bumping, or burning extremities
C. Daily pattern and amount of assistance needed for ADL and aids that can promote independence	C. Allows for care with control over situations

INTERVENTION	RATIONALE
IV. Perform/provide:	
A. Change position and turn q2h primarily on unaffected side alternating with affected side and supine without pillow under knees, avoid flexion of thigh when in sidelying position, limit prone position for 15 minutes using pillow under pelvis, avoid pulling on any paralyzed limb, support flaccid extremities	A. Prevents deformities if paralysis present by relieving pressure on parts
B. Place a trochanter roll to thigh area, support the paralyzed leg when changing position, and place a pillow between the legs when lying on unaffected side	B. Prevents external hip rotation by preventing the femur from rolling, provides support and maintains correct position to prevent flexion
C. Sitting up for short periods with support in a chair and feet on floor, apply a footboard or tennis shoes to maintain feet at 90-degree angle	C. Avoids footdrop, limiting sitting prevents prolonged hip flexion
D. Passive ROM to all limbs and progress to assistive and then active ROM in all joints four times/day	D. Promotes circulation, muscle tone, joint flexibility, prevents contractures and weakness

INTERVENTION	RATIONALE
E. Alignment of hand in supination with fingers flexed using hand roll and splint if needed to prevent flexion, pillow at axilla to abduct arm in slight flexion, elevate affected arm to prevent edema	E. Maintains joint function of upper extremities
F. Exercises such as gluteal and quadriceps setting 5 times q1–2h and progress to 10 to 20 times	F. Prepares for ambulation by muscle strengthening
G. Encourage to sit up and get out of bed when allowed, assist to slowly rise to a sitting position while supporting the head and paralyzed or flaccid extremities	G. Assists to regain balance and begin ambulation with security and safety, can be achieved with physical rehabilitation program
H. Place in wheel chair or on commode using transfer techniques, progressing to standing and walking with support or use of leg brace	H. Assists to begin transferring from bed to perform other activities, can be achieved with physical rehabilitation when condition has stabilized
I. Use assistive devices as appropriate (cane, walker) for ambulation, clothing with velcro and zipper closures, suction cups on personal hygiene articles for brushing teeth, shaving, combing hair, clothing that is easily managed to dress and undress (loose with opening in front, elastic waist bands)	I. Provides safe support for mobility and other self-care activities to promote independence

INTERVENTION	RATIONALE
J. Align arm and support, apply an arm and hand sling when out of bed	J. Prevents shoulder subluxation
K. Bed in low position with side rails up, place articles within reach on unaffected side, clear pathways of clutter or spills, provide rails, bath mats, shower chair, other aids as needed; remind to walk slowly and not to hurry	K. Prevents falls and possible injury from bumping, slipping, stumbling
L. Reinforce and encourage all activities achieved with rehabilitation (physical and occupational)	L. Promotes return to optimal mobility and self-care activities

NURSING DIAGNOSES

Sensory/perceptual alterations (visual) related to altered status of sense organ resulting from neurological deficit

Unilateral neglect related to effects of disturbed perceptual abilities (hemianopsia), neurological deficit or trauma causing inattention to stimuli on affected side

Impaired verbal communication related to decrease in circulation to brain resulting from stroke in the dominant hemisphere area causing aphasia, dysarthia, refusal to attempt speech

EXPECTED OUTCOMES

Adaptation to sensory, communication, and unilateral neglect evidenced by verbalizations of awareness of deficits (spatial, agnosia, apraxia, hemianopsia) and effect on daily functions and gradual reduction in impairments by rehabilitation and therapy or compensation for perceptual loss in safe performance of daily routines; optimize communication by development of and adaptation to effective method of communicating (understanding others and being understood)

INTERVENTION	RATIONALE
I. Assess for:	
A. Deficits in speech and language abilities, presence of slurring with partial or complete aphasia, ability to comprehend spoken and written language, English as a second language	A. Provides data to be used in promotion of communication
B. Facial grimaces or expressions, pointing at items or using hands to communicate (pantomine)	B. Nonverbal forms of communication that indicate feelings or needs
C. Degree of sensory deficits, factors that affect deficit, visual impairment, disregard for objects in visual field on affected side (hemianopsia), diplopia or double vision	C. Data regarding deficits and abilities related to sensory perception
IV. Perform/provide:	
A. Approach and interact with patient on unaffected side, place articles needed in view of unaffected side, place in view of affected side as condition improves	A. Promotes awareness of objects and people, allows for complete view of environment as visual impairment and hemianopsia warrants
B. Encourage to touch affected side, rub affected side, provide activities that enhance the use of affected side	B. Progressively improves body image if paralysis is neglected or denied

INTERVENTION	RATIONALE
C. Environment that is quiet and supportive, avoid unnecessary articles or clutter, least number of articles for food tray or when performing ADL	C. Decreases stimuli that add to confusion, gains attention and decreases distraction if verbal communication is affected
D. Supervision of all activities before allowing independence, maintain items in same positions, provide proper lighting and clear pathways	D. Prevents injury from falls if vision impaired
E. Eyepatch application over eye, alternate between affected and unaffected eye	E. Temporarily stops diplopia
F. Place mirror in room, describe room and furniture placement, assist to judge distances and use pathways	F. Promotes orientation to environment
G. Paper and pencil, magic slate, gestures, pictures, cards; reinforce established communication techniques	G. Promotes alternate method of communicating while providing a familiar or preferred technique
H. Anticipate and validate needs, answer call light immediately	H. Reduces frustration and facilitates communication

INTERVENTION	RATIONALE
I. Speak slowly and clearly, ask simple, direct questions that require short one-word answers, and allow time to process and organize a verbal response, avoid allowing family members to speak for patient	I. Eases process when vocal expression is difficult
J. Avoid interruptions, encourage to speak, but don't force attempts to communicate, avoid criticism and promote continued efforts to speak	J. Allows to speak and enhances self-confidence
K. Allow to practice speaking words slowly, avoid rushing, and display patience and calmness, allow time to attempt to speak words when confident that ready or able	K. Promotes and expands speech at own pace while preventing embarrassment or frustration
L. Encourage to control rate and number of words spoken, to separate each syllable, refer to speech pathologist if dysarthia present	L. Promotes comprehension of communication and instructs in oral and facial muscle exercises to improve speech

NURSING DIAGNOSES

Constipation related to less-than-adequate physical activity (immobility), less-than-adequate dietary/fluid intake (bulk, dysphagia), and neuromuscular impairment (lack of defecation impulse) resulting from CVA

Bowel incontinence related to perception or cognitive impairment resulting in involuntary passage of feces

Altered urinary elimination related to neuromuscular/sensory impairment resulting in poor bladder control causing incontinence, concern about avoidance of participation in sexual activity

Toileting self-care deficit related to neuromuscular impairment causing inability to carry out proper urinary and feces elimination independently using a commode or toilet

EXPECTED OUTCOMES
Reduction or resolution of urinary and bowel incontinence episodes, relief from constipation and incontinence evidenced by establishment of an effective elimination pattern without use of a urinary catheter and daily or usual frequency of bowel elimination of soft formed feces

INTERVENTION	RATIONALE
I. Assess for:	
A. Past urinary pattern, present continent and incontinent pattern, ability to sense bladder fullness, urinary urgency or frequency, ability to communicate need to void, mobility limitations that prevent ability to use commode or toilet, amount and timing of fluid intake/day	A. Provides data to devise bladder rehabilitation program
B. Past bowel elimination pattern, present bowel incontinence pattern, ability to sense rectal fullness and urge to defecate, mobility limitations that prevent use of commode or toilet, amount and time of defecation/day	B. Provides data to devise bowel rehabilitation program
C. Feces characteristics such as hard, dry, marble formed, fecal impaction check q2 days	C. Indicates constipation resulting from inadequate activity, intake of high-fiber foods and fluids caused by chewing and swallowing difficulties

INTERVENTION	RATIONALE
III. Administer:	
A. Sympathomimetics PO	A. Acts to reduce bladder spasms and increase urinary sphincter tone
B. Suppository stimulant REC	B. Acts to induce peristaltic contractions by stimulating sensory nerve endings in wall of colon
C. Stool softener PO	C. Acts to lower surface tension to permit water to penetrate and soften stool for easier passage
IV. Perform/provide:	
A. Paper and pencil or other means to reveal need for toileting	A. Provides method of communicating urge to void or defecate
B. Bedpan, urinal within easy reach, assist to use as needed or to use commode or bathroom	B. Provides access to toileting equipment
C. Offer toileting q2–3h, raise head of bed, place toilet paper and damp cloth within reach, adjust schedule to normal elimination pattern such as 30 minutes following breakfast and at bedtime, change schedule if needed to conform to patient needs	C. Allows for frequent elimination as this assists with bladder/bowel retraining by preventing incontinence if muscle function affected

INTERVENTION	RATIONALE
D. Increase fluid intake to 2 to 3 L/day if permitted, limit fluids at bedtime, avoid caffeine-containing beverages	D. Dilutes urine and promotes elimination, prevents constipation and possible incontinence at night and excessive diuresis caused by caffeine
E. Include fiber in daily diet	E. Provides bulk to feces to prevent constipation
F. Digital stimulation of rectum, remove fecal impaction if present	F. Promotes defecation at a regular time to prevent fecal incontinence or fecal impaction
G. Continence aids such as condom catheter, female incontinence pouch, waterproof pads or underwear	G. Preserves skin integrity until bladder control regained and embarrassment of incontinence soiling clothing
H. Perineal care following each incontinence episode, cleanse with mild soap and warm water and pat dry	H. Promotes cleanliness and preserves skin integrity
I. Indwelling catheter insertion and maintenance as a temporary measure, remove as soon as possible	I. Last resort effort to control urinary incontinence

NURSING DIAGNOSES

Knowledge deficit related to follow-up care, including medication regimen, changes in life-style, and precautions to prevent recurrent CVA, rehabilitation of sensory/motor/communication deficits, signs and symptoms to report to physician

Grieving, dysfunctional related to loss of physiopsychosocial well-being following CVA causing expression of anger, guilt, sadness, and interference with life functioning

EXPECTED OUTCOMES

Adequate knowledge of components of follow-up care evidenced by compliance with long-term therapeutic plan, progressive resolution of grieving process, absence of recurrence of signs and symptoms of CVA and adaptation to long-term rehabilitation regimen

INTERVENTION	RATIONALE
I. Assess for: 　A. Readiness, willingness, and motivation to learn, discharge care and life-style changes	A. Learning can best take place if client is receptive and compliance is more likely to occur
B. Health practices, health beliefs, ethnic identity (religion, diet, language), value orientations, family interactions and cooperation	B. Factors to incorporate into teaching plan to facilitate learning and compliance with long-term care
IV. Perform/provide: 　A. Acknowledgment of perceptions with a nonjudgmental attitude	A. Establishes nurse–patient relationship in an accepting environment
B. Explanations that are clear, accurate in understandable terms, small amount of information over time	B. Prevents misconceptions, erroneous attitudes and beliefs about disease
C. Environment conducive to learning with space, lighting, and proper equipment and supplies	C. Distractions or discomfort will interfere with learning

D. As much control over life-style change decisions as possible, include family in discharge planning

D. Allows power to be given or retained by patient

E. Teaching aids (pamphlets, video tapes, pictures, written instructions)

E. Reinforces learning

F. Team of resource personnel/professionals

F. Nutritionist, social worker, counselor, physical/occupational rehabilitation therapist, speech pathologist, and others can assist in teaching specific care and providing support for desired changes

V. Teach patient/family:

A. Anatomy and pathophysiology of disorder, nature of disease and possible recurrence

A. Promotes understanding of disease that facilitates compliance

B. Risk factors such as dietary intake of high-fat/-cholesterol foods, stress, smoking, exercise deficit, effect on body image and independence in self-care activities

B. Contributes to information about factors that can be modified with life-style changes

C. Dietary modification with sample menus for reduction in calories, fat and cholesterol, salt intake, list of foods to include and restrict in diet

C. Reduces risk factor associated with overweight, abnormal lipid panel, hypertension leading to CVA

INTERVENTION	RATIONALE
D. Administration and rationale of all prescribed medications (antihypertensives, anti-inflammatory, anticoagulant), written schedule of times and dosages, side effects to expect and report, drugs that can interact with prescribed medications, laboratory testing to monitor drug therapy	D. Promotes compliance of complete medication regimen
E. Demonstrate taking of BP and maintaining log of readings, allow for return demonstration and practices	E. Monitors for increases in BP to report
F. Grieving process and expected responses, allow for long period for resolution (varies with individuals and depending on changes to be made)	F. Allows for nonjudgmental movement through stages of grieving and need for support during this time
G. Progressive activity routine allowing for restrictions, use of extremity splints, rest periods when needed during activity, take steps to arrange or continue rehabilitation programs if ordered	G. Supports life-style change to maintain or improve motor status
H. Reinforce urinary and/or bowel training, use protective pads or underwear as needed	H. Promotes continued continence

INTERVENTION	RATIONALE
I. Suggest home modifications to support performance of ADL and mobility, secure and utilize aids to support and continue independence	I. Maintains activities and control of self-care, safe environment if deficits are present
J. Avoid stressful situations, consider counseling or stress-reduction program to assist in development of coping and problem-solving skills, smoking cessation groups, weight loss groups	J. Prevents risk factors associated with recurrence of CVA
K. Community resources such as American Heart Association and rehabilitation (sensory/motor/communication) agencies and professionals	K. Provides information, support, and equipment for home care
L. Report mobility difficulties, confusion, rise in BP, visual changes, speech changes, lethargy, irritability, to physician	L. Indicates possible recurrence or complication of CVA
M. Comply with scheduled physician and laboratory appointments, therapy sessions	M. Monitors improvement or need to adjust medications

intracranial/spinal infections
(brain abscess/encephalitis/meningitis)

DEFINITION
The invasion and multiplication of infectious micro-organisms that affect the brain and spinal cord. Brain abscess is a focal infection within the brain with a collection of pus caused by the spread of an infectious process from another area (mastoid or nasal sinus, lungs), by the introduction of the pathogens via brain trauma or surgery, or as a result of conditions such as AIDS. Encephalitis involves inflammation of the parenchyma of the brain caused by a variety of viruses. The agent can enter the body via bites from infected insects, respiratory, mouth or genitalia routes and invade the central nervous system. Meningitis is a bacterial, viral, or fungal infection affecting the arachnoid and pia meningeal layers and subarachnoid space of the brain and spinal cord. It can result from the spread of a systemic infection, introduction of the micro-organism via nearby cranial areas (fracture, invasive procedures), or as a result of immunodeficiency disorders. This plan includes care specific to these conditions and can also be used in association with the INTRACRANIAL TRAUMA and SEIZURE DISORDERS care plans

NURSING DIAGNOSES
Pain related to biologic injuring agent (pathogen) resulting in inflammation causing pressure by compression to areas in the brain or spinal column

Hyperthermia related to illness (infectious process) causing compression to the hypothalamic center and a febrile state

EXPECTED OUTCOMES
Control or reduction of headache, back pain evidenced by verbalization that pain relieved and ability to rest, afebrile state evidenced by temperature of <100°F (37.8°C) and absence of chills

INTERVENTION	RATIONALE
I. Assess for:	
A. Headache, back pain and severity, other characteristics or descriptors, especially location	A. Headache can range in severity of moderate to severe as a result of meningeal irritation, compression, or enlarging area of infectious process
B. Temperature elevation, chills, malaise, prostration, skin hot to touch	B. Associated with infectious process and can be high and difficult to control depending on type of infection
II. Monitor, describe, record:	
A. Temperature q2–4h	A. Provides data regarding febrile state
III. Administer:	
A. Antipyretic PO	A. Acts to reduce temperature
B. Analgesic PO, IM given with caution to prevent obscuring CNS findings	B. Acts to control mild-to-moderate-to-severe pain by decreasing neurotransmitter release
IV. Perform/provide:	
A. Environmental temperature at optimal level based on body temperature	A. Promotes comfort in presence of elevated temperature
B. Position of comfort with head of bed slightly elevated if tolerated	B. Promotes comfort and reduces pain
C. Cool compress/ice bag to head, cool bath or ice packs	C. Relieves headache and reduces temperature to prevent possible increase in intracranial pressure (ICP)

INTERVENTION	RATIONALE
D. Cooling blanket continuously	D. Reduces temperature and maintains desired body temperature
E. Change clothing and linens as needed if diaphoretic	E. Prevents chilling and shivering
F. Bed rest with minimal stimulation (noise, bumping bed, lights)	F. Increases pain if hypersensitivity present

NURSING DIAGNOSES

Risk for fluid volume deficit related to active excessive losses through normal routes resulting from vomiting, diuresis, hypermetabolic state from infectious process, and temperature elevation; deficits affecting intake of fluids resulting from impaired thirst mechanism

Altered nutrition: less than body requirements related to inability to ingest food resulting from nausea, vomiting, unconscious state

EXPECTED OUTCOMES

Adequate nutritional and fluid intake evidenced by I&O, weight, and caloric intake within baseline determinations as vomiting is controlled and level of consciousness returns to normal

INTERVENTION	RATIONALE
I. Assess for: A. Nausea, vomiting with amounts and frequency, urinary output, diaphoresis, and record as output	A. Sources of fluid loss leading to possible dehydration as areas of the brain are affected, projectile vomiting is caused by pressure on the medullary vomiting center
II. Monitor, describe, record: A. I&O q1–4h	A. Indicates fluid imbalance and fluid deficit

INTERVENTION	RATIONALE
B. Weight daily, same time, scale, and same clothing	B. Indicates fluid/nutritional deficit
III. Administer:	
A. Antiemetic IM	A. Acts to relieve nausea and vomiting
IV. Perform/provide:	
A. Fluids IV calculated to include losses from respirations and temperature elevation, vomiting	A. Replaces fluid loss and ensures fluid balance
B. Oral intake when allowed of calculated amount or 1 to 2 L/day progressing to 2 to 3 L/day if permitted	B. Maintains fluid intake and balance if fluid losses are excessive
C. Offer easily digested soft foods of high-protein/calorie value in six small meals/day when oral intake allowed	C. Maintains adequate nutrition via oral route as tolerated

NURSING DIAGNOSES

Risk for injury related to internal regulatory function resulting from local or spread of infection, sensory and integrative dysfunction and deficits causing seizure activity, neuromuscular, perceptual, cognitive, and speech impairments

Sensory/perceptual alterations (visual, auditory, kinesthetic, tactile) related to neurological disease, trauma, or deficit resulting from infectious process causing irritation and deficit to areas of the brain controlling sensory perception or injury to spinal nerves or nerve roots controlling motor function

EXPECTED OUTCOMES

Optimal sensory, motor, mental function evidenced by progressive return to baseline levels of functioning, participation in ADL with or without assistance or use of aids, utilizing aids or techniques to compensate for deficits

INTERVENTION	RATIONALE
I. Assess for: A. Confusion, drowsiness, change in mentation, neurological changes such as speech impairment or loss of movement on one side of the body, progressing to increased intracranial pressure (ICP) and seizures	A. Signs and symptoms of brain abscess caused by focal cerebral irritation depending on the area affected
B. Nuchal rigidity, positive Kernig's and Brudzinski's signs, spinal stiffness, photophobia, weakness, hyperalgesia, change in level of consciousness, and possible seizure activity	B. Signs and symptoms of meningitis caused by meningeal and spinal root irritation, infection, edema, and compression
C. Confusion, delirium, aphasia, hemiparesis, involuntary movements, asymmetric reflexes, hemiplegia, visual deficits and photophobia, and eventually stupor or coma	C. Signs and symptoms of encephalitis depending on causative agent that can lead to mental retardation, loss of sight, speech, and hearing
II. Monitor, describe, record: A. Neurological status q1h	A. Detects early signs of increasing ICP leading to seizure activity

INTERVENTION	RATIONALE
B. EEG	B. Diagnostic procedure to reveal the decrease in brain electrical activity in the presence of infection
C. CT scan, MRI	C. Reveals brain edema and necrosis, location and size of an abscess
D. Lumbar puncture fluid (CSF) analysis and pressure	D. Reveals causative agent and effects, increased pressure, WBC, and protein levels, decreased glucose levels all associated with infection
E. Serial blood, urine, sputum cultures, Gram stain	E. Identifies causative agent and identifies new or spread of infection
III. Administer:	
A. Antimicrobial PO, IV depending on type of infectious agent	A. Acts to destroy micro-organisms by interfering in cell wall synthesis
B. Anticonvulsive PO, IV	B. Acts to prevent or control seizures
C. Anti-inflammatory IV	C. Acts to control inflammation and cerebral edema

INTERVENTION	RATIONALE
IV. Perform/provide: A. Quiet, dim environment free of stimuli such as visitors, loud noises, avoid startling, loud noises or bumping bed, move gently with smooth movements, and refrain from moving head and neck when possible, speak in a quiet voice, and allow for bed rest with restricted activity	A. Prevents unnecessary stimulation that increases headache pain and can potentiate seizure activity
B. Orient to environment, where belongings are kept, assist or supervise as needed in obtaining and using articles, cover eye if appropriate	B. Assists if vision is impaired
C. Assist with ambulation or movement in bed, shaving or smoking	C. Prevents falls and trauma associated with sensory/ motor deficits
D. Seizure precautions such as padding side rails, supervision without restraint, equipment on hand for emergency care	D. Prevents injury if seizure occurs
E. Constant supervision if needed	E. Reduces risk of injury if confused, irritable, combative, bizarre behavior evident
F. Isolation precautions if necessary	F. Prevents disease transmission in meningitis

INTERVENTION	RATIONALE
G. Aseptic technique for performance of all procedures, including ICP monitoring, wound care	G. Prevents cross-contamination
H. Prepare and assist with lumbar puncture	H. Diagnostic procedure to obtain cerebrospinal fluid for analysis

NURSING DIAGNOSES

Anxiety related to threat of death and health status resulting from neurological deficits causing mental retardation, visual, auditory, or speech deficits

Bathing/hygiene and feeding self-care deficits related to neuromuscular, sensory-perceptual, and cognitive impairment causing inability to perform ADL

EXPECTED OUTCOMES

Anxiety reduced to manageable level and optimal participation in ADL evidenced by verbalizations that anxiety decreasing, fears and feelings expressed, and progressive independence in self-care with or without the use of aids as condition improves

INTERVENTION	RATIONALE
I. Assess for: A. Sensory/motor deficits, ability to bathe, brush teeth and hair, feed and dress self, use commode or bathroom, assume sitting, standing positions, and ambulate	A. Determines self-care deficits and amount of assistance or use of aids

INTERVENTION	RATIONALE
B. Anxiety level and expressed feelings and concerns, nonverbal behaviors, use of coping mechanisms	B. Provides information regarding level of fear and anxiety and ability to cope with illness and possible long-term deficits and rehabilitation needs

IV. Perform/provide:

INTERVENTION	RATIONALE
A. Calm, supportive, nonjudgmental environment	A. Encourages rapport and support for expression of anxiety
B. Allow for expression of feelings regarding deficits and behavioral alterations	B. Venting feelings reduces anxiety and fear
C. Remain during times of most acute anxiety episodes	C. Promotes support and understanding
D. Describe and explain all articles and aids used, how to use them, where they are stored	D. Promotes attempts at self-care if visual or motor deficits are present
E. Allow time to perform any aspect of self-care, assist as needed	E. Rushing causes frustration in the presence of impairments
F. Assist to compensate for deficits by use of aids, participation in rehabilitation therapy (speech, physical, occupational)	F. Encourages self-care and independence and maximizes perceptual abilities
G. Encourage and praise all attempts at self-care	G. Provides support by positive feedback

NURSING DIAGNOSIS

Knowledge deficit related to follow-up care regarding rehabilitation, medication regimen, health practices and measures to prevent complications of the disease, and signs and symptoms to report

EXPECTED OUTCOMES

Adequate knowledge evidenced by compliance with continuing care regimen and progressive resolution of deficits caused by brain/spinal column infection

INTERVENTION	RATIONALE
V. Teach patient/family:	
A. Methods to interact within family structure	A. Promotes independence
B. Type of neurological deficits and rehabilitation programs available for speech, occupational, and physical therapy, visual, hearing, and education services for mental deficits and procedure to obtain referral	B. Results from infection that can result in short- or long-term disabilities and services that can be utilized to resolve deficits
C. Medication regimen, especially antimicrobials including taking all the medication as prescribed, expected results, side effects to report	C. Promotes compliance in the treatment of specific types of infection
D. Preventive measures and care prior to or during seizure	D. Prevents injury or trauma resulting from seizure activity

INTERVENTION	RATIONALE
E. Use of assistive aids and techniques in ambulation, transfer, eating, bathing, grooming, dressing and un-dressing, toileting, allow to return demonstrations as appropriate, reinforce reha-bilitation/occupational ther-apy instruction	E. Promotes independence in ADL and control over situa-tions
F. Report behavior changes, mental changes, sensory/motor changes, seizure activity, persistent headache to physician	F. Provides for immediate in-terventions for spread or re-currence of infection
G. Counseling for relaxation, support system from com-munity groups	G. Reduces anxiety and pro-motes adjustment to long-term therapy

intracranial trauma
(contusion/laceration)

DEFINITION

Intracranial trauma or injury to the brain, also known as head injury, is the bruising (contusion) or tearing (laceration) of brain tissue. It is most commonly caused by car accidents, falls, sports or other contact injuries, and penetration by objects such as bullets or bone splinters from fracture of the skull. It can affect any area of the brain and cause edema, cerebral ischemia, hemorrhage, seizure activity, and altered flow of cerebrospinal fluid (CSF). Hematoma formation following a hemorrhage can be epidural or subdural in location. Trauma can be mild or severe resulting in respective damage with symptoms ranging from temporary loss of consciousness and amnesia, to partial or complete unconsciousness with motor/respiratory/temperature/mental/speech and other abnormalities depending on area affected. This plan includes interventions specific to brain injury and can be used in association with the SEIZURE DISORDERS, INTRACRANIAL/SPINAL INFECTIONS, and PREOPERATIVE CARE, POSTOPERATIVE CARE plans if surgery is indicated

NURSING DIAGNOSES

Ineffective individual coping related to situational crises of risk for or actual disabilities and psychophysiological changes (sensory, motor and communication), inability to manage stress, and cope with present and future life-style changes (possible transfer to long-term facility and/or rehabilitation)

Self-esteem disturbance related to neurological damage/deficits causing a loss in function and capabilities, and feelings of helplessness, depression

Anxiety related to threat to self-concept, change in health status resulting from temporary or possible permanent neurological deficits

EXPECTED OUTCOMES

Acknowledgment and progressive adaptation to changes in body functions and ability to cope evidenced by verbalization of positive statements about body changes and feeling less helpless and hopeless, development and utilization of coping skills, personal aids and assistance, return of interest in appearance and social participation, verbalization that feeling less anxious and more relaxed

INTERVENTION	RATIONALE
I. Assess for: A. Use of coping mechanisms, mechanisms, stated fears of uncertainty of disease outcome, life-style changes, reactions to loss of motor, sensory, speech, and mental function	A. Assists in identifying inappropriate use of coping skills and feelings of grief over losses associated with intracranial injury
B. Negative expressions about return of functions, self-worth, feelings of helplessness and uselessness, withdrawal behavior	B. Indicates difficulty in coping, and decrease in self-esteem
C. Personal resources to cope with stress of illness, and interest in learning to problem-solve	C. Support systems and personal strengths assist in developing coping skills
D. Feelings about inability to carry out role, participate in activities, and need to modify life-style	D. Decline in self-esteem common in those left with neurological deficits
IV. Perform/provide: A. Environment conducive to rest, expression of fears and concerns, avoid anxiety-producing situations	A. Decreases stimuli that cause stress, venting of feelings assist in coping with changes and reduces anxiety

INTERVENTION	RATIONALE
B. Listen and clarify perceptions and information given, correct misconceptions, and assist to understand condition	B. Promotes successful resolution of crisis and establishes positive coping mechanisms
C. Allow time to verbalize feelings of denial or anger, comments about appearance if head is shaved, possible loss of abilities in a nonjudgmental environment	C. Promotes temporary use of defense mechanisms to assist in reducing negative feelings
D. Discuss strengths and abilities with honesty, realistic expectations of what can be accomplished with specialized therapy	D. Promotes self-esteem and develops trust and rapport in the nurse–patient relationship
E. Suggest new methods to enhance coping skills and problem solving, allow to externalize and identify those that help	E. Offers alternative coping strategies that allow for release of anxiety and promote hope for optimal outcome
F. Encouragement and give positive feedback regarding progress made, focus on abilities and improvements rather than disabilities and losses (especially if permanent)	F. Provides support for adaptive behavior, promotes self-worth and responsibility for independence
G. Allow to participate in planning of care and to maintain usual routine activities when possible	G. Allows for some control over situations

INTERVENTION	RATIONALE
H. Support grieving for loss of life-style and restrictions in activities, changes in role, goals, needs	H. Provides assistance in adaptation to changes imposed by condition
I. Explain changes in behavior responses caused by brain injury and that improvement can be expected with time and physical care	I. Prevents feelings of guilt and shame regarding feelings and behaviors that are unfamiliar to the patient
J. Include family in information regarding condition and support participation in care when possible	J. Provides opportunity for involvement and understanding of care

NURSING DIAGNOSES

Altered cerebral tissue perfusion related to interruption of arterial or venous flow resulting from hemorrhage, infarction from pressure of hematoma in an injured area of the brain causing possible increase in intracranial pressure (ICP), loss of consciousness, and neurological deficits

Altered thought processes related to physiological changes resulting from reduced cerebral blood flow and cerebral hypoxia (intracranial hemorrhage or hematoma formation) causing impaired memory, reasoning, change in consciousness and confusion, sensory and speech deficits

Sensory/perceptual alterations (visual, auditory, kinesthetic, tactile, olfactory) related to neurological deficits resulting from trauma to areas of the brain containing optic, acoustic, olfactory, or other cranial nerves

EXPECTED OUTCOMES

Adequate or improved cerebral perfusion, return of sensory perception and thought processes evidenced by VS, ICP, temperature within baseline levels, improving level of consciousness and stability of Glasgow Coma Scale, motor, and mental functions, appropriate behavior pattern, absence of sensory deficits (visual, speech, hearing, smell)

INTERVENTION	RATIONALE
I. Assess for:	
A. Level of consciousness (LOC), dizziness, confusion, orientation, alertness, pupillary size, position, and reaction equality, extraocular movements	A. Neurological manifestations of reduced cerebral perfusion or increased intracranial pressure (ICP) caused by head injury
B. Cognitive status, spontaneous movements, response to painful stimuli and verbal communication	B. Indicates level of coma or brain function
C. Respiratory hyperventilation, bounding and slow pulse, increasing BP, vomiting, seizures, ICP of >15 mm Hg	C. Signs and symptoms of increasing ICP resulting from brain injury
D. Mental (memory, reasoning), motor or sensory deficits (visual, auditory, olfactory), speech impairment, behavior changes (agitation, confusion, irritability)	D. Deficits resulting from brain injury and causing changes in thought process and sensory perception
II. Monitor, describe, record:	
A. Glasgow Coma Scale, neurological checks, PERL q1–4h or as appropriate	A. Provides measurement of level of consciousness, pupil reaction and motor activity to determine deficits, stability, improvement, or expanding hematoma
B. VS q2–4h or as appropriate	B. Indicates rise in ICP, continued cerebral bleeding

INTERVENTION	RATIONALE
C. I&O q1–4h as appropriate	C. Indicates renal perfusion affecting urinary output
D. ICP per intraventricular catheter	D. Indicates ICP increases to determine interventions based on rises
E. Skull, cervical spine x rays	E. Identifies fractures
F. Brain scan, CT scan, MRI	F. Identifies areas of bleeding or shift in brain indicating pressure
G. EEG, ECG	G. Determines brain electrical activity and possible dysrhymias affecting cardiac output and perfusion
H. CSF analysis	H. Bloody fluid indicates hemorrhage in the subarachnoid space
I. Hb, Hct	I. Determines continued blood losses that cause decrease in brain perfusion

III. Administer:

A. Anticonvulsive, sedative IV	A. Acts to control seizure activity if present, restlessness, or delirium
B. Osmotic diuretic IV	B. Acts to reduce cerebral edema by osmotically extracting fluid from cerebral tissue, excessive fluid predisposes to ICP
C. Anti-inflammatory IV	C. Acts to reduce cerebral edema and inflammation

INTERVENTION	RATIONALE
D. Psychotherapeutic agent IV	D. Acts to reduce agitation that increases ICP
E. Blood or blood products IV	E. Replaces losses or maintains blood volume

IV. Perform/provide:

INTERVENTION	RATIONALE
A. Elevate head of bed to semi-Fowler's position if allowed, immobilize head and neck in midline position, avoid flexion, rotation of the head, use sandbag, cervical collar to immobilize head	A. Promotes cerebral drainage to prevent ICP, immobilizes neck until cervical fracture ruled out as this is a common injury associated with head trauma
B. Restrict fluid intake as ordered, or limit to 1 L/day and distribute over 24 hours	B. Prevents ICP by reducing fluids
C. Schedule care and activities to avoid excessive movement, anxiety, muscle tension, distended bladder, or constipation	C. Prevents increased ICP
D. Environment that is understanding and nonjudgmental as attempts are made to return to normalcy	D. Provides support and empathy for those experiencing behavior and other changes and promotes cooperation
E. As consciousness returns, reorient to environment, especially if mental deficit is present (confused or has memory loss)	E. Prevents disorientation and regression while maintaining reality of the situations

INTERVENTION	RATIONALE
F. Place familiar articles within reach, face patient, and speak slowly and clearly, use short sentences, and repeat words as needed	F. Promotes return of memory, attention span and orientation
G. Quiet, calm environment with minimal stimuli, use touch if acceptable to patient	G. Prevents ICP increases
H. Eye care with lubricant q2h, use steristrips to maintain closed eyes	H. Prevents corneal irritation, abrasion if corneal reflex diminished or absent

NURSING DIAGNOSES

Pain related to physical injuring agent of trauma causing cervical fracture, brain tissue irritation, and increased ICP

Sleep pattern disturbance related to internal factor of illness and pain causing frequent interruptions for assessment of neurological status

EXPECTED OUTCOMES

Pain relieved or controlled evidenced by verbalization that pain reduced and able to rest and sleep with reduced interruptions

INTERVENTION	RATIONALE
I. Assess for:	
A. Neck pain or stiffness, bruising in neck area	A. Indicates possible cervical fracture with pain caused by hemorrhage into the subarachnoid space
B. Headache with characteristics such as general or localized, aching, piercing, or pounding	B. Indicates tissue irritation and increasing ICP

INTERVENTION	RATIONALE
C. Sleep pattern, number and reason for interruptions	C. Provides data to be used to promote complete stages of sleep
III. Administer:	
A. Analgesic, short-acting and easily reversible non-narcotic PO	A. Acts on CNS with minimal effect to avoid obscuring neurological findings
IV. Perform/provide:	
A. Calm, quiet, supportive environment, dim lights, avoid speaking loudly	A. Reduces stimuli that increase pain and promotes sleep
B. Change position slowly and gently, avoid moving or bumping bed	B. Sudden movements can increase pain and ICP
C. Cool wet cloth to head	C. Promotes comfort
D. Schedule rest and sleep periods around assessments and other care	D. Allows uninterrupted sleep for full stages of sleep (usually about 90 minutes)

NURSING DIAGNOSES

Ineffective thermoregulation related to trauma to temperature-regulating center resulting from head injury

Ineffective airway clearance related to brain stem trauma and coma state resulting in inability to cough up blood or secretions in airway

EXPECTED OUTCOMES

Clear, patent airway with respiration rate, depth, ease and breath sounds within baseline parameters, temperature maintained in range of 98.6°F (37°C)

INTERVENTION	RATIONALE
I. Assess for:	
A. Respiratory rate, depth, ease, breath sounds, ability to raise and remove secretions, presence of dyspnea, use of accessory muscles	A. Respirations can be affected if respiratory center is involved in injury or airway obstructed by blood or secretions
B. Temperature elevation, hot and dry skin	B. Indicates injury to hypothalamus or edema near this area causing failure to the regulatory system that controls the body temperature
II. Monitor, describe, record:	
A. VS, temperature, breath sounds q2–4h or as needed	A. Indicates changes to allow for early interventions
B. ABGs, chest x ray	B. Indicates hypoxemia, lung infection, or other abnormality/injury associated with accident that caused head trauma
III. Administer:	
A. Oxygen via nasal cannula or face mask	A. Supplements oxygen based on ABG results
IV. Perform/provide:	
A. Semi-Fowlers, sidelying position in bed	A. Facilitates drainage of secretions and prevents aspiration
B. Suction airway, pharyngeal and tracheal q1–2h, PRN	B. Removes blood and secretions that obstruct airways
C. Cooling sponge bath with warm water	C. Provides external measure to reduce temperature

INTERVENTION	RATIONALE
D. Hypothermia blanket	D. Provides external measure to reduce temperature
E. Adjust environmental temperature to 70 to 75°F	E. Promotes comfort if body temperature elevated
F. Prepare for ventilatory support if needed, and assist with intubation	F. Maintains function in presence of respiratory insufficiency

NURSING DIAGNOSES

Impaired physical mobility related to neuromuscular and perceptual or cognitive impairments (coma state) resulting in immobility and causing motor activity deficits, contractures, loss of muscle strength and mass

Risk for impaired skin impairment related to immobility resulting from coma state, mucous membrane impairment resulting from nasogastric tube, and corneal damage, eye irritation resulting from absence of corneal reflex

Bathing/hygiene, dressing/grooming: self-care deficit related to impaired physical mobility and sensory/perceptual alterations resulting from LOC status and neurological deficits

EXPECTED OUTCOMES

Progressive adequate physical activity evidenced by optimal ROM in all joints and gradual participation in ADL with or without assistance leading to self-care within limitations, absence of weakness, contractures, and no evidence of skin, mucous membrane breakdown, or eye irritation or damage

INTERVENTION	RATIONALE
I. Assess for:	
A. Degree and type of mobility or joint impairment, reflexes, paralysis, paresis, ability to perform activities (ADL)	A. Provides data regarding mobility and ability to perform activities within limitations without injury or frustration

B. Sensory deficits affecting mobility such as visual, auditory perception

B. Affects ability to protect self from injury by falling, bumping into objects

C. Amount of assistance needed for ADL and aids that can promote independence

C. Allows for care with control over situations

D. Corneal reflex, eyes for dryness, irritation, inflammation

D. Absence of reflex causes loss of protection from injury, infection

E. Nasal and oral mucous membranes for redness, breaks, dryness, stomatitis, infection

E. Permits early identification of inflammatory conditions caused by nasogastric tube, antibiotic therapy, NPO status

IV. Perform/provide:
A. Change position and turn q2h, align body parts when positioning, ROM to all joints

A. Prevents deformities if immobile or paralysis present, maintains joint mobility and muscle strength and tone

B. Apply footboard to maintain feet at 90 degree angle

B. Avoids footdrop, limiting sitting prevents prolonged hip flexion

C. Pad bony prominences and massage if color is normal

C. Promotes blood circulation to areas and prevents pressure on susceptible areas

D. Mouth care q4h, artificial saliva to mouth, artificial tears to eyes and tape in closed position if needed

D. Prevents dryness and irritation to mucous membranes and eyes

INTERVENTION	RATIONALE
E. Use assistive devices as appropriate (cane, walker) for ambulation, clothing with velcro and zipper closures, suction cups on personal hygiene articles for brushing teeth, shaving, combing hair, clothing that is easily managed to dress and undress (loose with opening in front, elastic waist bands)	E. Provides safe support for mobility and other self-care activities to promote independence
F. Bed in low position with side rails up, place articles within reach, clear pathways of clutter or spills, provide rails, bath mats, shower chair, other aids as needed	F. Prevents falls and possible injury from bumping, slipping, stumbling
G. Reinforce and encourage all activities achieved with rehabilitation (physical and occupational)	G. Promotes return to optimal mobility and self-care activities

NURSING DIAGNOSES

Altered nutrition: less than body requirements related to inability to oral ingestion of food resulting from coma state and risk for aspiration

Risk for fluid volume deficit related to coma state affecting access to and oral intake of fluids

EXPECTED OUTCOMES

Adequate oral fluid (IV) and nutritional intake (tube feedings) evidenced by stable weight with dietary and fluid intake

INTERVENTION	RATIONALE
I. Assess for:	
A. Total daily amount of oral intake of food and fluid, anorexia, ability to feed self as condition improves	A. Provides data about nutritional and fluid status and needs, route of intake, or assistance in oral feedings to avoid frustration caused by eating difficulties
B. Method of providing calculated caloric and fluids needs, amounts and frequency established	B. Usually provided by formula feedings via nasogastric tube and IV infusion of fluids and electrolytes (K) if ordered
II. Monitor, describe, record:	
A. Weight daily or as needed at same time, on same scale, same clothing	A. Reveals losses that can result from inadequate intake of food and fluid
B. I&O ratio q8h	B. Determines fluid balance and need for increased or decreased intake
IV. Perform/provide:	
A. Quiet, clean environment during feedings	A. Promotes digestion without additional stimuli that can cause nausea
B. Place in sitting, upright position for feedings and maintain the position for 30 minutes	B. Permits gravity flow of food and fluid to prevent aspiration
C. Formula feedings of 2000 to 3000 calories/day that includes 60 g protein	C. Additional calories needed to enhance healing

INTERVENTION	RATIONALE
D. Fluid intake of 1 to 2 L/day as allowed or indicated by I&O, add to tube feedings if needed to provide adequate intake	D. Ensures fluid balance and avoids dehydration, especially if temperature is elevated
E. Soft foods and advance diet as condition and mentation warrant	E. Provides nutrients as ability to tolerate oral intake improves
F. Assist to eat and use assistive aids/utensils if appropriate	F. Promotes self-feeding and independence

NURSING DIAGNOSES

Constipation related to less-than-adequate physical activity (immobility), less-than-adequate dietary/fluid intake (bulk), neuromuscular impairment (lack of reflexes)

Altered urinary elimination related to coma state, neuromuscular/sensory impairment resulting in poor bladder control causing incontinence and infection

Toileting self-care deficit related to coma state causing inability to carry out proper urinary and feces elimination independently using a commode or toilet

EXPECTED OUTCOMES

Reduction or relief from constipation and urinary incontinence evidenced by return of an adequate and regular bowel and urinary elimination output with absence of distention, infection, or impaction

INTERVENTION	RATIONALE
I. Assess for:	
A. Past urinary pattern, present continent and incontinent pattern, ability to sense bladder fullness, bladder distention, retention, overflow conditions, coma state or ability to communicate urge to void, amount and timing of fluid intake/day	A. Provides data to determine urinary elimination abnormality
B. Characteristics of urine such as cloudy, foul-smelling, need for catheterization to empty bladder	B. Indicates urinary bladder infection
C. Past bowel elimination pattern, ability to sense rectal fullness and urge to defecate (coma), bowel sounds, distention, amount and time of defecation	C. Provides data to determine bowel elimination abnormalities caused by decrease or loss of reflex activity and muscle tone
D. Feces characteristics such as hard, dry, marble formed, fecal impaction check q2days	D. Indicates constipation resulting from immobility, lack of fiber and fluids
II. Monitor, describe, record:	
A. I&O q4–8h	A. Provides data regarding fluid balance, output in particular
III. Administer:	
A. Suppository stimulant REC	A. Acts to induce peristaltic contractions by stimulating sensory nerve endings in wall of colon

INTERVENTION	RATIONALE
B. Stool softener PO	B. Acts to lower surface tension to permit water to penetrate and soften stool for easier passage

IV. Perform/provide:

A. Bedpan, urinal within easy reach, assist to use as needed or to use commode or bathroom	A. Provides access to toileting equipment if conscious and aware of urge to void or defecate
B. Intermittent catheterization for bladder distention	B. Preferred over indwelling catheter, which predisposes to bladder infection
C. Increase fluid intake if permitted, limit fluids at bedtime	C. Dilutes urine and promotes elimination, prevents constipation
D. Bladder training to regain continence when feasible	D. Promotes control and independence in urinary elimination
E. Enema if medication is not successful	E. Promotes bowel evacuation and prevents impaction
F. Remove fecal impaction if present	F. Necessary in the comatose patient, as urge to defecate is absent
G. Include fiber in diet when appropriate	G. Provides bulk to feces to prevent constipation
H. Continence aids such as condom catheter, female incontinence pouch, waterproof pads or underwear	H. Preserves skin integrity until bladder control regained

INTERVENTION	RATIONALE
I. Perineal care following each incontinence episode, cleanse with mild soap and warm water and pat dry	I. Promotes cleanliness and preserves skin integrity

NURSING DIAGNOSES

Knowledge deficit related to follow-up care, including medication regimen, changes in life-style and rehabilitation of sensory/motor/speech/mental deficits, signs and symptoms to report to physician

Grieving, dysfunctional related to loss of physiopsychosocial well-being following brain trauma causing difficulty in adjustment to deficits and maintenance of health

EXPECTED OUTCOMES

Adequate knowledge of follow-up care evidenced by compliance with and adaptation to long-term rehabilitation plan, progressive resolution of grieving process

INTERVENTION	RATIONALE
I. Assess for:	
A. Readiness, willingness, and motivation to learn discharge plan and life-style changes	A. Learning can best take place if client is receptive and compliance is more likely to occur
B. Health practices, health beliefs, ethnic identity (religion, diet, language), value orientations, family interactions and cooperation	B. Factors to incorporate into teaching plan to facilitate learning and compliance with long-term care
IV. Perform/provide:	
A. Acknowledgment of perceptions with a nonjudgmental attitude	A. Establishes nurse–patient relationship in an accepting environment

INTERVENTION	RATIONALE
B. Explanations that are clear, accurate in understandable terms, small amount of information over time	B. Prevents misconceptions, erroneous attitudes and beliefs about disease
C. Environment conducive to learning with space, lighting, and proper equipment and supplies	C. Distractions or discomfort will interfere with learning
D. As much control over lifestyle change decisions as possible, include family in discharge planning	D. Allows power to be given or retained by patient
E. Teaching aids (pamphlets, video tapes, pictures, written instructions)	E. Reinforces learning
F. Team of resource personnel/professionals	F. Nutritionist, social worker, counselor, physical/occupational rehabilitation therapist, speech pathologist, and others can assist in teaching specific care and providing support for desired changes
V. Teach patient/family:	
A. Anatomy and pathophysiology of disorder, nature of deficits	A. Promotes understanding of disease that facilitates compliance

INTERVENTION	RATIONALE
B. Rehabilitation program for at least 6 months that can include speech therapy, cognitive therapy, physical and occupational therapy, development of social and recreational skills	B. Promotes maximum function in areas of deficit to ensure an optimal productive life
C. Dietary and fluid daily intake	C. Ensures adequate nutritional and fluid requirements for general health
D. Grieving process and expected responses, to allow time for resolution (varies with individuals and depends on changes to be made)	D. Allows for nonjudgmental movement through stages of grieving and need for support during this time
E. Suggest home modifications to support performance of ADL, secure and utilize aids to support and continue independence	E. Maintains activities and control of self-care, safe environment if deficits are present
F. Community resources such as agencies and support groups for health maintenance	F. Provides information, support, and equipment for home care
G. Comply with scheduled physician appointments and therapy sessions	G. Monitors improvement or need to adjust therapy

seizure disorders

DEFINITION

Seizures are paroxysmal episodes of excessive and erratic neuronal discharges in the gray matter of the brain. As the discharges become more intense and reach a threshold, they spread to the entire cortex, basal ganglia, brain stem, and thalamus. They are classified as partial (involves one portion of the brain and begins locally) or generalized (widespread bilaterally and diffuse without local onset). Considered a symptom, the causes include diseases or conditions associated with cerebral irritation such as brain tumor, craniocerebral trauma, cerebrovascular accident, central nervous system infections, toxic substances and drugs, cerebral hypoxia, degenerative brain disorders, congenital malformations or brain defects, all of which lower the seizure threshold. Epilepsy is defined as seizures that are spontaneously recurring with the first seizure usually occurring before the age of 20. This plan includes care specific to this condition and can be used in association with the INTRACRANIAL/SPINAL INFECTIONS and INTRACRANIAL TRAUMA care plans

NURSING DIAGNOSES

Anxiety related to change in health status, threat to self-concept resulting from unpredictable nature and embarrassment of seizure occurring with behavior changes and possible injury causing self-consciousness and depression

Self-esteem disturbance related to poor self-image resulting from recurring seizures causing anger, guilt, shame, and feelings of inferiority and helplessness regarding long-term therapy

Social isolation related to altered state of wellness and unaccepted social behavior resulting from seizure activity and stigma attached to this disorder

EXPECTED OUTCOMES

Anxiety controlled or within manageable levels and improved self-esteem, increased ability to engage in social and personal relationships evidenced by verbalizations that feeling more relaxed, embarrassment and feelings of rejection/indifference and loneliness reduced, importance of social and family interactions and activities, and increasing ability to cope with and develop appropriate social and problem-solving skills

INTERVENTION	RATIONALE
I. Assess for: A. Level of anxiety, use of coping mechanisms, stated fears of uncertainty about seizures, feelings about public attitudes about seizures, misconceptions about the disorder	A. Anxiety can range from mild to severe, assists in identifying level of anxiety associated with future seizures
B. Restlessness, complaining, joking, withdrawal, talkativeness, increased P and R	B. Nonverbal expressions of anxiety when not able to communicate feelings
C. Personal resources to cope with stress, anxiety; appropriate use of coping mechanisms such as denial, rationalization	C. Support systems and personal strengths assist to manage anxiety and defense mechanisms offers temporary coping with seizure activity
D. Feelings and expressions of shame or guilt, self-consciousness, anger, negative remarks about self, and legal restrictions imposed, activity restrictions imposed (driving, occupational, dangerous recreational activities)	D. Changes in body image and self-esteem constitutes a common and serious problem as social attitudes impose life-style restrictions and, in some cases, social rejection and isolation

INTERVENTION	RATIONALE
IV. Perform/provide:	
A. Environment conducive to rest, expression of fears and anxiety, personal views by others, anger about diagnosis and how it can impact on life-style, avoid anxiety-producing situations	A. Decreases stimuli that cause stress/anxiety, venting of feelings decreases anxiety and hostility
B. Suggest new methods to enhance coping skills and problem solving, allow to externalize and identify those that help	B. Offers alternative coping strategies that allow for release of anxiety and fear
C. Allow time to verbalize effect on social interactions, mental status and preference to be alone, insecurity in public	C. Reduces anxiety that can lead to social isolation thought to be imposed by social values and expectations
D. Allow to participate in planning of care to maintain usual activities when possible and maintenance of social relationships	D. Allows for some control over situations and prevents social withdrawal
E. Aid in developing strategies to reduce anxiety such as relaxation techniques and exercises, reading, music, guided imagery	E. Develops coping skills to reduce stress and reestablish relationships

NURSING DIAGNOSIS

Risk for injury related to internal factor of regulatory function resulting in seizure activity (uncontrolled movements, changes in consciousness) causing physical trauma

EXPECTED OUTCOMES
Prevention of seizure and trauma prior to, during, or following occurrence of seizure activity evidenced by control of seizure, absence of bruising or breaks to bones, skin or soft tissues, trauma to mouth and tongue

INTERVENTION	RATIONALE
I. Assess for:	
A. Age at onset of seizures, history of type and frequency of seizures experienced, precipitating factors and diseases that can cause seizure activity, mental status	A. Provides information regarding the status of the disorder, risk for occurrence
B. All aspects of the seizure such as predisposing event, onset and length of each phase, activity that occurred during each phase and sequence of body part(s) affected, loss of consciousness and length, clonic or tonic movements (stiffening/twitching/jerking), tongue or lip biting, loss of muscle tone, falling to the floor, flushing color or cyanosis, diaphoresis or salivation, incontinence	B. Description of seizure activity essential for appropriate treatment, can last for minutes or hours, can include sensory experiences at the onset such as dizziness, weakness, numbness, odor, twitching depending on focus of the brain from which the seizure originates, signs and symptoms depend on whether generalized or partial and phase of seizure activity
C. Level of consciousness, sleep period, memory loss, muscle soreness, aphasia, weakness or paralysis, (include duration of each post-seizure effect)	C. Indicates possible effects following seizure activity that can result in physical injury or mental/motor changes

INTERVENTION	RATIONALE
II. Monitor, describe, record: A. Electroencephalography (EEG)	A. Diagnostic procedure to identify focus of discharges, type of seizure, diagnose epilepsy
B. Computerized tomography (CT)	B. Diagnostic procedure to identify congenital or tumor causes of seizures
C. Anticonvulsive drug level	C. Maintains therapeutic level for optimal drug effect or to determine potential for toxicity
III. Administer: A. Anticonvulsive PO, IV based on type of seizures	A. Acts to reduce voltage and spread of electrical discharges in the motor cortex to prevent seizure activity
IV. Perform/provide: A. Pad side rails and maintain in raised position, bed in low position, oral airway and suctioning equipment at bedside, remove harmful objects from the immediate environment	A. Precautions taken to prevent injury during seizure

INTERVENTION	RATIONALE
B. Remain until seizure concludes, avoid restraining or attempting to open mouth and insert anything if teeth clenched, carefully ease to floor at onset if not in bed and place a pillow or towel under the head or place head in lap, loosen clothing, turn head to the side to allow secretions to drain, insert airway, or suction to ensure patent airway or to prevent aspiration	B. Provides support and prevents injury during a seizure
C. Reorient to events, quiet, calm and reassuring environment, cleanse oral cavity and sponge face with damp cloth	C. Promotes comfort, rest, and relaxation following seizure

NURSING DIAGNOSIS

Knowledge deficit related to follow-up long-term care regarding medication regimen, dietary, fluid, sleep, and activity pattern, measures to take to prevent seizures or injury during seizure, rehabilitation needs

EXPECTED OUTCOMES

Adequate knowledge of general and specific follow-up care evidenced by compliance with long-term medication regimen and measures to restrict stimulating activities (absence of seizure activity), and measures to ensure safety (absence of injury during seizure activity)

INTERVENTION	RATIONALE
V. Teach patient/family:	
A. Cause and pathophysiology of seizures, chronicity of disorder, and need for long-term therapy, use of denial as a coping mechanism	A. Provides information about the disorder for better understanding and compliance of medical regimen
B. Medication regimen, probably for life to include action in controlling seizures, use of calendar or other reminders, to take anticonvulsant even if not having seizures, avoiding nonprescribed medications	B. Compliance important to prevent seizures and avoidance of other drugs that can interact with anticonvulsant therapy
C. Nutritional dietary and fluid intake daily, moderate recreational and occupational activities	C. Promotes health status and general felling of well-being
D. Caution against physical and emotional stress, kinds of stimulation to avoid triggering seizure such as noise, lights, flickering shadows	D. Measures to prevent seizure activity
E. Modification of environment by removing sharp objects, measures to take if seizure occurs such as loosening clothing, position on side, remain until consciousness returns, avoid restraining, when to call emergency service	E. Prevents injury if seizure occurs

INTERVENTION	RATIONALE
F. Legal restrictions, antidis- crimination laws	F. Protects those with epilepsy from denial of rights and services and allows for ex- posure to education of dri- ving restrictions, employ- ment difficulties
G. Wear medication alert bracelet, or identification in purse or wallet	G. Identifies condition in case of emergency, although can be a burden or cause stigma depending on the patient
H. Availability of support groups in the community, National Epilepsy League, vocational rehabilitation, psychological counseling if needed	H. Provides information, sup- port, and social interaction

spinal cord trauma

DEFINITION

Injury to the spinal cord ranges from a mild to severe trauma at the cervical, thoracic, or lumbar level that determines the motor and sensory loss and severity of disability. The types of injury can be flexion-rotation or dislocation (cervical), extension/hyperextension (neck injury from diving, driving), compression (lower thoracic and lumbar), or complete transection (any area). Most common areas of injury are the cervical (area of first, second, and sixth), thoracic (area of eleventh), and lumbar (area of second). Quadriplegia results from cervical injury, and paraplegia results from thoracic or lumbar injury. Causes of spinal cord injury are motor accidents, gunshot or other penetrating wounds, sports or other contact injuries, falls, and diseases such as osteoporosis, tumors, vascular disorders, spondylosis, and myelitis leading to cord abnormalities. This plan includes care specific to cord trauma and can be used in association with the INTRACRANIAL/SPINAL INFECTIONS (ENCEPHALITIS/MENINGITIS) care plans

NURSING DIAGNOSES

Ineffective individual coping related to situational crises and personal vulnerability to the risk for or actual disabilities and psychophysiological changes (sensory and motor), inability to manage stress and cope with present and future life-style changes (possible transfer to long-term facility and/or rehabilitation)

Ineffective family coping: compromised: related to temporary family disorganization and role changes, prolonged disease or disability progression resulting in exhaustive supportive capacity of significant people in care of family member

Self-esteem disturbance related to neurological damage/deficits causing a loss in function and capabilities (quadriplegia, paraplegia), and feelings of helplessness, depression

Anxiety related to threat to self-concept, change in health status resulting from temporary or possible permanent neurological deficits

EXPECTED OUTCOMES

Acknowledgment and progressive adaptation to changes in body functions and ability to cope evidenced by verbalization of positive statements about body changes and feeling less helpless and hopeless, development and utilization of coping skills, personal aids and assistance, return of interest in appearance and social participation, verbalization that feeling less anxious, more relaxed, and able to request assistance

INTERVENTION	RATIONALE
I. Assess for:	
A. Use of coping mechanisms, mechanisms, stated fears of uncertainty of disease outcome, life-style changes, reactions to loss of motor and sensory function, family responses to crisis situation	A. Assists in identifying inappropriate use of coping skills, feelings of grief over losses associated with intracranial injury
B. Negative expressions about return of functions, self-worth, feelings of helplessness and uselessness, withdrawal behavior	B. Indicates difficulty in coping and decrease in self-esteem
C. Personal resources to cope with stress of injury, and interest in learning to problem-solve	C. Support systems and personal strengths assist to develop coping skills
D. Family strengths, willingness to assist and support patient	D. Identifies how family members manage stress and crisis situations
E. Feelings about inability to carry out role, participate in activities and need to modify life-style	E. Decline in self-esteem common in those left with neuromuscular and neurosensory deficits

INTERVENTION	RATIONALE
IV. Perform/provide:	
A. Environment conducive to rest, expression of fears and concerns, avoid anxiety-producing situations	A. Decreases stimuli that cause stress, venting of feelings assists in coping with changes and reduces anxiety
B. Listen and clarify perceptions and information given, correct misconceptions and assist to understand condition	B. Promotes successful resolution of crisis and establishes positive coping mechanisms
C. Allow time to verbalize feelings of denial or anger, comments about loss of abilities, negative feelings about possible disabilities in a nonjudgmental environment	C. Promotes temporary use of defense mechanisms to assist in reducing negative feelings
D. Discuss strengths and abilities with honesty, realistic expectations of what can be accomplished with specialized therapy	D. Promotes self-esteem and develops trust and rapport in the nurse–patient relationship
E. Suggest new methods to enhance coping skills and problem solving, allow to externalize and identify those that help	E. Offers alternative coping strategies that allow for release of anxiety and promotes hope for optimal outcome
F. Encouragement and give positive feedback regarding progress made, focus on abilities and improvements rather than disabilities	F. Provides support for adaptive behavior, promotes self-worth and responsibility for independence

INTERVENTION	RATIONALE
G. Allow to participate in planning of care and to maintain usual routine activities when possible	G. Allows for some control over situations
H. Support grieving for loss of life-style and restrictions, changes in role, goals, needs	H. Provides assistance in adaptation to changes imposed by injury
I. Include family in information regarding condition and support participation in care when possible	I. Provides opportunity for involvement and understanding of care

NURSING DIAGNOSES

Ineffective airway clearance related to trauma to spinal cord with paralysis of muscles needed for breathing resulting in inability to cough up secretions causing tracheobronchial obstruction and stasis of secretions

Ineffective breathing pattern related to neuromuscular impairment resulting in paralysis of muscles needed for breathing resulting in decreased chest expansion and compromised ventilation

Risk for aspiration related to depressed cough and gag reflexes resulting in ineffective ability to remove secretions from the airway and possible reflux of gastric contents causing high risk for aspiration pneumonia

EXPECTED OUTCOMES

Clear, patent airway and effective breathing pattern evidenced by respiration rate, depth, ease and breath sounds within baseline parameters, secretions mobilized and removed by coughing or suctioning, ABGs within normal ranges, temperature maintained in range of 98.6°F (37°C) with absence of atelectasis and pneumonia

INTERVENTION	RATIONALE
I. Assess for:	
A. Respiratory rate, depth, ease, breath sounds, ability to raise and remove secretions, presence of dyspnea, use of accessory muscles	A. Respirations are affected if spinal cord is injured and edema that results can cause respiratory compromise that can be short or long term
B. Temperature elevation, hot and dry skin	B. Indicates infectious process that can result from aspiration of secretions into the lungs
II. Monitor, describe, record:	
A. VS, temperature, breath sounds q2–4h or as needed	A. Indicates changes to allow for early interventions
B. ABGs, pulse oximetry, chest x ray	B. Indicates hypoxemia, lung infection or other abnormality/injury associated with accident that caused cord injury
C. ECG	C. Determines presence of dysrhythmias during suctioning in the most acute phase of the injury
D. Sputum culture	D. Indicates and identifies pulmonary infectious agent
III. Administer:	
A. Oxygen via nasal cannula or face mask	A. Supplements oxygen based on ABG or oximetry results
IV. Perform/provide:	
A. Bed rest in flat position, especially during coughing	A. Facilitates removal of secretions to promote airway patency and prevents aspiration

INTERVENTION	RATIONALE
B. Suction airway, pharyngeal and tracheal q1–2h, PRN	B. Removes secretions that obstruct airways during acute phase of treatment
C. Diaphragmatic breathing exercises with incentive spirometry, assist as needed	C. Promotes chest expansion and improves ventilation (vital capacity)
D. Prepare for ventilatory support if needed and assist with intubation	D. Maintains function in presence of respiratory insufficiency

NURSING DIAGNOSES

Pain related to physical injuring agent of trauma to nerve root irritation and stress on neck, arm and shoulder muscles resulting from return to activities following enforced immobility

Sleep pattern disturbance related to internal factor of illness and pain resulting from devices used to immobilize spine and frequent interruptions for assessment of neurological status

Dysreflexia related to cord injury above thoracic 7 resulting in autonomic nervous system loss or dysfunction

EXPECTED OUTCOMES

Pain relieved or controlled evidenced by pain reduced, adaptation to halo and turning frame devices, and reduced interruptions for assessments with increased ability to rest and sleep; dysreflexia prevented or reduced evidenced by ongoing assessment and immediate response to signs and symptoms of reflex activity to prevent dysreflexia

INTERVENTION	RATIONALE
I. Assess for: A. Neck pain, pain in shoulders or arms, headache, pain that radiates at spinal nerves in area and at the level of injury	A. Indicates response to strain of muscles following immobility of body parts and spinal root reaction at the site of cord injury

INTERVENTION	RATIONALE
B. Headache with characteristics such as throbbing and of extreme severity, can be diffuse in various areas of the head	B. Indicates manifestation of autonomic dysreflexia
C. Sleep pattern, number and reason for interruptions	C. Provides data to be used to promote beneficial sleep and rest pattern
II. Monitor, describe, record: A. VS q2–4h or as appropriate	A. Hypertension of as high as 300 mm Hg systolic, bradycardia, and associated diaphoresis, flushing of skin above injury area, blurred vision, and stuffy nose indicate autonomic dysreflexia
III. Administer: A. Analgesic, non-narcotic PO	A. Acts on CNS with minimal effect, avoids respiratory depression
B. Antihypertensive IV	B. Acts to reduce severe hypertension associated with presence of dysreflexia
C. Muscle relaxant PO, IV	C. Acts to control muscle spasms that cause pain by depressing nerve transmission through pathways in the spinal cord and brain
IV. Perform/provide: A. Calm, quiet, supportive environment, dim lights, avoid speaking loudly	A. Reduces stimuli that increase pain and promote sleep

INTERVENTION	RATIONALE
B. Change position slowly and gently, avoid moving or bumping bed, avoid movement or contact with tongs, pins, traction weights, or halo frame	B. Sudden movements can increase pain and disrupt rest
C. Cool wet cloth to head	C. Promotes comfort for headache
D. Schedule rest and sleep periods around assessments and other care, allow for position preferred for sleep within restrictions imposed by immobilization device	D. Allows uninterrupted sleep for full stages of sleep (usually about 90 minutes)
E. Support neck and shoulder when changing position without pushing or pulling of these body parts, use turning sheet and additional staff to move patient	E. Prevents pain to these areas
F. Application of cervical collar after immobilization to spine	F. Relieves pain and continues support
G. Massage arms and shoulders following stabilization of condition	G. Relives stiffness resulting from immobilization during acute stage of injury

INTERVENTION	RATIONALE
H. Application of anesthetic lubricant prior to enema, impaction removal, catheterization, avoid performing care, stimuli such as cold or heat, or allowing pressure on body parts applied below level of injury	H. Prevents stimuli that can trigger dysreflexia response

NURSING DIAGNOSES

Impaired physical mobility related to neuromuscular impairment (paralysis caused by spinal cord disruption) resulting in immobility and pain causing motor activity deficits, contractures, loss of muscle strength and mass

Bathing/hygiene, dressing/grooming, feeding, toileting self-care deficit related to physical functional impairment resulting from paralysis, muscle spasms, imposed immobility status

EXPECTED OUTCOMES

Progressive adequate physical activity within planned treatment protocol evidenced by gradual and optimal mobility and participation in ADL with or without assistance or aids leading to self-care within limitations, absence of contractures, shortening of muscles, or other joint or muscle complication

INTERVENTION	RATIONALE
I. Assess for: A. Degree and type of mobility or joint impairment, paralysis, spasms, sensorimotor strengths/abilities, ADL abilities, fatigue level	A. Provides data regarding mobility and ability to perform activities based on effect of injury, paraplegic, quadriplegic

INTERVENTION	RATIONALE
B. Sensory deficits affecting mobility such as visual, tactile perception	B. Affects ability to perceive sensation caused by injury to spinal pathways, head/neck immobilization limits visual field
C. Amount of assistance needed for ADL and aids that can promote independence	C. Allows for care with control over situations when condition warrants this, usually during or following rehabilitation therapy program

IV. Perform/provide:

A. Change position and turn q2h, align body parts when positioning, passive ROM to all joints below the level of injury q2–4h	A. Prevents deformities (contractures, ankylosis, muscle shortening), maintains joint mobility and muscle strength and tone
B. Shoulder, arm, hand exercises, massage, electrical stimulation to the areas	B. Prevents pain and reflex dystrophy, increases muscle strength to prepare for future transfer and ambulatory activities
C. Splints, removable casts, placing upper extremities away from the body, flex knees when in supine position, prone positioning for limited time	C. Prevents complications associated with loss of functional abilities
D. Avoid stimuli to extremities such as touch or pressure on areas, bumping or jarring the bed	D. Reduces spasms associated with cord injury affecting muscles

E. Place feet in dorsiflexion, apply tennis shoes to maintain feet at a 90-degree angle, splint to arm when in bed and a sling when out of bed

E. Prevents footdrop and wrist-drop

F. Use assistive devices as appropriate (crutches, walker) for ambulation, wheelchair, clothing with velcro or zipper closures, suction cups on personal hygiene articles for brushing teeth, shaving, combing hair, clothing that is easily managed to dress and undress (loose with opening in front, elastic waist bands), padded handled or swiveling eating utensils

F. Provides safe support for mobility and other self-care activities to promote independence with assistance as needed

G. Reinforce and encourage all activities achieved with rehabilitation (physical and occupational), assist to apply brace, corset prior to getting out of bed

G. Promotes return to optimal mobility and self-care activities

NURSING DIAGNOSES

Constipation related to less-than-adequate physical activity (immobility), neuromuscular impairment (autonomic system functional loss at the level below the cord injury), less-than-adequate intake of fiber and fluids resulting in decreased defecation and possible fecal impaction

Bowel incontinence related to neuromuscular involvement (autonomic system functional loss at the level below the cord injury) resulting in involuntary passage of feces

Total incontinence related to trauma affecting spinal cord nerves resulting in atonic bladder (neurogenic) causing problem with bladder control and possible infection

EXPECTED OUTCOMES
Reduction or relief from constipation, fecal and urinary incontinence evidenced by return of an adequate and regular bowel and urinary elimination output with absence of incontinence, distention, infection, or impaction

INTERVENTION	RATIONALE
I. Assess for:	
A. Past urinary pattern, present continent and incontinent pattern, ability to sense bladder fullness, bladder distention, or incontinence, residual urine, amount and timing of fluid intake/day	A. Provides data to determine urinary elimination dysfunction
B. Characteristics of urine such as cloudy, foul-smelling, urgency, frequency, need for catheterization to empty bladder (retention and distention)	B. Indicates urinary bladder infection
C. Past bowel elimination pattern, ability to sense rectal fullness and urge to defecate, bowel sounds, distention, amount and time of defecation	C. Provides data to determine bowel elimination abnormalities caused by decrease or loss of reflex activity and muscle tone
D. Feces characteristics such as hard, dry, marble formed, fecal impaction check q2days	D. Indicates constipation resulting from immobility, lack of fiber and fluids

INTERVENTION	RATIONALE
II. Monitor, describe, record:	
A. I&O q4–8h	A. Determines ratio and fluid balance
B. Urine culture	B. Reveals bacterial count of >10,000/mL indicating infection
III. Administer:	
A. Suppository stimulant REC	A. Acts to induce peristaltic contractions by stimulating sensory nerve endings in wall of colon
B. Stool softener PO	B. Acts to lower surface tension to permit water to penetrate and soften stool for easier passage
C. Urinary antiseptic PO	C. Acts to prevent urinary tract infection and as long-term prophylaxis in presence of neurogenic bladder
IV. Perform/provide:	
A. Intermittent catheterization for bladder distention q4–6h, indwelling catheter initially during atony	A. Preferred over indwelling catheter, which predisposes to bladder infection
B. Increase fluid intake if permitted, spread over daytime hours, limit fluids at bedtime	B. Dilutes urine and promotes elimination while preventing distention, prevents constipation

INTERVENTION	RATIONALE
C. Bladder training to regain continence when feasible to include allowing to sit on toilet or commode when possible, tap suprapubic area or massage the abdominal area	C. Promotes control and independence in urinary elimination by stimulating reflex arc to assist in voiding
D. Participation in urinary elimination by performing Credé or Valsalva maneuver, rectal stretch by inserting a finger into the anus during the Valsalva maneuver to relax perineal floor; assist to practice these methods to empty the bladder	D. Methods to promote urination by increasing intra-abdominal pressure against the bladder to force emptying of urine
E. Enema if medication is not successful with precautions to avoid overdistention of the bowel with fluid, oil retention enema can be given to soften feces	E. Promotes bowel evacuation and prevents impaction
F. Remove fecal impaction if present	F. Necessary if obstipation occurs
G. Include fiber in diet when appropriate	G. Provides bulk to feces to prevent constipation
H. Perineal care following each incontinence episode, cleanse with mild soap and warm water and pat dry	H. Promotes cleanliness and preserves skin integrity

INTERVENTION	RATIONALE
I. Bowel training to include digital stimulation or insert rectal tube, offer opportunity $\frac{1}{2}$ to 1 hour after a meal in a sitting position and provide privacy, avoid rushing through an attempt at bowel continence	I. Stimulates peristalsis and reflex evacuation, program to ensure daily bowel elimination depends on the conditioning of reflex activity

NURSING DIAGNOSES

Risk for impaired skin integrity related to immobility resulting from cord injury and loss of reflexes causing prolonged pressure on vulnerable areas, excretions and secretions resulting from urinary and/or fecal incontinence causing irritation and maceration, altered sensation resulting from tactile perception deficit causing burns or trauma

Altered oral mucous membrane related to NPO, mouth breathing resulting from cord injury causing inability to swallow, dry mucous membrane

EXPECTED OUTCOMES

Skin and oral mucous membranes intact evidenced by absence of redness, irritation, lesions, disruptions, burns, or trauma

INTERVENTION	RATIONALE
I. Assess for:	
A. Skin changes at pressure sites, vest edges, tong insertion sites, and perineal/buttocks areas if incontinent	A. Provides data regarding potential skin breakdown
B. Oral cavity for dryness, lesions, bleeding, pain	B. Indicates abnormalities of mucosa of oral cavity if NPO and mouth breathing is present and continues

INTERVENTION	RATIONALE
IV. Perform/provide:	
A. Special bed or mattress to reduce pressure (Stryker frame, Roto-Rest, alternating air pressure mattress)	A. Prevents skin breakdown caused by prolonged immobilization
B. Massage pressure sites q4h	B. Promotes circulation to vulnerable body parts
C. Pad vest and cover rough edges with tape, maintain dryness and cleanliness of shirt worn under the vest	C. Prevents irritation of skin and risk for breakdown
D. Bed free of wrinkles and debris	D. Prevents pressure or irritation to skin
E. Cleanse and dry area exposed to urinary or fecal incontinence and apply a protective ointment, protective pads or underwear	E. Prevents irritations from excretions
F. Adjust weight frequently when sitting in a chair	F. Distributes the pressure on the skin to prevent vasoconstriction and reduction in circulation to tissues
G. Adequate fluid and nutritional intake, avoid hot foods if tactile perception has been lost	G. Promotes healthy skin and prevents burns
H. Oral care TID with a brush or toothettes, frequent rinsing or wiping with diluted mouthwash	H. Cleanses and moisturizes mouth if dry and uncomfortable

INTERVENTION	RATIONALE
I. Bathing with water that is tepid, check that water is not too hot, avoid use of heating pad or hot water bottle	I. Prevents burns in presence of sensory loss (tactile)
J. Ensure that clothing and shoes are not tight and con-strictive	J. Prevents pressure on areas in which sensory perception has been altered or lost (tactile)

NURSING DIAGNOSIS

Sexual dysfunction related to altered body function (spinal trauma) re-sulting in loss of motor/sensory function causing alteration in erection, ejaculation and sexual satisfaction

EXPECTED OUTCOMES

Adaptation to changes in sexual function evidenced by verbalization and practice of satisfying alternative methods in achieving sexual expression

INTERVENTION	RATIONALE
I. Assess for:	
A. Feelings about limitations or disability in achieving sexual satisfaction, change in role performance or change in relationship with sexual partner	A. Provides information about status of sexual dysfunction caused by cord injury and degree of disability
B. Feelings about discussing the subject of sexual con-cerns such as embarrass-ment, difficulty in approach-ing the subject	B. Provides information about comfort level in expressing personal problems or need to refer to an agency or therapist for assistance

INTERVENTION	RATIONALE
C. Knowledge of injury and impact on sexuality, reproductive ability	C. Promotes rationale for sexual dysfunction and lost or remaining functions
IV. Perform/provide:	
A. Quiet, accepting, uninterrupted environment to explain sexual limitations, what can be achieved and what cannot be achieved, allow time to express concerns, denial, and anger in a nonjudgmental manner	A. Facilitates trust and provides information and clarification of questions, allows temporary use of defense mechanisms
B. Explain type of lesion and sexual capabilities, possible reflex or psychogenic erection, ejaculation in men, possible reflux or psychogenic lubrication and stimulation in women	B. Promotes sexual and reproductive function with upper neuron lesions that allow reflex erections and reflux lubrication, or lower lesions resulting in an absence of reflex or psychogenic erection if complete, but present if incomplete with psychogenic lubrication and stimulation
C. Discuss alternate methods of attaining sexual satisfaction such as touching, caressing, massage, exploring erogenous areas	C. Promotes acceptance of belief that psychological response is not the only expression of sexuality
D. Bowel and urinary elimination and taping catheter tubing prior to intercourse	D. Promotes a more optimal situation in preparation for a sexual encounter

INTERVENTION	RATIONALE
E. Suggestion to see physician regarding a penile implant	E. Assists in maintaining an erection
F. Offer films of positions, other procedures to facilitate sexual intercourse	F. Promotes successful intercourse with sexual satisfaction
G. Include significant other in all information and planning	G. Promotes relationship and gains assistance from partner when needed
H. Suggest sexual therapy, support group, counseling	H. Provides support and maximizes potential for sexual functioning
I. Suggest referral to fertility specialist	I. Provides information and support for reproductive potential

NURSING DIAGNOSES

Grieving, dysfunctional related to loss of physiopsychosocial well-being following spinal cord injury causing difficulty in adjustment to deficits and maintenance of health

Powerlessness related to illness-related regimen and life-style of helplessness resulting in dependence, loss of control over situations, apathy causing depression, frustration, and dissatisfaction with life

EXPECTED OUTCOMES

Progressive resolution of grief and control over daily situations evidenced by verbalization of losses and effect on life, denial, guilt, sorrow, and anger about loss; reduced frustration, dissatisfaction, doubt and dependence about control of and participation in own care

INTERVENTION	RATIONALE

I. Assess for:

A. Withdrawal behavior, denial, insomnia, expression of sadness, anger, guilt

    A. Signs and symptoms of grief

B. Expression of no control or influence over situation or outcome, depression, dissatisfaction, frustration, anger over dependence on others for body functions and care

    B. Indicates feelings of powerlessness to affect events in life and eventual outcome

IV. Perform/provide:

A. Grieving process and expected responses, allow time for resolution (varies with individuals and depends on changes to be made)

    A. Allows for nonjudgmental movement through stages of grieving and need for support during this time

B. Accepting environment to express phases of grief process with time as needed for resolution

    B. Allows for temporary use of defense mechanisms to support progressive movement through grieving process

C. Answer all questions honestly and sincerely, obtain information when needed

    C. Promotes trust in nurse–patient relationship

D. Maintain environment that is convenient to access belongings, comfortable with all needed articles/supplies/equipment needed for progressive self-care

    D. Reduces frustrations while promoting self-reliance to prevent constant requests for assistance

E. Allow for a visit from one who has had a similar injury

E. Promotes understanding from one who can relate to the consequences of cord trauma and associated feelings

F. Encourage participation in care planning and choice of assistive aids, assist with care only if needed or requested

F. Reduces dependence and feelings of helplessness

G. Encourage to review literature regarding the latest devices available and laws/legal resources to assist the physical disabled

G. Promotes independence by utilizing electronic devices, protecting against discrimination

H. Remind to continue with rehabilitation program

H. Promotes ongoing progress leading to independent lifestyle

NURSING DIAGNOSES

Knowledge deficit related to follow-up care including use and care of assistive devices, urinary and bowel management, changes in life-style and rehabilitation of sensory/motor deficits, signs and symptoms to report to physician

EXPECTED OUTCOMES

Adequate knowledge of follow-up care evidenced by compliance with and adaptation to long-term disabilities and rehabilitation plan (physical, occupational, vocational, elimination, sexual)

INTERVENTION	RATIONALE
I. Assess for:	
A. Readiness, willingness, and motivation to learn, discharge plan and lifestyle changes	A. Learning can best take place if client is receptive and compliance is more likely to occur
B. Health practices, health beliefs, ethnic identity (religion, diet, language), value orientations, family interactions and cooperation	B. Factors to incorporate into teaching plan to facilitate learning and compliance with long-term care
IV. Perform/provide:	
A. Acknowledgment of perceptions with a nonjudgmental attitude	A. Establishes nurse–patient relationship in an accepting environment
B. Explanations that are clear, accurate in understandable terms, small amount of information over time	B. Prevents misconceptions, erroneous attitudes and beliefs about disease
C. Environment conducive to learning with space, lighting, and proper equipment and supplies	C. Distractions or discomfort will interfere with learning
D. As much control over lifestyle change decisions as possible, include family in discharge planning	D. Allows power to be given or retained by patient
E. Teaching aids (pamphlets, videotapes, pictures, written instructions)	E. Reinforces learning

INTERVENTION	RATIONALE
F. Team of resource personnel/professionals	F. Nutritionist, social worker, counselor, physical/occupational/sexual rehabilitation therapists, and others can assist in teaching specific care and providing support for desired changes

V. Teach patient/family:

INTERVENTION	RATIONALE
A. Anatomy and pathophysiology of cord injury, nature of deficits	A. Promotes understanding of disorder that facilitates compliance
B. Rehabilitation program that can include physical and occupational therapy, development of alternative sexual, social, and recreational skills, vocational counseling, and counseling to assist in mental/emotional adaptation to disabilities	B. Promotes maximum function in areas of deficit to ensure an optimal productive life
C. Dietary and fluid daily intake	C. Ensures adequate nutritional and fluid requirements for general health
D. Measures to prevent skin breakdown, circulatory problems, muscle spasms or contractures, fatigue, burns, trauma	D. Prevents complications of immobilization and reduced motor/sensory deficits

INTERVENTION	RATIONALE
E. Elevate legs, avoid chilling or hot water or heaters nearby, avoid smoking alone, avoid hot foods and drinks, continue ROM and coughing exercises, correct positioning and alignment with protective padding/protectors to important parts (heels, elbows, pressure points)	E. Prevents complications associated with motor/sensory deficits
F. Intermittent catheterization and reinforcement of bowel and urinary retraining procedures, allow to demonstrate and practice	F. Manages bowel and bladder function
G. Community agencies to provide aids/supplies/equipment to rent or purchase, repair when needed	G. Ensures correct and functioning aids needed to function independently
H. Report temperature, cloudy, foul-smelling urine, vomiting, redness or irritation of skin, cough with yellow or greenish sputum, change in joint or muscle motion or swelling	H. Indicates infection or other complications to ensure early intervention
I. Stages of grieving process and expected responses, to allow time for resolution (varies with individuals and depends on changes to be made and extent of losses)	I. Allows for nonjudgmental movement through stages of grieving and need for support during this time

INTERVENTION	RATIONALE
J. Suggest home modifications to support performance of ADL, secure and utilize aids to support and continue independence, remove hazards that can cause falls	J. Maintains activities and control of self-care, safe environment if deficits are present
K. Community resources such as agencies and support groups for health maintenance	K. Provides information, support, and equipment for home care
L. Comply with scheduled physician appointments and therapy sessions	L. Monitors improvement or need to adjust therapy

transient ischemic attacks/carotid endarterectomy

DEFINITION
Transient ischemic attacks (TIAs) are temporary and short episodes of cerebral ischemia or cerebrovascular insufficiency caused by occlusion of the blood supply to an area of the brain. The most common site of occlusion is the carotid arterial system. Often referred to as "mini stroke," it is differentiated from cerebrovascular accident by its briefness (15 minutes to 1 hour) and transiency of the neurological symptoms (sensory and motor, mental changes). The most frequent surgical procedure performed to correct this condition is the carotid endarterectomy to remove the artherosclerotic plaque from the intima of the arteries to restore cerebral blood flow. This plan includes care specific to both the medical and surgical aspects of this condition and can be used in association with the PREOPERATIVE CARE, POSTOPERATIVE CARE, HYPERTENSION, and CEREBROVASCULAR ACCIDENT care plans

NURSING DIAGNOSES
Altered cerebral tissue perfusion related to interruption of arterial flow resulting in cerebral ischemia causing TIAs preoperatively and inability to tolerate clamping of artery during surgery, possible embolus or thrombosis at endarterectomy site postoperatively

Risk for injury related to internal factors of sensory and motor dysfunction resulting from TIAs (cerebral ischemia) causing possible physical trauma from falls preoperatively, temporary nerve damage postoperatively

EXPECTED OUTCOMES
Adequate cerebral perfusion and functional cerebral abilities retained evidenced by control of TIAs and associated symptoms of visual, auditory, mental deficits responsible for falls preoperatively, or postoperative embolus, hematoma or thrombosis at surgical site; absence of cranial nerve damage to facial, spinal accessory, hypoglossal, vagus nerves evidenced by return of taste perception, chewing and swallowing (saliva control and tongue deviation), speech (vocal cord paralysis) deficits

INTERVENTION	RATIONALE
I. Assess for:	
A. Headache, slowing mental processes and loss of consciousness, dizziness, motor or sensory changes (visual, auditory, vestibular disturbances, speech, seizures), number of episodes, frequency, length	A. Signs and symptoms of TIAs based on the area of brain lacking perfusion caused by inadequate blood flow to the brain
B. Lethargy, agitation, dizziness, diplopia, aphasia or slurred speech, paresthesia, hemiplegia, confusion, pupil reactions, level of consciousness	B. Indicates possible carotid arterial occlusion and cerebral ischemia preoperatively and postoperatively
C. Neurological function of cranial nerves VII (facial) causing ptosis or gustatory perception changes, X (vagus) causing swallowing or speech difficulty, XI (spinal accessory) causing shoulder sag, XII (hypoglossal) causing tongue biting or deviation, difficulty managing saliva and swallowing	C. Trauma and edema causing pressure to nerves as a result of close proximity to surgical site
D. Hematoma formation, amount of bleeding from wound or drain	D. Indicates bleeding excess at surgical site during first 24 hours postoperatively
II. Monitor, describe, record:	
A. Doppler carotid arterial studies, CT, carotid bruit auscultated	A. Procedures to diagnose risk for or presence of TIAs

INTERVENTION	RATIONALE
B. VS, especially blood pressure for levels of at least 120 mm Hg systolic	B. Maintains cerebral tissue perfusion postoperatively as surgical manipulation can interfere with baroreceptors in the carotid causing hypotension
C. Temporal pulse by palpation and auscultation by Doppler q4h for 24 hours	C. Determines internal carotid patency postoperatively
III. Administer: A. Antihypertensive PO	A. Acts to reduce blood pressure to prevent progression of TIAs, can be withheld prior to surgery to prevent hypotension postoperatively
B. Anticoagulant, antiplatelet PO	B. Acts to prevent clot formation
C. Anti-inflammatory IV	C. Acts to reduce edema at surgical site
IV. Perform/provide: A. Bed rest in flat position for TIAs or elevated to semi-Fowler's position if allowed postoperatively	A. Prevents cerebral ischemia during TIAs or to reduce edema at operative site
B. Application of cold locally	B. Reduces edema at surgical site
C. Support head during position changes and advise to use hands to hold head and neck when moving	C. Reduces pressure or stress on operative site

INTERVENTION	RATIONALE
D. Drainage system patency at surgical site	D. Prevents hematoma formation that causes compression of vessels to the brain
E. Withhold or offer foods that are easily chewed and swallowed, fluids that are thickened, moistened foods, when reflexes return or if temporary nerve damage evident	E. Prevents gagging or choking and possible aspiration following trauma to nerves that affect eating during surgery
F. Parenteral or tube feedings if necessary	F. Provides nutrition until oral intake permitted
G. Exercises and ROM to shoulder such as shrugs and finger climbing as appropriate to nerve impairment	G. Prevents atrophy of muscle and joint contracture

V. Teach patient/family:

A. Neurological status is usually normal between TIAs	A. Promotes understanding of the disorder to allay anxiety
B. Nerve damage is temporary and resolution time varies from days to months	B. Offers information and support to allay anxiety

NURSING DIAGNOSIS

Ineffective breathing pattern related to tracheobronchial obstruction resulting from surgical trauma and edema causing tracheal compression

EXPECTED OUTCOMES

Respiratory status maintained evidenced by rate, ease, depth within baseline determinations, absence of restlessness, stridor, neck muscle retraction, and tachypnea following surgery

INTERVENTION	RATIONALE
I. Assess for:	
A. Neck size increases, deviation of trachea from midline, difficulty swallowing, changes in respirations	A. Indicates edema, hematoma formation that have potential to cause tracheal obstruction
B. Deviation of the cricoid cartilage to the nonoperative side	B. Indicates progressive tracheal obstruction by an enlarging surgical site
II. Monitor, describe, record:	
A. Respiratory rate, depth, ease q2–4h, tachypnea, stridor, cyanosis, restlessness, agitation	A. Changes indicate respiratory distress or compromised respiratory status
B. ABGs, pulse oximetry	B. Determines abnormalities in oxygen level and need for supplemental oxygen
III. Administer:	
A. Oxygen via nasal cannula	A. Supplements oxygen based on results of blood gases and oximetry
IV. Perform/provide:	
A. Head of bed elevated 30 degrees	A. Reduces neck edema
B. Head and neck in alignment, avoid head rotation, neck flexion, hyperextension, moving head with abrupt movements	B. Prevents added tension or pressure on operative site
C. Loosen dressing on neck if tight	C. Prevents added pressure on wound

INTERVENTION	RATIONALE
D. Encourage coughing, deep breathing, incentive spirometry when risk of intracranial hypertension or rebleeding has subsided	D. Enhances ventilation and airway clearance
E. Tracheostomy tray and emergency supplies at bedside	E. Provides equipment for intervention if airway becomes obstructed

NURSING DIAGNOSIS

Knowledge deficit related to care requirements for TIAs and follow-up care for postoperative management of medication, wound care, dietary, and activity regimens

EXPECTED OUTCOMES

Adequate knowledge of preventive measures to treat TIAs and postoperative follow-up care evidenced by compliance with long-term antihypertensive therapy, specific measures for nerve damage if present, verbalization of signs and symptoms to report

INTERVENTION	RATIONALE
V. Teach patient/family:	
A. Cause and pathophysiology of TIAs, reason and expected effect of carotid endarterectomy	A. Provides information about the disorder and surgical intervention for better understanding and compliance of medical regimen
B. Medications regimen, probably for life to include action, dose, frequency, time, side effects	B. Compliance important to control TIAs and prevent a stroke

INTERVENTION	RATIONALE
C. Taking blood pressure and to record in a log, allow for return demonstration and practices of performing the procedure	C. Monitors effectiveness of therapy
D. Dietary information for low fat/cholesterol/sodium intake, and offer menus and meal planning assistance	D. Reduces progression of atherosclerosis
E. Foods that are easy to chew and swallow, sitting position for meals, thick fluids and moisten dry foods, add spices and sweetener for taste enhancement	E. Promotes dietary intake if nerve damage present
F. Exercises for shoulder, number of times and frequency/day	F. Promotes muscle function if nerve damage present
G. Report changes in appearance in wound (edema, discoloration), visual or speech changes, dizziness, weakness, irritability, confusion	G. Signs and symptoms of possible complications of surgery
H. Referral to nutritionist, speech pathologist, counseling as needed	H. Provides support and information to assist in convalescence
I. Keep appointments with physician as scheduled	I. Provides monitoring of pre- and postoperative condition and need to change therapeutic regimen

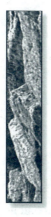

Hematologic/Immunologic Systems Standards

hematologic/immunologic systems data base

acquired immunodeficiency syndrome

anemia (hypovolemic/iron or folic acid deficiency/pernicious)

hemophilia

polycythemia (vera/secondary)

thrombocytopenia/splenectomy

hematologic/immunologic systems data base

HISTORICAL DATA REVIEW
Past events:
1. Acute and/or chronic blood and blood-forming organ disease or disorders, presence of other diseases that affect hematopoiesis and hemostasis
2. Signs and symptoms related to hematologic/immunologic disorders (bleeding episodes from any site, bruising, petechiae, enlarged nodes, fatigue, weakness, pallor, fever, chills)
3. Bleeding disorders or blood dyscrasias of family members
4. Allergies that can affect blood transfusions
5. Tobacco/alcohol use, exposure to toxic environmental agents
6. Treatments, transfusions, dietary habits (vitamin deficiency)
7. Medications (prescription and over-the-counter)
8. Hospitalizations and feelings about care, surgery associated with or affecting the hematologic system

Present events:
1. Medical diagnoses associated with or affecting hematologic/immunologic function
2. Vital signs (pulse and blood pressure) and changes related to blood loss or anemia
3. Abnormal skin changes such as small or large hemorrhages, jaundice
4. Prolonged bleeding from any mucous membrane site or into joints, delayed wound healing, night sweats, lethargy, malaise, fever, heat intolerance
5. Bone and joint pain, oral pain, lymph node pain, headache
6. Mentation or behavior changes, anxiety and coping difficulty
7. Responses to anemias (fatigue, weakness, dizziness, pallor, dyspnea, paresthesia, confusion, edema, and redness of oral cavity)
8. Tolerance for activities of daily living, ongoing treatments for chronic, long-term disorder

PHYSICAL ASSESSMENT DATA REVIEW

1. General appearance for dehydration, cachexia, ecchymoses or petechiae, bleeding from mucous membrane site
2. Liver and spleen size
3. Lymph nodes for size, location, tenderness, movement
4. Physical examination of systems associated with abnormalities

NURSING DIAGNOSES CONSIDERATIONS

1. Altered nutrition: Less than body requirements
2. Altered protection
3. Altered tissue perfusion
4. Fatigue
5. Fluid volume deficit
6. Risk for infection
7. Risk for injury
8. Impaired tissue integrity
9. Knowledge deficit
10. Pain

GERIATRIC CONSIDERATIONS

Hematologic changes in geriatric patients depend on the effect that the aging process has on nutritional intake and common chronic diseases in this population that can be related to blood abnormalities. Immunologic changes depend on the effect that the aging process has on the body's ability to protect itself from infection and neoplastic disorders. Hematologic and immunologic changes associated with aging that should be considered when assessing the geriatric patient include:

1. Atrophy of lymphoid tissue and gradual degeneration of thymus gland resulting in decreased immunity
2. Decreased capacity of bone marrow to produce blood cells resulting in a poor response to infection and anemia
3. Decreased antibodies resulting in a reduced response to antigens, reduced production of T-lymphocytes resulting in reduced ability to respond to antigens in tumor formation
4. Decreased immunocompetence resulting in reduced potential for survival from disease

5. Increased auto-antibodies resulting in susceptibility to autoimmune diseases
6. Impaired function of gastric cells causing a deficiency of intrinsic factor leading to pernicious anemia
7. Chewing, swallowing, anorexia, taste and smell deficits resulting in dietary intake deficiencies that can lead to nutritional anemias

DIAGNOSTIC LABORATORY TESTS AND PROCEDURES

1. Bone marrow aspiration and examination, gastrointestinal endoscopy if bleeding suspected, gastric analysis
2. Complete blood count with RBC, WBC, differential, red cell indices, Hct, Hb, platelets (CBC), blood smear, hemoglobin electrophoresis, prothrombin time (PT), partial thromboplastin time (PTT), thrombin time, fibrinogen, iron, iron-combining capacity, bleeding time, clot retraction, fibrin split products, capillary fragility, direct and indirect antiglobulin (Coombs'), coagulation factors, reticulocytes, bilirubin, blood typing and Rh factor, compatibility tests, Schilling test, heterophil antibody test, sickledex, enzyme-linked immunosorbent assay (ELISA), Western blot

MEDICATIONS

1. Anti-anemics: ferrous sulfate, ferrous gluconate, iron-dextran, cyanocobalamin, folic acid
2. Antimicrobials (AIDS): trimethoprim/sulfamethoxazole, dapsone, acyclovir, sulfadiazine/pyrimethamine, zidovudine, miconazole, ketoconazole, fluconazole, amphotericin B, zidovudine, retrovir
3. Corticosteroids: prednisone
4. Transfusions: whole blood, packed red blood cells, cryoprecipitate, coagulation factor VIII or IX concentrates, fresh frozen plasma or albumin/plasma protein fraction, platelet concentrates

acquired immunodeficiency syndrome

DEFINITION

Acquired immunodeficiency syndrome (AIDS), also known as human immunodeficiency virus (HIV), is a disease of the immune system. It is caused by a retrovirus that mostly affects T-helper lymphocytes (T4 lymphocytes), but also B cells, macrophages, and the cells of the brain, lymph nodes, spleen, and lungs. The virus causes eventual destruction of the T-helper lymphocytes and impairs cell-mediated immunity leading to profound immunosuppression. This leaves the infected individual prone to diseases such as opportunistic infections, malignancies, neurological disease, and general physical wasting. The virus can be found in the blood, cerebrospinal, and amniotic fluids, as well as the secretions of semen, vagina, breast milk, urine, saliva, and tears. The known routes of transmission include parenteral, sexual contact, pregnancy, and possibly breastfeeding. The disease is not known to be transmitted by casual contact with individuals, although there are societal fears that this is also a possibility. Those most at risk include participants in high-risk sexual practices, sharers of contaminated needles in drug addicts or an accidental needle stick, and recipients of transfusions of blood or blood products. New programs of blood testing prior to transfusion and public education for safe sexual conduct have been implemented to reduce the incidence of the disease. Following initial exposure, the disease follows a course identified by the Centers for Disease Control (CDC) that includes mild symptoms or acute infections and progresses to persistent symptoms and severe infections and finally end-stage severe diseases associated with HIV. This plan attempts to include care of the presenting symptomology and the complications associated with various stages of the disease

NURSING DIAGNOSES

Anxiety related to threat to or change in health status (seropositive for HIV), threat of death (poor prognosis and no effective treatment to prevent death), threat to self-concept, and interpersonal transmission of HIV (fear of exposure/transmission to family or partners) causing inability to manage feelings of uncertainty about outcome of the illness and apprehension regarding potential situation crisis

Ineffective individual coping related to inability to cope with illness (poor prognosis), personal vulnerability (rejection by others and inadequate support system), and life-style and role changes resulting in chronic anxiety, depression and worry, inability to problem-solve and meet basic needs

Powerlessness related to hospitalization and treatments, lack of control over illness or self-care resulting in increased apprehension and tension, feelings of helplessness and hopelessness as condition deteriorates, dependence on others for care

EXPECTED OUTCOMES

Anxiety and fear within manageable levels, development of coping and problem-solving skills, verbalizations that anxiety is decreasing, optimal participation and receptive attitude in planning for ongoing care and life-style changes needed to manage disease and chronic anxiety

INTERVENTION	RATIONALE
I. Assess for:	
A. Level of anxiety, use of coping mechanisms, stated fears of disease outcome, life-style changes, feelings of hopelessness	A. Anxiety can range from mild to severe, verbalizations assist to identify feelings and inappropriate use of coping skills
B. Restlessness, complaining, joking, withdrawal, talkativeness	B. Nonverbal expressions of anxiety when not able to communicate feelings
C. Personal resources to cope with stress, anxiety, and interest in learning to problem-solve	C. Support systems and personal strengths assist in developing coping skills

INTERVENTION	RATIONALE
D. Feelings and response to change in life-style, declining ability to carry out role and participate in activities, change in appearance as disease progresses	D. Changes in body image and self-concept common problem associated with AIDS
E. Expressed feelings of anger, fear, hostility, apathy, hopelessness	E. Results from feelings of powerlessness as disease progresses leading to increased debilitation and finally death

II. Monitor, describe, record:

A. ELISA (enzyme linked immunosorbent assay) performed twice	A. Reveals HIV antibody indicating exposure if positive
B. Western blot	B. Confirms presence of HIV

III. Administer:

A. Anti-anxiety agent PO	A. Acts to reduce anxiety level and provides calming effect and rest, depresses subcortical levels of CNS, limbic system

IV. Perform/provide:

A. Environment conducive to rest, and expressions of fear and anxiety, avoid anxiety-producing situations	A. Decreases stimuli that cause stress/anxiety, venting of feelings decreases anxiety
B. Orient to hospital room, staff, equipment, routines, and policies regarding visiting hours, others	B. Reduces anxiety and provides comfort and adjustment to a new situation

INTERVENTION	RATIONALE
C. Suggest new methods to enhance coping skills and problem solving, allow to externalize and identify those that help	C. Offers alternative coping strategies that allow for release of anxiety and fear
D. Positive feedback regarding progress made, focus on abilities rather than inabilities	D. Provides support for adaptive behavior, promotes self-worth and responsibility
E. Diversional activities such as relaxation exercises, TV, radio, music, reading, tapes, guided imagery	E. Reduces anxiety and promotes comfort
F. Allow visitors according to desire and condition, avoid stressful situations	F. Promotes support from significant others/family to decrease anxiety
G. Allow to participate in planning of care to maintain usual activities when possible	G. Allows for some control over situations
H. Support grieving for loss of life-style and restrictions in activities, changes in physical appearance	H. Provides assistance in adaptation to changes imposed by disease
I. Information about economic/legal/social resources, recent research and treatments available, hotlines, task forces, AIDS projects	I. Provides information and promotes control over present and future life-style changes, assists with finances, discrimination, living arrangements, medical care

NURSING DIAGNOSES

Social isolation related to unaccepted social behavior (drug abuse, sexual preference), inability to engage in satisfying personal relationship resulting from stigma associated with HIV-positive status, fear of exposure/transmission of disease, loss of confidentiality about HIV

Impaired social interaction related to therapeutic isolation (immunosuppressed state), available significant others (stigma associated with AIDS), altered thought processes (opportunistic brain infection) resulting in dysfunctional relationship with friends, family, significant others

Altered sexuality patterns related to conflicts with sexual orientation or preference, fear of acquiring or transmitting AIDS resulting in need to change and/or place limitations on sexual behaviors or activities (use of condoms)

EXPECTED OUTCOMES

Improved quality and quantity of social interactions and relationships with significant others and those in the community, reduced fear of sexual expression and feelings of rejection and loneliness evidenced by verbalization of understanding about the effect of HIV on sexual behavior and need for modification acceptable to partner

INTERVENTION	RATIONALE
I. Assess for:	
A. Immunosuppressed state and need for therapeutic isolation based on results of laboratory tests and health status	A. Determines need for protective care to reduce risk of transmission of infective organisms to the host
B. Decreased interest in social interactions, relationships, hostility and sadness, verbalizations of depression, rejection, loneliness	B. Indicates decreasing social activities with negative emotional responses

INTERVENTION	RATIONALE
C. Sexual preference and behavior, knowledge of HIV transmission and limitations of behavior	C. Provides information regarding need for information to promote relationships
D. Feelings of insecurity in public, indifference of significant others, and effect on life-style, work, social activities	D. Responses of public opinion about AIDS

IV. Perform/provide:

INTERVENTION	RATIONALE
A. Private room and supplies to support protective isolation	A. Prevents transmission of infectious agents to immunosuppressed patient
B. Procedures including use of gowns, mask, gloves, care of linen, used articles and supplies, handwash prior to and after contact	B. Reduces risk for infection by carrying out universal precautions
C. Special care in treatment of all information with confidentiality, inform of rights regarding testing results and discrimination laws	C. Protects from job and insurability losses, rejection by society
D. Encourage to continue relationships with those that are accepting and feel comfortable with, such as physician, clergy, staff, AIDS volunteers	D. Decreases social isolation
E. Contact with friends and family by telephone, visits as appropriate using touch and assisting with care	E. Promotes contact and prevents feelings of rejection

INTERVENTION	RATIONALE
F. Precautions to take during intercourse (condoms), using clean needles for drug injections, informing sexual partner of HIV status prior to intercourse	F. Prevents transmission by semen or blood and reduces fear of acquiring or transmitting the disease
G. Include partner in discussions of changes in sexual patterns, some activities to express sexuality to prevent transmission	G. Provides other methods to meet sexual needs based on level of weakness and fear of contracting or transmitting disease

NURSING DIAGNOSES

Altered role performance related to family planning, parenting ability, change in physical ability to perform role(s) resulting in role conflict, role denial, and rejection of responsibility

Altered family processes related to situational crisis of disclosure or fear of disclosure of AIDS diagnosis of/to family member resulting in fear of contracting the disease, change in role and decision making in the family and anticipatory grief associated with debilitation and early death

EXPECTED OUTCOMES

Adaption to role changes as a parent, spouse, and usual responsibilities, family participation in meeting physical, emotional, and spiritual needs of member with AIDS evidenced by verbalization of acceptance of diagnosis, ability to make decisions to deal with the crisis and become involved in care and community activities

INTERVENTION	RATIONALE
I. Assess for:	
A. Personal status regarding nuclear and extended family, marital status, significant others, varied roles established, role failure, loss, or conflict	A. Reveals personal and family present and future relationships and responsibilities

INTERVENTION	RATIONALE
B. Feelings about role changes, changes in roles of family members, feelings of family about diagnosis and participation in care through the stages of the disease, cultural factors influencing role of family members	B. Reveals information about capacity to assume or resume role, family ability to provide care and support

IV. Perform/provide

INTERVENTION	RATIONALE
A. Environment that is supportive and nonjudgmental and allows expression about loss of roles and physical health	A. Promotes comfort and rapport of nurse–patient relationship
B. Assistance to identify and use strategies to deal with role changes; assist family to adjust to changes in lifestyle and interactions of members	B. Allows for progressive adaptation to changes by patient and family
C. Assistance to family to become more flexible and change behaviors during stressful times, set priorities for important activities when needed	C. Allows for improved family relationships and adjustment to situations
D. Information regarding disease and transmission, plan of care, and possible changes in family structure to provide support and care	D. Facilitates family's understanding of the diagnosis and permits formulation of goals to care for family member

INTERVENTION	RATIONALE
E. Inclusion of family members and significant others in decisions and planning of care	E. Provides support for interactions among family and and promotes participation in care

NURSING DIAGNOSES

Activity intolerance related to generalized weakness, fatigue, symptoms of opportunistic infection (dyspnea, fever, chills, arthralgia, malnutrition) resulting in decreased endurance, and inability to perform ADL

Sleep pattern disturbance related to internal factors of illness (night sweats, chills, dyspnea, pruritis), drug withdrawal resulting in psychological stress (anxiety, fear, depression), inability to sleep (insomnia)

Bathing/hygiene, dressing/grooming, toileting self-care deficit related to weakness, fatigue, pain, impaired mobility resulting in inability to wash, dress, get to the toilet, perform personal hygiene tasks

EXPECTED OUTCOMES

Progressive increase in activity tolerance and improved sleep and rest pattern with reduction in fatigue level evidenced by increased performance of ADL activities with or without assistance and within limitations, decreased symptoms of infectious process, increased energy and endurance, VS stable before, during, and after activity, uninterrupted sleep with verbalizations that feeling more rested and less anxious

INTERVENTION	RATIONALE
I. Assess for:	
A. Level of fatigue, weakness, and potential for activity progression, effect of dyspnea, temperature, pain on activity	A. Provides baseline and allows for planning activities and need for assistance (dependent on stage of illness)
B. Interest and ability in performing ADL with or without assistance	B. Readiness and increased energy level necessary for successful program

INTERVENTION	RATIONALE
C. Sleep/rest pattern, wakefulness during night, irritability, lethargy	C. Optimal rest and sleep necessary to reduce fatigue and increase strength
D. R >20/minute, P >120/bpm and not returning to preactivity level within 3 minutes, palpitations, dyspnea, dizziness, weakness, and stopping activity if symptoms appear	D. Signs and symptoms of activity intolerance leading to fatigue

III. Administer:

INTERVENTION	RATIONALE
A. Sedative PO, unless respirations <12/minute	A. Acts on limbic and subcortical levels of CNS and increases sleep time
B. Oxygen via nasal cannula	B. Supplements oxygen during daily activities and sleep as needed
C. Whole blood, packed RBC via IV transfusion	C. Increases oxygen-carrying capacity if anemic to improve activity tolerance

IV. Perform/provide:

INTERVENTION	RATIONALE
A. Bed rest in a position of comfort with body parts supported with pillows, restricted activities as ordered	A. Conserves energy and provides needed rest

INTERVENTION	RATIONALE
B. Perform or assist in ADL and other activities as needed, place all articles and call light within reach to use as desired, utilize self-care aids as appropriate	B. Conserves energy while preserving as much control and independence as possible
C. Increase activities gradually from sitting up in bed, in chair, walking in room, to bathroom, and in hall with daily increase in distance and ADL, suggest deep breathing during activities	C. Progressive change in activities increases with endurance and energy level and prevents symptoms of activity intolerance (dependent on stage of illness)
D. Organize activities around rest periods in a quiet, calm, dimly lit, environment free of stimuli	D. Permits rest without interruptions
E. Assist to assume preferred position for sleep, offer backrub, oral care, extra pillows, use of bathroom, other activities based on sleep pattern	E. Provides for usual bedtime rituals to ensure comfort and sleep
F. Restrict visitors and limit time of visit with patient's acceptance	F. Prevents additional stimuli that interferes with rest, causes fatigue

NURSING DIAGNOSES

Altered nutrition: Less than body requirements related to inability to ingest or absorb nutrients because of biologic factors (anorexia, diarrhea, opportunistic infection of upper or lower gastrointestinal tract) resulting in malnutrition, wasting in later stages

Risk for fluid volume deficit related to excessive losses through normal routes (diarrhea, diaphoresis, temperature elevation) resulting in possible dehydration

EXPECTED OUTCOMES

Adequate nutrition and fluid intake evidenced by daily ingestion of fluid/caloric requirements, absence of diarrhea, temperature, and oral/pharyngeal/esophageal/gastroenteric infection, weight and I&O within baseline determinations

INTERVENTION	RATIONALE
I. Assess for:	
A. Dietary pattern and intake including calories, basic four, vitamins and minerals	A. Provides baseline data for possible nutritional deficiencies
B. Anorexia, dysphagia, stomatitis, oral pain, periodontitis, effect on eating	B. Indicates changes caused by inflammatory process resulting in decreased intake
C. Diarrhea, amount and frequency, possible losses from other routes	C. Source of active fluid loss
D. Fluid daily intake, preferred fluids, calculated daily fluid need	D. Determines if adjustment in fluid intake is needed
E. Dry skin and mucous membrane, thirst, poor skin turgor, decreased urinary output	E. Indicates risk for dehydration
II. Monitor, describe, record:	
A. I&O q4–8h depending on illness stage	A. Reveals fluid balance or need to adjust the ratio
B. Weight on same scale, same time, same clothing daily/weekly	B. Monitors gains and losses indicating nutritional deficiencies, losses in advanced stage resulting in wasting syndrome

INTERVENTION	RATIONALE
C. Electrolytes	C. Decreases indicate losses caused by diarrhea
D. Feces, oral, throat cultures	D. Identifies infectious agent causing diarrhea, stomatitis, pharyngitis

III. Administer:

INTERVENTION	RATIONALE
A. Antidiarrheal PO	A. Acts to control diarrhea by decreasing intestinal spasms and motility
B. Hormone antineoplastic agent PO	B. Acts to stimulate appetite and weight gain in AIDS

IV. Perform/provide:

INTERVENTION	RATIONALE
A. Dietary supplements and food inclusions (high caloric) based on deficiency, restrictions based on sore mouth and throat	A. Provides foods to treat deficiencies, prevents malnutrition
B. Small, frequent meals of soft foods, high-calorie liquid supplements such as Ensure	B. Provides optimal nutritional intake while preventing discomfort of chewing or swallowing
C. Oral care with soft brush, mouth rinses prior to and after meals with saline or hydrogen peroxide solution, position dentures in place if needed for meals	C. Prevents irritation of oral mucosa and promotes comfort
D. Fluid intake increased to 2 to 3 L/day, avoid hot, acid, carbonated liquids that could irritate oral cavity	D. Provides fluid replacement

INTERVENTION	RATIONALE
E. Initiate tube feedings or total parenteral nutrition (TPN)	E. Maintains nutritional needs as condition changes
F. Referral to nutritionist	F. Assists to modify diet to correct deficiencies

NURSING DIAGNOSES

Risk for infection related to inadequate secondary defenses (immunodeficiency) resulting from disease (HIV) causing opportunistic infections (lungs, brain, skin, oral cavity)

Hyperthermia related to illness (opportunistic infectious process)

EXPECTED OUTCOMES

Infection-free status or resolution of opportunistic infection and temperature elevation evidenced by temperature, WBC, cultures within normal levels, and absence of signs and symptoms of infection at susceptible sites

INTERVENTION	RATIONALE
I. Assess for:	
A. Dyspnea or other respiratory changes, decreased breath sounds and crackles auscultated, pleuritic pain, cough with yellowish to greenish sputum and increased tenaciousness	A. Signs and symptoms of pulmonary infection, upper or lower tract (*Pneumocystis carinii* pneumonia)
B. Skin eruptions, pruritus, herpes simplex or zoster, impetigo, abscess, histoplasmosis, others (malignancies)	B. Indicates cutaneous infections common to AIDS with more than one skin infection present, possible Kaposi's sarcoma
C. Cloudy, foul-smelling urine, urgency, frequency, dysuria	C. Indicates urinary tract infection

INTERVENTION	RATIONALE
D. Oral mucosa inflammation, lesions, irritation, pain, dysphagia, periodontitis, mucositis, cheesy white vaginal discharge, lesions, irritation of rectal area	D. Indicates fungus infection of upper gastrointestinal system or vagina/rectum (*Candida albicans*)
E. Changes in mentation, memory, disorientation, headache, lethargy, delirium, seizures	E. Indicates infection of the central nervous system (*Toxoplasmosis gondii*)
F. Temperature elevation, chills, excess diaphoresis, night sweats	F. Indicates presence of infection in any organ of the body
II. Monitor, describe, record: A. Temperature q4h and PRN, and VS q4h if pulmonary infection present or suspected	A. Elevations in temperature, pulse, and respirations indicate infection
B. Neurological checks q4–8h	B. Notes changes indicating progressive neurological deficit
C. WBC and differential	C. WBC of >12,000/mm^3 indicates infectious process
D. Sputum, urine, feces, skin, blood, oral, vaginal/anal cultures	D. Identifies infectious agent and evaluates antimicrobial therapy
E. Chest x ray	E. Reveals areas of consolidation in diagnosis of pneumonia

INTERVENTION	RATIONALE
III. Administer:	
A. Antimicrobial PO, IV	A. Acts to prevent cell-wall synthesis to destroy microorganisms in the treatment of acute infection
B. Corticosteroid PO, IV, TOP	B. Acts as an anti-inflammatory agent to reduce inflammation and increase body defenses in acute infection
C. Antipyretic PO	C. Acts to reduce temperature
D. Antiviral agent PO	D. Acts to prevent or treat opportunistic infection by preventing replication of HIV
E. Immunologic agent IM, SC	E. Acts to reduce viral and proliferative activity in Kaposi's sarcoma
F. Oxygen via nasal cannula	F. Provides supplemental oxygen in pulmonary complication
IV. Perform/provide:	
A. Environment with optimal temperature, humidity, and ventilation	A. Promotes comfort and respiratory ease
B. Handwash prior to and after giving care, inform to wash hands after using bathroom, before meals	B. Prevents transmission of pathogens

INTERVENTION	RATIONALE
C. Calm, restful environment with warm blankets and change of damp linens or clothing	C. Prevents stimuli that decreases rest and prevents chilling associated with fever
D. Backrub, sponge bath, relaxation techniques	D. Cooling measures to decrease temperature and promote comfort
E. Fluid intake of 2 to 3 L/day as permitted, warm fluids if chilled	E. Replaces fluid lost from diaphoresis as temperature increases or persists
F. Adequate nutritional intake of high-calorie, high-protein diet	F. Ensures nutritional status to prevent infection and maintain health status
G. Change position q2h, encourage deep-breathing and coughing exercises, semi-Fowler's position	G. Measures to prevent pulmonary secretion stasis and facilitate ventilation
H. Avoid exposure to visitors or staff with upper respiratory infection	H. Prevents transmission of infectious agents
I. Void as soon as urge is present and wipe from front to back	I. Prevents urinary stasis leading to infection
J. Cleanse perineal area with warm water and mild soap, pat dry following each diarrhea or incontinence episode	J. Prevents skin irritation and breakdown
K. Bathwater with cornstarch, baking soda for itching, cream or oil to dry skin	K. Allays pruritis, moisturizes skin if needed

INTERVENTION	RATIONALE
L. Offer mouth care of saline or baking soda solution rinses q4h, apply oil or petrolatum to lips, use soft toothbrush or damp cloth to cleanse teeth	L. Soothes and cleanses oral mucous membranes and lubricates lips to maintain integrity
M. Sterile technique for all invasive procedures and intravenous site care, change tubings, dressings, catheters according to policy	M. Prevents introduction of pathogens
N. Reorient, repeat words as needed, reduce stimuli, allow time to perform activity or speak, assist when needed	N. Provides attention to changes in mental competency/thought processes and reassurance if confused or slow to respond
O. Cleansing and disinfection of equipment, disposal of supplies used in treatments according to universal precautions	O. Prevents transmission of infectious agent

NURSING DIAGNOSES

Anticipatory grieving related to loss of physiopsychosocial well-being, losses of position in society and family (work, housing, friends and associates, independence, personal possessions), and loss of life (fatal illness)

Spiritual distress related to effects on life caused by disease and early or approaching death, lack of support system

EXPECTED OUTCOMES

Progressive movement toward resolution of grieving and improved spiritual well-being evidenced by verbalizations of support from belief system and awareness of the disease and loss of health

INTERVENTION	RATIONALE
I. Assess for:	
A. Feelings about life and comfort with belief system, participation in formal religious affiliation	A. Provides data about spiritual status
B. Expression of feelings about loss of health and life, anger, denial, withdrawal, appetite, energy, sleep	B. Identifies emotional reactions regarding grieving
IV. Perform/provide:	
A. Accepting environment to express anger, fear, and concerns	A. Facilitates grieving process, allows to externalize feelings to acknowledge the diagnosis and potential losses
B. Time to progress through stages of grief without judgment or criticisms, inform of the different stages of grieving and what to expect	B. Individuals vary in time needed to resolve each stage of the process before acceptance of loss and develop constructive strategies to cope with losses
C. Support for behaviors expressing grief, encourage established relationships and communication	C. Assists to adapt to losses, maintains support system
D. Positive attitude in assisting to recognize strengths, clarify information about present and future losses	D. Provides guidance to develop realistic goals for changes in life-style
E. Rituals, quiet time, clergy of choice if requested	E. Enhances spiritual well-being

INTERVENTION	RATIONALE
F. Referral to spiritual or psychological counseling	F. Provides professional support if appropriate

NURSING DIAGNOSIS
Knowledge deficit related to information regarding the disease AIDS, treatments, preventive measures for transmission and opportunistic infections, medical monitoring of disease

EXPECTED OUTCOMES
Adequate knowledge of follow-up regimen evidenced by compliance with preventive information, absence of infections, verbalization of signs and symptoms to report

INTERVENTION	RATIONALE
I. Assess for:	
A. Readiness, willingness, and motivation to learn, perform discharge care and life-style changes	A. Learning can best take place if client is receptive and compliance is more likely to occur
B. Health practices, health beliefs, ethnic identity, value orientations, family interactions and cooperation	B. Factors to incorporate into teaching to facilitate learning and compliance with long-term care
C. Home for kitchen, bathroom, and laundry provisions	C. Provides information about safety precautions regarding falls and sanitary practices
IV. Perform/provide:	
A. Acknowledgment of perceptions with a nonjudgmental attitude	A. Establishes nurse–patient relationship in an accepting manner

INTERVENTION	RATIONALE
B. Explanations that are clear, accurate in understandable terms, small amount of information over time	B. Prevents erroneous information, allows for patience, time, and understanding of new procedures to learn for regulation of the disease
C. Environment conducive to learning with space, lighting, and proper equipment and supplies	C. Distractions or discomfort will interfere with learning
D. As much control over lifestyle change decisions as possible, include family in discharge planning	D. Allows power to be given or retained by patient
E. Teaching aids (pamphlets, video tapes, pictures, written instructions)	E. Reinforces learning
F. Demonstration of procedures and time for return demonstration and practices with encouragement	F. Hands-on experience enhances and reinforces learning
V. Teach patient/family:	
A. Pathophysiology of the disease, changes in the immune system, risk for or presence of AIDS, high-risk groups, mode of transmission	A. Promotes understanding of disease and risk factors for transmission prior to or early in the disease
B. Inform of reactions of others toward those with AIDS, and explore ways to deal with these if they occur, inform that confidentiality will be honored if desired	B. Lack of knowledge or misinformation has resulted in stigma against AIDS population

INTERVENTION	RATIONALE
C. Inform of use of condom, refrain from giving blood or semen for artificial insemination, sex with prostitutes or those with multiple sexual partners or use of drugs	C. Prevents transmission to sexual partner, receivers of blood transfusion, newborns, or drug users
D. Precautionary measures if sexually active, including: a. Avoid pregnancy b. Select HIV-negative sexual partners c. Avoid unsafe sexual activities (improper use of condom, allowing body fluids or secretions to come in contact with breaks in skin or mucosa d. Avoid unsafe IV drug use (sharing needles, not cleaning skin and needles well)	D. Prevents spread of HIV
E. Precautionary measures for infections, including: a. Wash hands after contact with body fluids or secretions using liquid soap b. Disinfect kitchen and bathroom and any areas with spills or soiled with blood or body fluids c. Avoid sharing eating, personal hygiene articles	E. Prevents risk for opportunistic infections

   d. Maintain nutritional/fluid
      intake and a rest/activity
      schedule

   e. Wash clothes and linens
      with bleach if soiled

   f. Dressings, tampons, arti-
      cles used for care dis-
      posed of in a plastic bag
      and then placed in a la-
      beled container

F. Medication regimen to include drug name, action
   and why prescribed, dos-
   age, frequency and when
   to take, signs and symptoms
   to report, provide written
   instructions for drug administration, avoid over-the-
   counter medications unless
   advised by physician

F. Promotes compliance with
   proper administration for
   each drug taken to treat
   AIDS

G. Report fever, chills,
   headache, changes in
   breathing, urine, skin, diarrhea, sore mouth, weakness,
   visual changes, dizziness,
   weight loss, and any other
   questionable complaints

G. Indicates infection and allows for early interventions
   if needed

H. Importance of follow-up appointments with physician,
   professional referrals such
   as counseling, social
   worker, lawyer, others

H. Encourages compliance with
   physician visits to monitor
   disease

INTERVENTION

I. Inform of support groups for AIDS such as hotlines, networks, foundations, CDC, public health services, hospice services, buddy programs

RATIONALE

I. Provides community resources for assistance if needed

anemia
(hypovolemic/iron or folic acid deficiency/pernicious)

DEFINITION
Anemia is a condition or manifestation of a condition characterized by a decrease in red blood cells (RBC), or erythrocytes, resulting in a reduction in the transport of oxygen to all cells of the body. The condition also involves a decrease in hemoglobin (Hb) and hematocrit (Hct). Its reduced oxygen-carrying capacity causes hypoxia and its associated signs and symptoms related to all systems. Types of anemias included in this plan include acquired anemias caused by a reduced red cell production (iron or folic acid deficiency, pernicious anemia) and by blood loss or hemorrhage (hypovolemic). Increased metabolic needs or inadequate intake of iron and folic acid or deficiency of intrinsic factor needed to absorb B_{12} cause a reduction in RBC production. Chronic or acute blood loss cause excessive loss of RBCs.

NURSING DIAGNOSES
Impaired gas exchange related to altered oxygen-carrying capacity of blood resulting from reduced numbers of RBCs, Hb causing hypoxia

Ineffective breathing pattern related to decreased energy and fatigue resulting from hypoxia and causing dyspnea, tachypnea

Activity intolerance related to imbalance between oxygen supply and demand resulting from decreased RBC, Hb causing hypoxia, weakness, and fatigue

EXPECTED OUTCOMES
Adequate ventilation and tissue oxygenation with improvement in activity tolerance evidenced by respiration rate, depth, and ease, RBC, Hb within baseline determinations as anemic state resolves, absence of exertional dyspnea, weakness, and verbalization that energy and endurance increased

INTERVENTION	RATIONALE
I. Assess for:	
A. Respiratory rate, depth, ease, exertional dyspnea, palpitations, tachycardia, dizziness	A. Indicates severity of anemia and associated hypoxia
B. Activity level and tolerance, pattern of activities, ability to perform ADL, factors that precipitate fatigue, amount of sleep/rest	B. Provides baseline data for planning assistive care to prevent fatigue
II. Monitor, describe, record:	
A. VS q4h and PRN	A. Indicates changes in status resulting from increased oxygen need and cardiac output
B. RBC, Hb for decreases, red cell indices	B. Range of Hb for mild anemia is 10 to 14 g/dL, moderate anemia is 6 to 10 g/dL, severe anemia is <6 g/dL, RBC decreased to <4,000,000/cu mm; abnormally large sized RBC indicates pernicious or folic acid deficiency anemia
C. Schilling test	C. Indicates pernicious anemia with a positive test of 5% or less tagged vitamin B_{12}
III. Administer:	
A. Oxygen via nasal cannula	A. Provides supplemental tissue oxygenation if needed

INTERVENTION	RATIONALE
IV. Perform/provide:	
A. Position for comfort, semi- or high Fowler's in chair or bed	A. Facilitates breathing if dyspnea is present
B. Assist with ADL when needed, refrain from activities that cause fatigue or increased weakness	B. Conserves energy and prevents fatigue
C. Schedule rest periods around activities	C. Allows for uninterrupted rest periods
D. Progressive increases in self-care and ambulation as tolerated	D. Increases endurance and sense of independence and control
E. Energy-saving techniques and aids for ADL, place articles within reach, and anticipate needs when possible	E. Conserves energy while maintaining independence

NURSING DIAGNOSIS

Altered nutrition: Less than body requirements related to inability to ingest foods containing iron and folate, to biologic factor of lack of intrinsic factor in the stomach to allow absorption of B_{12} resulting in anemia

EXPECTED OUTCOMES

Adequate nutritional intake of iron, folate with deficiency resolved evidenced by iron, total iron binding capacity, folic acid, ferritin within normal ranges, absence of signs and symptoms of anemia

INTERVENTION	RATIONALE
I. Assess for:	
A. Dietary pattern and intake including calories, basic four, vitamins and minerals	A. Provides baseline data for possible nutritional deficiencies
B. Anorexia, nausea, vomiting, feeling of fullness, discomfort in epigastric region	B. Indicates gastrointestinal changes in any of the anemias
C. Oral mucosa for lesions, glossy red tongue, stomatitis, painful and burning tongue	C. Indicates nutritional deficiency of iron
II. Monitor, describe, record:	
A. Serum iron, total iron binding capacity (TIBC), folic acid, ferritin	A. Iron or folic acid deficiency anemia indicated by decreases of <50 mcg/dL TIBC, <4 ng/dL folic acid, <2.5 ng/dL iron
B. Weight on same scale, same time and same clothing daily/weekly	B. Monitors gains and losses indicating nutritional deficiencies
III. Administer:	
A. Iron supplement PO, IM (Z-track if appropriate)	A. Acts to replace iron deficiency anemia
B. Folic acid PO, IM, Vitamin C PO	B. Acts to replace folic acid deficiency anemia
C. Cyanocobalamin IM	C. Acts to provide vitamin B_{12} in pernicious anemia

INTERVENTION	RATIONALE
IV. Perform/provide:	
A. Dietary supplements and food inclusions based on deficiency, restrictions based on sore mouth and tongue	A. Provides foods to treat deficiencies
B. Small, frequent meals	B. Provides optimal nutritional intake while preventing early satiety, nausea, vomiting, indigestion, bloating
C. Oral care with soft brush, mouth rinses prior to and after meals with saline or hydrogen peroxide solution	C. Prevents irritation of oral mucosa and promotes comfort
D. Apply artificial saliva to mouth, vaseline to lips	D. Treats dry mouth and prevents dry, cracking lips
E. Referral to nutritionist	E. Assists to modify diet to correct deficiencies

NURSING DIAGNOSES

Altered tissue perfusion (all systems) related to hypovolemia resulting from blood loss causing reduced cardiac output and risk for shock state

Fluid volume deficit related to active loss resulting from chronic or acute blood loss causing anemic response or possible hypovolemic shock

EXPECTED OUTCOMES

Adequate tissue and organ perfusion and blood volume evidenced by VS, skin color, quality, and temperature, urinary output, mentation within baseline parameters

INTERVENTION	RATIONALE
I. Assess for:	
A. Exertional dyspnea, weakness, palpitations, dizziness	A. Symptoms associated with anemia caused by chronic bleeding
B. Tachypnea, tachycardia, decreased BP, pallor and clammy skin	B. Indicates reduced cardiac output and cardiopulmonary hypoxia of impending shock caused by acute blood loss
C. Dizziness, headache, faintness, changes in mentation	C. Indicates decreased cerebral perfusion and symptoms of chronic or acute blood loss
D. Numbness, tingling, coldness of extremities, peripheral pulses capillary refill	D. Indicates decreased peripheral perfusion
E. Urinary output of <30 mL/hr	E. Indicates decreased renal perfusion
II. Monitor, describe, record:	
A. BP, P, R, temperature q15 minutes to q1h as appropriate	A. Indicates changes leading to shock state
III. Administer:	
A. Albumin, dextran, Ringer's lactate IV	A. Replaces fluid and electrolyte losses
B. Whole blood, packed RBC transfusion IV	B. Immediate replacement of blood loss or RBCs depending on need
IV. Perform/provide:	
A. Bed rest, assistance with activities if weak	A. Promotes rest to prevent fatigue

INTERVENTION	RATIONALE
B. Increased oral fluids if allowed	B. Replaced deficit in chronic blood loss
C. Place flat in bed, elevate legs, initiate oxygen and IV fluids/blood, continuous monitoring of VS and ECG	C. Emergency treatment in hypovolemic shock
D. Discontinue transfusion in presence of dyspnea, wheezing, temperature, chills	D. Indicates reaction to transfusion and possible impending anaphylactic shock

NURSING DIAGNOSIS

Knowledge deficit related to resolution of anemia and ongoing care including nutritional and medication regimens, signs and symptoms to report

EXPECTED OUTCOMES

Compliance with instructions and performance of treatments to correct anemia and prevent recurrence

INTERVENTION	RATIONALE
V. Teach patient/family: A. Condition of the anemia, causes, pathophysiology of symptomology	A. Basic information to promote understanding of anemia
B. Administration of oral medications including action, dose, time, frequency, expected results, side effects to report, color change of feces if iron is administered	B. Promotes recovery from nutritional deficiency

INTERVENTION	RATIONALE
C. Maintain schedule of medication IM administration, lifelong injections for pernicious anemia, instruct family member if appropriate	C. Promotes recovery and maintains status
D. High-fiber diet, stool softener	D. Acts to treat or prevent constipation during iron therapy
E. Dietary modifications to include a. Whole-grain breads/cereals, organ meats, green vegetables, eggs, legumes, oysters, or	E. Supplements diet with deficient nutrients Foods rich in iron
b. Meats, whole-grain breads/cereals, nuts, fruits, fish, legumes, green leafy vegetables, or	Foods rich in folate
c. Organ meats, eggs, pork, milk, chicken, oysters	Foods rich in B_{12}
F. Avoid hot, spicy, irritating foods and smoking, select soothing foods such as ice cream and popsicles	F. Irritates oral mucosa
G. Remind to keep laboratory tests appointments, offer a written schedule of dates and times	G. Determines if anemia is resolved and that it does not predispose to severe complications such as heart failure from low Hb levels
H. Report dyspnea, dizziness, black tarry feces, slow, long-term bleeding from any source caused by medications such as anticoagulants, aspirin	H. Signs and symptoms to report

hemophilia

DEFINITION

Hemophilia is a congenital disorder affecting blood coagulation capability. Hemophilia A, the most common type, is caused by a deficiency in factor VIII, the antihemophilic globulin coagulation factor. Hemophilia B is caused by a deficiency in factor IX, the plasma thromboplastin coagulation factor. The severity of the disease (slow persistent bleeding to hemorrhage and hematoma formation) depends on the degree of activity of the coagulation factor.

NURSING DIAGNOSES

Altered protection related to abnormal blood profile (coagulation) resulting from disease causing altered clotting and hemorrhagic conditions

   Pain related to physical injuring agent of pressure of hematoma on peripheral nerves and bleeding into joints (hemarthrosis)

EXPECTED OUTCOMES

Pain relieved or controlled and management of bleeding episodes maintained evidenced by verbalization that pain reduced with analgesic, and minimal or absence of internal or external hemorrhage

INTERVENTION	RATIONALE
I. Assess for: A. Pain in areas of hematoma formation, joints such as knees, elbows, wrists, hips, shoulder, others	A. Provides pain descriptors for analgesic and other pain-reducing care, administration of factor to control bleeding

INTERVENTION	RATIONALE
B. Bleeding from mouth and gums, hematemesis, hemoptysis, epistaxis, hematuria, neck or joint swelling, hematomas in subcutaneous tissue, following dental extraction, any small cuts or open injury to the skin	B. Common sites of bleeding from trauma or spontaneous hemorrhage
II. Monitor, describe, record: A. VS when bleeding occurs	A. Excessive bleeding can predispose to hypovolemic shock and causing increased P and decreased BP
B. Coagulation factor assay	B. Reveals absent factor VIII or IX of up to 1 to 3% indicating severe state or up to 25% indicating mild to moderate deficiency
C. PTT, bleeding time, clotting time, platelet count	C. Reveals prolonged time of >6 minutes for bleeding time, more than 2 minutes for clotting time, more than 1 minute for PTT, normal platelet count
III. Administer: A. Analgesic PO, avoid aspirin and injection administration	A. Acts to reduce pain caused by compression of hematoma or blood accumulation in tissues or joints
B. Anti-inflammatory PO	B. Acts to reduce joint pain and edema

INTERVENTION	RATIONALE
C. Packed red or white blood cells IV	C. Replaces blood volume in severe hemorrhage
D. Cryoprecipitate (AHF therapy) IV for factor VIII, fresh-frozen plasma IV for factor IX, AHF therapy derived from animal sources with development of anti-AHF (auto-immune antibodies)	D. Replaces clotting factors and acts to maintain adequate levels of clotting factors
E. Antidiuretic hormone IV, SC	E. Acts to control bleeding by increasing factor VIII activity

IV. Perform/provide:

INTERVENTION	RATIONALE
A. Rest and elevation of painful extremity or body part, avoid weight bearing and excessive movement of limb or area when giving care	A. Reduces pain and swelling during bleeding episode and prevents joint deformity and possible disability with repeated episodes
B. Ice pack around painful joint	B. Produces vasoconstriction that reduces pain
C. Protect areas of hematomas from heavy linens, trauma, and handle gently to prevent extension of hematoma	C. Continued pressure from hematoma can result in nerve damage and paralysis
D. Apply pressure to blood oozing from small cuts or breaks in skin	D. Prevents continued bleeding that can result in increasing blood loss

INTERVENTION	RATIONALE
E. Soft toothbrush, avoid flossing, electric razor, avoid blowing nose or straining on defecation and exposure to other skin injury	E. Prevents trauma that can initiate a bleeding episode

NURSING DIAGNOSES

Risk for injury and trauma related to internal factor of altered clotting factors, lack of safety education and precautions resulting in hemorrhage

Knowledge deficit related to disease and complications, safety measures, and treatment regimen in prevention or treatment of bleeding episode

EXPECTED OUTCOMES

Adequate information to prevent or control bleeding episodes and their complications evidenced by compliance with safety measures and self-administration of medication regimen, avoiding unsafe practices and activities and minimal or absence of trauma or injury

INTERVENTION	RATIONALE
V. Teach patient/family:	
A. Disease process, cause, and course and what to expect, including lifelong treatment	A. Promotes information about what care is needed and changes necessary
B. Importance of treating any bleeding immediately	B. Critical to intervene early to prevent severe complications
C. Preparation and administration of factor concentrate IV	C. Prevents or treats factor deficiency prior to procedures or following trauma or injury

INTERVENTION	RATIONALE
D. Techniques to control bleeding such as applying pressure to an area, application of cold or ice to area immobilizing an area	D. Slows or stops bleeding
E. Inform of which conditions to treat at home and which to bring to the hospital	E. Prevents risk for emergency situations that can be life-threatening
F. Avoid contact sports or traumatizing play, use soft toothbrush, avoid safety razor, walking barefoot, falling or bumping into objects, protect hands by wearing gloves when working, and inform of other safety measures specific to patient	F. Prevents trauma that can initiate bleeding
G. Consider genetic counseling if appropriate	G. Promotes support and understanding of inherited aspects of the disease
H. Carry or wear identification in wallet or as a bracelet	H. Informs of bleeding condition prior to administering emergency care
I. Refer to community agencies such as National Hemophilia Society, counseling support groups	I. Provides information and support to patient and families (legal, economic, social)

polycythemia
(vera/secondary)

DEFINITION

Polycythemia vera is an increase in the number of erythrocytes (RBC) and an associated increase in hemoglobin (Hb) causing increased blood viscosity, hypervolemia, and a congestion of blood in the body tissues. Secondary polycythemia is a compensatory response to hypoxia associated with disorders that increase the body's demand for oxygen such as chronic obstructive pulmonary disease, heart defect, tumor, and residing in high altitudes. Polycythemia caused by fluid deficit resulting in loss of plasma and concentration of RBCs is known as relative polycythemia and is usually corrected by the return of fluid balance. This plan is specific to this condition and can be used in association with the NEOPLASM (CHEMOTHERAPY/EXTERNAL and INTERNAL RADIATION) care plan if radiation therapy is done.

NURSING DIAGNOSES

Altered renal, cerebral, cardiopulmonary, peripheral, gastro-intestinal tissue perfusion related to interruption of blood flow and hypervolemia resulting from increased production of RBCs causing increased viscosity and congestion of organ tissues

Pain related to biologic injuring agent of increased RBCs resulting in altered circulation and discomfort

EXPECTED OUTCOMES

Adequate circulation and perfusion with pain relieved or controlled evidenced by verbalizations the pain and manifestations resulting from hypervolemia and hyperviscosity are reduced or absent

INTERVENTION	RATIONALE
I. Assess for:	
A. Headache or fullness in head, joint pain, especially in toes	A. Signs and symptoms of polycythemia including circulatory abnormality and increases in uric acid
B. Dizziness, tinnitus, visual change, dyspnea, orthopnea, redness of mucosa, skin of ruddy color, bleeding caused by rupture of vessels, splenomegaly and hepatomegaly	B. Signs and symptoms of organ systems affected by increased RBCs
II. Monitor, describe, record:	
A. VS q4h	A. Hypertension, respiratory changes, and gastrointestinal bleeding can result from polycythemia
B. RBC, Hb, Hct, platelet count, uric acid, ABGs	B. RBC can increase to 6,000,000 to 10,000,000/mm^3, Hb >18 g/dL, Hct >25%, platelet count >350,000/mm^3, three to four times increase in uric acid, and normal ABGs unless hypoxia severe
C. I&O q4–8h	C. Monitors fluid balance and need for increase or decrease intake based on need to increase or decrease viscosity
III. Administer:	
A. Analgesic PO	A. Acts to reduce pain by interfering with CNS pathways

INTERVENTION	RATIONALE
B. Myelosuppressive PO	B. Acts to destroy bone marrow activity in the suppression of RBC production
C. Radioactive phosphorus therapy	C. Acts to inhibit bone marrow activity
D. Anticoagulant PO	D. Acts to decrease blood clotting that can lead to cerebrovascular accident or myocardial infarction
IV. Perform/provide: A. Encourage fluid intake to 2 to 3 L/day, 500 to 750 mL following phlebotomy	A. Reduces blood viscosity, replaces lost volume to prevent hypovolemia
B. Encourage activity, ambulation, ROM to extremities	B. Prevents thrombus formation caused by circulatory stasis
C. Place extremities in elevated position when seated and apply support hose	C. Promotes return circulation
D. Assist with phlebotomy to remove 500 to 2000 mL of blood, observe during the procedure to prevent shock state	D. Reduces blood volume until Hct of 40 to 45% is maintained

NURSING DIAGNOSIS
Knowledge deficit related to lack of information about follow-up and ongoing care including medication and phlebotomy regimen, fluid/nutritional requirements, radiation therapy precautions

EXPECTED OUTCOMES

Compliance with instructions for follow-up care evidenced by verbalization and correct performance of activities to maintain circulatory competence and prevent manifestation of the disorder

INTERVENTION	RATIONALE
V. Teach patient/family:	
A. Schedule of activities, ROM to joints daily	A. Prevents circulatory stasis
B. High-protein and caloric dietary intake, avoid iron-containing foods	B. Provides and maintains nutritional status, iron can increase RBC production
C. Phlebotomy as scheduled	C. Procedure can vary from q2–3 months to 2–3/year
D. Care of body fluids if radiation therapy administered (see Internal Radiation Therapy)	D. Contamination considered to be presence for 2 weeks with urine, blood, vomitus, saliva, perspiration affected
E. Importance of keeping scheduled physician and laboratory appointments	E. Monitors effects of or need for change in therapy

thrombocytopenia/splenectomy

DEFINITION

Splenectomy is a surgical procedure to remove the spleen. It is most commonly performed for the rupture of the spleen that results in hemorrhage following trauma from accidents, penetrating wounds, or diseases affecting the spleen such as idiopathic thrombocytopenic purpura, congenital spherocytosis causing primary hypersplenism, and lymphomas, leukemias, infections, polycythemia, liver cirrhosis causing secondary hypersplenism. This plan is specific to this procedure and can be used in association with the NEOPLASM, PREOPERATIVE CARE, and POSTOPERATIVE CARE plans

NURSING DIAGNOSES

Altered tissue perfusion (all organ systems) related to hypovolemia resulting from hemorrhage following trauma, idiopathic thrombocytopenia purpura preoperatively, and hemorrhage postoperatively if surgery for thrombocytopenia is performed causing risk for shock state

Decreased cardiac output related to altered preload postoperatively resulting from reduced workload since output is shunted through the spleen

EXPECTED OUTCOMES

Adequate perfusion and cardiac output pre- and postoperatively evidenced by absence of signs and symptoms of shock with vital signs, ECG, skin condition, and urinary output within baseline parameters, absence of petechiae, ecchymosis, or bleeding from mucous membranes

INTERVENTION	RATIONALE
I. Assess for:	
A. Pain in upper abdomen or general abdomen and left shoulder	A. Signs and symptoms of splenic injury and rupture preoperatively
B. Decreased BP, tachycardia with pulse that is weak and thready, cold and clammy skin, decreases in peripheral pulses, pallor or cyanosis, reduced urinary output, restlessness, confusion	B. Signs and symptoms of impending or actual shock state as result of blood loss
C. Bleeding or oozing of blood from mucous membranes of mouth, nose, urinary or gastrointestinal tract, easy bruising, petechiae, ecchymosis	C. Indicates bleeding into mucous membranes and tissues caused by thrombocytopenia
II. Monitor, describe, record:	
A. VS q15min to 1h as appropriate	A. Indicates potential shock state
B. ECG for dysrhythmias or changes	B. Results from changes in cardiac output and workload
C. Platelet count, Hct, Hb	C. Platelets $<150,000/mm^3$ indicates thrombocytopenia, decreases in Hct and Hb are associated with blood loss; platelets $<20,000/mm^3$ indicates the possibility of spontaneous bleeding

INTERVENTION	RATIONALE
D. Abdominal girth	D. Indicates distention caused by hemorrhage into the abdomen if spleen has ruptured
III. Administer: A. Anti-inflammatory PO	A. Acts to suppress phago-cytic response of macrophages from the spleen
B. Immunosuppresive agent	B. Possible use in refractory conditions
C. Platelet transfusion IV	C. Administered for thrombo-cytopenia pre- and postop-eratively based on platelet count
D. Blood transfusion, volume expanders, fluids IV	D. Increases blood volume to prevent or treat hypo-volemia
IV. Perform/provide: A. Place on bed rest in a quiet, calm environment	A. Reduces unnecessary stim-uli
B. Place in flat position with legs elevated	B. Promotes return of blood to the heart in impending shock
C. Prepare for surgery if ap-propriate	C. Splenectomy performed to treat conditions associated with hypersplenism as a cure or palliative treat-ment depending on cause

NURSING DIAGNOSES

Pain related to biologic injuring agent of bleeding into tissues resulting from decreased platelet count in thrombocytopenia

Risk for injury related to internal factor of bleeding resulting in excessive blood loss and impaired skin integrity

EXPECTED OUTCOMES

Absence of injury to organ, skin, and mucous membrane tissues evidenced by effective treatment of bleeding abnormality

INTERVENTION	RATIONALE
I. Assess for: A. Prolonged oozing or spontaneous bleeding into joints, from gums, nose, and presence of petechiae, ecchymosis on skin, hemorrhage from the urinary or gastrointestinal tracts	A. Indicates lowering levels of platelets in idiopathic thrombocytopenic purpura
III. Administer: A. Analgesic PO	A. Acts to relieve pain by interfering with CNS pathways
IV. Perform/provide: A. Ice application or pressure application to area	A. Promotes hemostasis by controlling bleeding and relieves pain
B. Place bed cradle, light covers over painful areas	B. Relieves any pressure on extremities that increases discomfort

INTERVENTION	RATIONALE
C. Refrain from administering injections, anticoagulants, and use soft toothbrush without flossing, electric instead of safety razor, and to avoid exertion during defecation	C. Increases bleeding tendency if platelet count is low

NURSING DIAGNOSIS
Risk for infection related to inadequate secondary defense (leukopenia) resulting in reduced macrophage activity in destroying pathogens and decreased antibodies and resistance to infection following splenectomy

EXPECTED OUTCOMES
Absence of infection evidenced by temperature, WBC, cultures, respiratory rate, depth, and ease, within baseline determinations, wound incision dry and healing

INTERVENTION	RATIONALE
I. Assess for:	
A. Temperature elevation above 101°F (38.3°C), chills, pulse >100/bpm	A. Low-grade temperature common following splenectomy for 7 to 10 days but, if persistent, can indicate infection
B. Tachypnea, crackles on auscultation, cough, foul-smelling urine with urgency and frequency, irritation or ulceration of oral, vaginal or other mucous membranes, redness, swelling, drainage from wound or invasive sites, increased WBC for extended time following surgery	B. Indicates pulmonary infection or an overwhelming infection as phagocytic ability of the spleen to destroy pathogens is decreased

INTERVENTION	RATIONALE
C. Abdominal pain, extension of the pain to other areas such as back or upper abdomen, nausea, vomiting, headache, increasing temperature	C. Indicates postoperative infectious complications such as pancreatitis, abscess, or sepsis
III. Administer:	
A. Antibiotic PO	A. Acts as a prophylaxis or treatment of infection by destroying pathogens by preventing synthesis of cell wall
B. Antipyretic PO	B. Acts on hypothalamus to reduce temperature
IV. Perform/provide:	
A. Handwash prior to any care	A. Prevents cross-contamination
B. Aseptic technique for all procedures (invasive)	B. Prevents introduction of infectious agents
C. Increase fluid intake to 2000 to 2500 mL/day, adequate daily nutritional intake	C. Maintains support to prevent susceptibility to infection and prevent stasis of urine
D. Meticulous mouth and perineal care	D. Promotes comfort and care to areas susceptible to infection
E. Encourage to deep-breath and cough, change position q2h	E. Promotes ventilation and prevents stasis of secretions leading to infection

NURSING DIAGNOSIS
Knowledge deficit related to postoperative follow-up care, measures to prevent infections, medications, signs and symptoms to report to physician

EXPECTED OUTCOMES
Adequate knowledge of care regimen evidenced by compliance with instruction, absence of infections, verbalization of signs and symptoms to report

INTERVENTION	RATIONALE
V. Teach patient/family:	
A. That prone to infection for a period of weeks postoperatively	A. Time needed for body to adjust and compensate for loss of spleen and its function
B. Avoid contact with others that have infections	B. Prevents exposure to upper respiratory infection or other contagion
C. Advise to have pneumonia and flu immunization	C. Prevents pulmonary infection
D. Antibiotic regimen and other medications, including action, dose, frequency, side effects	D. Promotes correct and effective administration of medications
E. Fluid, nutritional, activity requirements	E. Reinforces health status during convalescence
F. Report temperature, changes in breathing, urinary pattern, mentation, wound redness and drainage	F. Indicates possible infection and allows for early intervention

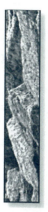

Endocrine System Standards

endocrine system data base

HISTORICAL DATA REVIEW
Past events:
1. Acute and/or chronic endocrine/hormonal disease or disorders
2. Signs and symptoms related to endocrine gland structure or function (body growth delay or acceleration, palpitations, tremors, appetite and hydration changes, weakness, fatigue, weight changes, menstrual cycle disturbances, impotence, infertility, constipation, excess hair and texture changes, skin color and texture changes, exophthalmos, bone complaints, muscle cramps, visual disturbances)
3. Endocrine disorders in family members
4. Anxiety and tolerance to stress and coping, exercise and sleep patterns, tobacco/alcohol use, dietary habits and special dietary restrictions/inclusions
5. Medications (prescription and over-the-counter), especially use of hormones
6. Hospitalizations and feelings about care, surgery associated with or affecting the endocrine system

Present events:
1. Medical diagnoses associated with or affecting hormonal function
2. Vital signs for changes in temperature, pulse, and respirations
3. Mentation changes (lability, mood, depression, nervousness)
4. Bone/joint aching or pain, headache
5. System changes and complaints resulting from endocrine gland dysfunction
6. Activities of daily living and effect on life-style, activity intolerance, fatigue, insomnia, self-esteem

PHYSICAL ASSESSMENT DATA REVIEW

1. General appearance for growth and development of abnormalities, alertness or level of consciousness
2. Thyroid gland/neck palpation for symmetry, enlargement or bulging, nodes or nodules
3. Physical examination of systems associated with abnormalities

NURSING DIAGNOSES CONSIDERATIONS

1. Activity intolerance
2. Altered nutrition: More/Less than body requirements
3. Altered thought processes
4. Constipation
5. Fatigue
6. Risk for impaired skin integrity
7. Risk for infection
8. Risk for injury
9. Hyperthermia/Hypothermia
10. Knowledge deficit
11. Sexual dysfunction

GERIATRIC CONSIDERATIONS

Endocrine changes in geriatric patients depend on central endocrine deficiencies that affect the ability of the body to maintain homokinesis. Chronic over- or underproduction of hormones cause changes in the structure and function of the ductless glands. Function can be disturbed when the elderly patient is stressed. Endocrine changes associated with aging that should be considered when assessing the geriatric patient include:

1. Thyroid gland fibrosis and follicular distention, parathyroid gland atrophy, decreased vascularity of pituitary gland with an increased amount of connective tissue, pancreatic alveolar degeneration and obstruction of ducts
2. Decreased number of insulin receptors on cells, amount of insulin secreted, and glucose tolerance deterioration resulting in diabetes mellitus, type II

3. Decreased thyroid secretion of triiodothyronine resulting in reduced metabolic rate
4. Increased follicle-stimulating hormone by pituitary in menopause, cessation of estrogen at menopause resulting in uterus, vaginal, and ovarian atrophy, continued production of testosterone in menopause
5. Decreased adrenal secretion of cortisol and reduced rate of excretion by kidneys, decreased adrenal androgen excretion
6. Decreased excretion of aldosterone resulting in reduced concentration in the blood
7. Decreased gonad production of anabolic steroid resulting in muscle loss, decreased ovarian, testes, and adrenal gland production of progesterone
8. Decreased production and excretion of testosterone in males resulting in a decline in muscle strength, genital tissue, and sexual energy

DIAGNOSTIC LABORATORY TESTS AND PROCEDURES

1. Skull x ray, computerized tomography (CT), magnetic resonance imaging (MRI), nuclear scan, basal metabolic rate (BMR)
2. Thyroxine (T_4), triiodothyronine (T_3), thyroid stimulating hormone (TSH), iodine[131] uptake, triiodothyronine uptake, thyrotropin-releasing stimulation, antithyroid antibodies, calcitonin, parathyroid hormone (PTH), growth hormone (GH), growth hormone stimulation, antidiuretic hormone (ADH), cortisol, cortisone suppression, adrenocorticotropic hormone (ACTH), ACTH stimulation, catecholamines, urinary catecholamines and metabolites, aldosterone, follicle stimulating hormone (FSH), estrogens, progesterone, testosterone, glucose, luteinizing hormine (LH), 2-hour postprandial, glycosylated hemoglobin, glucose tolerance (OGT), glucagon, blood and urinary ketones, routine urinalysis (UA), complete blood count (CBC), electrolytes (calcium, phosphorus, sodium, potassium)

MEDICATIONS

1. Antidiabetics: insulin (rapid, intermediate, long-acting), glucagon, glipzide, tolbutamide
2. Anti-inflammatory agents: ibuprofen, indomethacin
3. Bone resorption agents: mithramycin, gallium nitrate, calcitonin
4. Diuretics: furosemide (loop)

5. Hormones/antihormones: levothyroxine sodium, liotrix, propylthio-uracil (thyroid), cortisone, prednisone, beclomethasone, fludrocorti-sone acetate, mitotane, trilostane (adrenal), bromocriptine, soma-tropin, vasopressin (pituitary)
6. Vitamins/minerals: calcium gluconate, vitamin D

diabetes mellitus

DEFINITION
Diabetes mellitus is a metabolic disorder characterized by the absence of or insufficient secretion of insulin causing an imbalance between the insulin availability and need in the metabolism of carbohydrates (decrease in utilization of glucose), proteins (increase in utilization of protein), and fats (increase in fat utilization). Two types of diabetes are type I or insulin-dependent diabetes mellitus (IDDM) and type II or non-insulin-dependent diabetes mellitus (NIDDM). The disease is associated with hyperglycemia that eventually affects the blood vessels and nerves resulting in impaired circulation and nerve conduction. Classic signs and symptoms of diabetes include polyuria, polydipsia, polyphagia, and decrease in weight. The disease is incurable, and treatment concentrates on regulation of glucose levels and prevention of complications associated with increased or decreased glucose levels. This plan includes initial and ongoing care of the newly diagnosed person with diabetes

NURSING DIAGNOSES
Ineffective individual coping related to knowledge deficit regarding diabetes mellitus and associated psychophysiological changes, inability to manage stress and cope with long-term illness and uncertainty about present and future life-style changes resulting in chronic anxiety and worry, emotional tension, and inability to comply with medical protocol to regulate the disease

Anxiety related to threat to self-concept, change in health status resulting from new diagnosis of incurable but treatable disease (diabetes mellitus) causing difficulty in its regulation and control (hyperglycemia, hypoglycemia), feelings of helplessness and apprehension

EXPECTED OUTCOMES
Acknowledgment and progressive adaptation to changes in life-style caused by diabetes and ability to cope evidenced by verbalization of positive statements about changes in daily routine and life-style, and feeling

less helpless and hopeless about long-term care, development and use of coping skills, interest in managing and participating in own care, and that feeling less anxious and more relaxed

INTERVENTION	RATIONALE
I. Assess for:	
A. Anxiety level, stated feelings of uncertainty, distress, helplessness	A. Anxiety can range from mild to severe with a higher level expected with a new diagnosis of diabetes that eventually should diminish to a moderate level as adaptation to change in life-style progresses
B. Restlessness, irritability, complaining, joking, withdrawal, talkativeness, increased P and R	B. Nonverbal expressions of anxiety when not able to communicate feelings
C. Use of coping mechanisms, mechanisms, stated fears of uncertainty of disease outcome, life-style changes, reactions to long-term complications	C. Assists to identify inappropriate use of coping skills, feelings of personal vulnerability associated with chronic long-term illness
D. Negative expressions about changes in daily routines, self-worth, feelings of helplessness and uselessness, withdrawal behavior	D. Indicates difficulty in coping and decrease in self-esteem
E. Personal resources to cope with stress of disease and interest in learning to problem-solve	E. Support systems and personal strengths assist to develop coping skills

INTERVENTION	RATIONALE
F. Feelings about inability to carry out role, participate in activities, and to modify life-style	F. Decline in self-esteem common in those left with chronic disease
IV. Perform/provide:	
A. Environment conducive to expression of fears and concerns, avoid anxiety-producing situations	A. Decreases stress caused by new diagnosis, venting of feelings assists in reducing anxiety
B. Listen and clarify perceptions and information given, correct misconceptions and assist to understand disease and required care	B. Promotes successful resolution of uncertainty and establishes positive coping mechanisms
C. Allow time to verbalize feelings of denial or anger, comments in a nonjudgmental manner	C. Promotes temporary use of defense mechanisms to assist in reducing negative feelings
D. Discuss strengths and abilities with honesty, suggest new methods to enhance coping skills and problem solving, allow to externalize and identify coping skills that help	D. Promotes self-esteem and develops trust and rapport in the nurse–patient relationship, offers alternative coping strategies that allow for release of anxiety
E. Encourage and give positive feedback regarding ability to manage stress and changes in life-style	E. Provides support for adaptive behavior, promotes self-worth and independence

F. Allow to participate in planning of care and integrate into usual routine activities when possible

F. Allows for some control over situations

G. Include family in information regarding disease and support participation in care/teaching when possible

G. Provides opportunity for involvement and understanding of needs and care

V. Teach patient/family:
   A. Disease process, cause, pathophysiology, chronic and acute complications, type of lifelong care needed

A. Informs of basic information about the conditions to reduce anxiety and fear of the unknown

B. Recent advances in the study and research findings regarding the disease, investigational surgical procedure and medical protocols to correct and/or prevent complications

B. Promotes hope without false reassurance

NURSING DIAGNOSES

Altered nutrition: Less than body requirements related to inability to metabolize nutrients because of biologic factor (insulin deficiency) resulting in hyperglycemia

Knowledge deficit related to special dietary requirements (protein, carbohydrate, fat) associated with activity, replacement medications (insulin injection, oral hypoglycemic), results of blood and urine glucose levels

EXPECTED OUTCOMES

Adequate knowledge and understanding of initial and follow-up care involving dietary intake evidenced by compliance of daily meals properly calculated and ingested within prescribed caloric and food group inclusions, and blood glucose maintained within normal range (70–110 mg/dL)

INTERVENTION	RATIONALE
I. Assess for:	
A. Weight loss/obesity, 48-hour intake with amount, preferred foods, eating pattern, cultural or ethnic differences, appetite, weakness	A. Provides basic information about nutritional pattern to integrate into dietary regimen in managing diabetes
B. Daily exercise routine, when it increases, when at rest or more sedentary, special activities that require more energy	B. Control depends on the interrelationship among nutritional intake, medications to control glucose level, and exercise/activity/occupation
C. Ability and motivation to learn, adjust, and develop discipline to conform to essential dietary regimen	C. Adaptation to lifelong changes requires maturity and independence, willingness and readiness to learn
D. Calculated daily nutritional and caloric requirements for age, weight, activity, and insulin or hypoglycemic dosage	D. Diabetic diet usually consists of 50 to 60% carbohydrate, 12 to 20% protein, 30% fat, can be individualized according to patient's needs
II. Monitor, describe, record:	
A. Glucose level, glycosated hemoglobin	A. Provides information of compliance with regimen and glucose levels to determine need for change in dietary intake, medication, or activities
B. Wt q week	B. Monitors weight loss when calories reduced for overweight patient

INTERVENTION	RATIONALE

IV. Perform/provide:

A. Environment conducive to learning with space, lighting, teaching aids such as charts, diagrams, books and pamphlets of menus and exchange lists

    A. Promotes learning, prevents distractions

V. Teach patient/family:

A. Importance of regulated diet, nature of the disease and seriousness of increases or decreases in glucose levels

    A. Diet is one of the most important factors in maintaining normoglycemia

B. Daily exercise routine 1–2 hours after meals usually for 30 minutes, three to four times/week or as appropriate in diabetes management

    B. Exercise is an important component, and diet should be modified according to changes in exercise, program should be based on age, other medical problem or disability

C. Calculation and planning of menus, assist to write sample meals for 3 days, allow to practice estimating or measuring amounts of foods, and use exchange lists that consider cultural aspects and preferred foods to comply with American Dietetic and Diabetes Association recommendations

    C. Promotes adequate nutrition while adjusting intake to other factors in controlling diabetes, promotes caloric intake for weight loss of 1 to 2 lb/week if appropriate

INTERVENTION	RATIONALE
D. Eat three meals/day with possible snacks, avoid skipping meals and fad diets for weight loss, if complete meal is not eaten, increase more calories in the snack	D. Provides strategy for successful dietary management
E. Correlate meal schedule with insulin administration and activities, adjust caloric intake prior to prolonged or excessive activities	E. Promotes compliance by adapting regimen with daily routines
F. Avoid sweets such as candy, jellies, pastries and desserts, canned fruits, sugar in beverages, high-cholesterol and unsaturated fats, alcohol unless substituted for another carbohydrate	F. Concentrated sweets are usually restricted, but some sucrose can be included in meals occasionally, alcohol inhibits gluconeogenesis
G. Report any illness, vomiting, or anorexia to readjust medication administration	G. Prevents fluctuating glucose levels leading to hypoglycemia
H. Referral to nutritionist	H. Provides professional assistance for diabetic meal planning

NURSING DIAGNOSIS

Knowledge deficit related to initial and follow-up care that includes administration of insulin or oral hypoglycemic, testing for blood glucose and/or urine glucose and ketone levels and their relation to dietary intake and exercise/activities

EXPECTED OUTCOMES

Appropriate preparation and performance of oral or subcutaneous administration of medication ordered, periodic self glucose testing evidenced by demonstration of correct and accurate medication administration, correct procedure and interpretation of glucose testing

INTERVENTION	RATIONALE
I. Assess for:	
A. Readiness, willingness, and motivation to learn, discharge care and lifestyle changes	A. Learning can best take place if client is receptive and compliance is more likely to occur
B. Health practices, health beliefs, ethnic identity, value orientations, family interactions and cooperation	B. Factors to incorporate into teaching to facilitate learning and compliance with long-term care
IV. Perform/provide:	
A. Acknowledgment of perceptions with a nonjudgmental attitude	A. Establishes nurse–patient relationship in an accepting manner
B. Explanations that are clear, accurate in understandable terms, small amount of information over time	B. Prevents erroneous information, allows for patience, time, and understanding of new procedures to learn for regulation of the disease
C. Environment conducive to learning with space, lighting, and proper equipment and supplies	C. Distractions or discomfort will interfere with learning

INTERVENTION	RATIONALE
D. As much control over life-style change decisions as possible, include family in discharge planning	D. Allows power to be given or retained by patient
E. Teaching aids (pamphlets, video tapes, pictures, written instructions)	E. Reinforces learning
F. Demonstration of procedures and time for return demonstration and practices with encouragement	F. Hands-on experience enhances and reinforces learning

V. Teach patient/family:

INTERVENTION	RATIONALE
A. Administration and rationale of oral hypoglycemic to include a written schedule of times and dosages, side effects (hypoglycemia, rash, gastrointestinal complaints) to expect and report, effect of taking chlorpropamide or alcohol with this medication	A. Sulfonylureas act to lower glucose levels in NIDDM by stimulating the beta cells in the pancreas to release insulin and increasing the number of receptor sites to enhance the action of the insulin
B. Administration and rationale of insulin, including type, action, onset, peak, and duration, dosage, when and where to administer injections, expected results, storage and care of vials according to specific actions as follows:	B. Insulin SC injections administered for IDDM type, information, and instruction promotes confidence and accuracy in self-preparation and administration, insulin is available in U-100 concentration and prepared and given in U-100 syringes containing one or two types as prescribed

INTERVENTION	RATIONALE
a. Store insulin at room temperature if unopened, refrigerate if opened, check for cloudiness or discoloration, expiration date	
b. Wash hands	b. Prevents transmission of pathogens
c. Assemble supplies and gently roll insulin vials in palm of hands	c. Prevents destruction of molecules while warming insulin to room temperature
d. Check for correct type and cleanse top of vial with alcohol swab	d. Prevents contamination of needle, matching units of insulin should match syringe units to prevent errors in measurement
e. Remove cover from needle and withdraw measured amount of air and inject into vial, withdraw correct amount of insulin, remove from vial and replace needle cover	e. Sterile technique prevents contamination of needle and medication
f. If two insulins are mixed in one syringe, inject air equal to amounts to be withdrawn from both vials and withdraw the fast-acting (clear) type first, intermediate or long-acting type second	

INTERVENTION	RATIONALE
g. Administer 30 minutes prior to breakfast or meals and adjust dosage with test results	
h. Inject SC following cleansing with alcohol at angle according to agency policy (usually 90 degrees)	h. Oranges can be used for practice, angle should ensure reaching subcutaneous tissue for proper absorption
i. Rotate sites for injections, use a chart to monitor sites (thighs, arms, abdomen, back), allow 1 inch between injection sites	i. Prevents atrophy or hypertrophy of tissues
j. Apply pressure to area, refrain from rubbing site following withdrawal of needle	
C. Avoid over-the-counter drugs, alcohol, unless advised by physician	C. Prevents interaction of drug with insulin or intolerance to alcohol intake
D. Instruct in dosage adjustments outlined by physician, exercise reduction if blood glucose is >300 mg/dL	D. Dosage will be based on blood glucose test results, illness that causes anorexia, vomiting, exercise can raise the glucose level by release of glycogen
E. Advise to adjust or avoid exercise during insulin peak level and if blood glucose is >250 mg/dL	E. More energy and insulin utilization needed during exercise

INTERVENTION	RATIONALE
F. Inform to carry glucose tablets, hard candy, or other fast-acting carbohydrate to take if weakness, shakiness, visual changes, sweating, or mentation changes occur, report to physician if symptoms persist	F. Immediate treatment for symptoms of hypoglycemia
G. If IDDM, inform to carry insulin and supplies in purse, have glucagon kit on hand and instruct in use	G. Provides supplies for emergency if needed
H. Administration of insulin via a syringe-type pump that infuses the medication continuously through an indwelling catheter with sites changed daily, care of the device and risks for complications	H. Portable pumps worn externally to allow for self-administration of short-acting insulin to control glucose levels
I. Blood testing technique and rationale, when and how to perform the test, use and care of blood glucose equipment or test strips as follows:	I. Provides instruction in glucose self-monitoring used as a basis for evaluation of therapy
a. Follow instructions that accompany the glucometer for use and care and to calibrate the meter	a. Many types of meters are available, and the patient should be involved in selecting the appropriate one
b. Wash hands prior to the procedure	

INTERVENTION	RATIONALE
c. Perform the test prior to meals or medication morning and evening	c. Frequency is advised by physician and varies with individuals, can be as often as q4h if illness present
d. Cleanse the side of the finger and prick with the sterile lancet	d. Offers a site with more available blood and less painful
e. Apply blood sample to strip for reading or inserting into meter for analysis	
f. Maintain a record of results for comparison and evaluation with laboratory testing for accuracy	f. Results are basis for treatment regimen
J. Urine testing and rationale, when how to perform as follows:	J. Urine testing is usually reserved for ketones if blood glucose is >250 mg/dL or if patient has an illness; presence of ketones can indicate ketoacidosis
a. Obtain urine specimen and test with dipstick or tablet	
b. Compare results with chart colors to determine presence and level of ketones present	
K. Wear or carry identification of disease, medications, physician to contact, in purse or wallet or worn as a bracelet	K. Provides information needed in an emergency situation

INTERVENTION	RATIONALE
L. Community resources such as American Diabetic Association	L. Provides support, information, and educational literature

NURSING DIAGNOSES

Risk for impaired skin integrity related to internal factor of altered circulation (atherosclerosis), neuropathy (nerve degeneration) causing pain, tissue fragility, infection, and diabetic skin lesions and gangrene of the extremities

Knowledge deficit related to skin care, foot care, and prevention of disruption in skin surfaces or layers

EXPECTED OUTCOMES

Skin integrity maintained evidenced by absence of redness, irritation, pressure, breakdown, necrosis, adequate knowledge of skin care evidenced by verbalization of foot care and skin procedures, preventive measures to protect vulnerable body areas

INTERVENTION	RATIONALE
I. Assess for:	
A. Bony prominences, perianal area and contact with body secretions for redness, irritation, breaks in skin	A. Areas prone to be affected by prolonged pressure, irritation from urinary incontinence or diarrhea caused by autonomic neuropathy
B. Skin on feet and legs, space between toes for redness, pallor, blister, ulcer, or other break, ingrown toenails, loss of sensation in extremities	B. Areas vulnerable to impairment resulting from circulatory deficiency and neuropathy

INTERVENTION	RATIONALE
C. Neck, axillae, groin, under breasts for redness, rawness, odor, soreness	C. Common sites for development of yeast infections
D. Numbness, pain or tingling in extremities, intermittent claudication	D. Indicates peripheral neuropathy or peripheral vascular disease resulting from long-term diabetes

IV. Perform/provide:

A. Position change q2h if in bed or sitting in chair	A. Prevents prolonged pressure on vulnerable body parts
B. Bathe skin with mild soap and warm water, pat dry, cleanse perineal area following any exposure to urine or feces	B. Promotes cleanliness of skin and comfort
C. Wash feet daily with mild soap and warm water, pat dry while examining the skin between toes, soles of feet for irritation or breaks	C. Promotes cleanliness and prevents skin impairment of extremities or toes
D. Apply moisturizer to feet or small amount of powder to feet, lamb's wool between toes	D. Prevents drying of skin, maintains skin integrity by protecting skin between toes
E. Apply clean socks daily (cotton preferred) that are not too large or tight, well-fitting leather shoes	E. Promotes cleanliness and prevents pressure on feet, protects feet from injury

INTERVENTION	RATIONALE
F. Cut toenails straight across following bath, have patient see podiatrist for trimming, care of corns and calluses	F. Prevents accidental cuts or nicks in skin
G. Cleanse areas that are injured or areas that are infected gently with mild soap and water, pat dry and apply a sterile dressing (avoid taping or using antiseptic cleansing agents)	G. Promotes cleanliness without irritation of already impaired area

V. Teach patient/family:

INTERVENTION	RATIONALE
A. Avoid soaking feet unless advised by physician, going barefoot, use hot water bottles or heating pads, shoes with pointed toes or seams in the inside, and tight garters, shoes, or socks	A. Practices that can cause injury to skin and possible breakdown
B. Check bath water temperature, proper light and removal of clutter in pathways, proper warmth for feet in cold weather	B. Prevents burns and injury from falls or frostbite if neuropathy present
C. Report any skin changes and any minor injury or break in the skin of extremities or feet that becomes red and does not show signs of healing	C. Prevents more severe complications with early treatment

NURSING DIAGNOSES

Risk for infection related to chronic disease resulting in increased glucose levels, inadequate primary defenses of skin breaks that are difficult to heal, stasis of body fluids such as urine and pulmonary secretions if mobility affected, periodontal disease and pyrorrhea

Risk for injury related to internal factor of regulatory function of metabolism resulting in hyperglycemia (ketoacidosis) or hypoglycemia (insulin reaction)

EXPECTED OUTCOMES

Absence of infection, hyperglycemia, hypoglycemia evidenced by temperature, urine, vaginal/oral mucosa, respiratory status, and WBC within normal parameters

INTERVENTION	RATIONALE
I. Assess for:	
A. Elevated temperature, chills, adventitious breath sounds, sputum color changing to yellow or greenish, positive sputum culture	A. Indicates pulmonary infection caused by stasis of secretions in the presence of increased glucose level and change in mobility status
B. Cloudy, foul-smelling urine, positive urine culture, burning, urgency, and frequency	B. Indicates urinary infection caused by stasis of urine, high glucose levels that provides medium for infectious agents
C. Pain, redness, swelling, drainage from gums, vagina, positive culture	C. Indicates infection of mucous membranes
D. Weakness, fatigue, shakiness, hunger, diaphoresis	D. Symptoms of mild hypoglycemia that can result from excess medication and exercise, decreased dietary intake

INTERVENTION	RATIONALE
E. Thirst, increased urinary output, warm skin, weakness, nausea	E. Symptoms of hyperglycemia that can result from infection, excess dietary intake, noncompliance with medication regimen

II. Monitor, describe, record:

A. Blood glucose when symptoms appear, urine testing for ketones	A. Levels of blood glucose <50 mg/dL indicate hypoglycemia, >300 mg/dL with urinary ketones present indicate hyperglycemia
B. Culture of body secretions, excretions, and blood	B. Indicates presence of and identifies pathogens
C. WBC, differential	C. Increases in presence of infection, although does not function effectively in preventing infection unless glucose levels are regulated

III. Administer:

A. Antibiotic PO	A. Acts to destroy pathogens by inhibiting cell-wall synthesis
B. Insulin SC, hypoglycemic PO	B. Acts to reduce glucose levels in the presence of hyperglycemia
C. Glucose 50% or glucagon IV	C. Acts to treat severe hypoglycemia

INTERVENTION	RATIONALE
IV. Perform/provide:	
A. Careful handwash technique prior to performing any care or treatment	A. Prevents transmission of micro-organisms
B. Comply with sterile technique standards for all invasive procedures	B. Prevents introduction of pathogens to susceptible areas
C. Oral care including brushing and flossing of teeth at least BID	C. Promotes cleanliness of oral mucous membranes
D. Increase fluid intake to 2 to 3 L/day if allowed	D. Dilutes urine and prevents stasis of urine in the bladder
E. Deep-breathing and coughing exercises as appropriate	E. Promotes ventilation, removal of secretions to prevent stasis
F. Rapid-acting carbohydrate (10–15 g) such as orange juice, glucose tablets or gel q15 minutes until symptoms disappear, follow with longer-acting carbohydrate such as crackers, skim milk, glucose IV for severe hypoglycemia	F. Acts to treat mild hypoglycemic episode with continued treatment if moderate or severe episode
G. Insulin SC or IV with saline, electrolytes as glucose levels decrease	G. Acts to treat hyperglycemia and ketoacidosis if present

INTERVENTION	RATIONALE
H. Refer to nutritionist and physician for evaluation of medication and diet to prevent subsequent hypoglycemia or hyperglycemia episodes	H. Corrects possible imbalance in management of diabetes

V. Teach patient/family:

A. Review preventive measures to take to avoid infection and hypoglycemia, hyperglycemia	A. Reinforces information given as this care is provided
B. Encourage to carry fast-acting carbohydrate, insulin and supplies for administration	B. Treatments that may be needed when away from home
C. Factors that cause hyper or hypoglycemia, signs and symptoms to report to physician	C. Provides early interventions and prevents acute complications
D. Immediate actions to take if symptoms appear (medications, carbohydrate, reduced exercise)	D. Prevents more severe condition that can lead to life-threatening state
E. Report changes in breathing, nausea, temperature, vaginal itching or drainage, change in urine characteristics, other persistent complaints	E. Indicates possible infection
F. Avoid exposure to those with infections	F. Prevents transmission of pathogens to patients

INTERVENTION	RATIONALE
G. Periodic dental examination, comply with physician and laboratory appointments	G. Provides ongoing monitoring of disease and its manifestations

NURSING DIAGNOSES

Risk for injury related to the complications of long-term diabetes (micro- and macro-angiopathy, peripheral and autonomic neuropathy) resulting in cardiac, renal, visual, sexual, and gastrointestinal dysfunction

Knowledge deficit related to information regarding measures to prevent or adapt to long-term system manifestations of diabetes

EXPECTED OUTCOMES

Limited progression of complications associated with diabetes evidenced by optimal ongoing management of glucose levels and absence or control of signs and symptoms related to the organs/systems affected and/or adaptation to deficits present

INTERVENTION	RATIONALE
I. Assess for:	
A. Visual impairment, cataract formation, retinal hemorrhage, glaucoma	A. Result of diabetic retinopathy caused by micro-angiopathy with changes in the retinal vessels that can lead to blindness
B. Hypertension, fluid accumulation, fatigue and weakness, albuminuria	B. Result of diabetic nephropathy caused by micro-angiography with changes in the capillaries of the renal glomerulus that can lead to renal failure

INTERVENTION	RATIONALE
C. Hypotension, angina, syncope, pain in extremities, increased P, mentation changes	C. Result of coronary artery, cerebral and peripheral vascular atherosclerosis that can lead to paralysis or loss of an extremity
D. Constipation, diarrhea, nausea, gastric fullness, heartburn	D. Result of autonomic neuropathy (gastroparesis) as digestion slows, causing gas and fluid accumulation
E. Pain, tingling or numbness in the extremities	E. Result of peripheral neuropathy causing peripheral nerve degeneration resulting in loss of sensation
F. Male impotence, vaginal dryness, decreased libido	F. Result of autonomic neuropathy that controls erection, decreased blood flow to sexual organs that can lead to sexual dissatisfaction and possible fertility problems
V. Teach patient/family:	
A. Reinforce dietary, exercise, medication regimens to control glucose levels, treat underlying conditions (hypertension, atherosclerosis, infections, other condition), *See prior nursing diagnoses for specific teaching content*	A. Prevents or delays long-term complications
B. Home modifications based on motor/sensory deficits	B. Prevents trauma from falls and burns in presence of neuropathy and macro- or micro-angiopathy

INTERVENTION

C. Resources such as American Diabetic Association, counseling, sexual therapist, nutritionist, dentist, specialized physicians to monitor specific organ function

RATIONALE

C. Assists to manage and adapt to diabetes and long-term implications

hyperthyroidism/hypothyroidism

DEFINITION

Hyperthyroidism is the increase in secretion and circulating thyroid hormones causing an increased metabolic and body functional state. It also affects pituitary, gonadal, and hypothalamic hormone secretion and metabolism. Hypothyroidism is the deficiency or absence of secretion and circulating thyroid hormones causing a decreased metabolic and body functional state. It also causes behavior and personality changes. Hormones associated with these conditions are those secreted by the thyroid gland (calcitonin, thyroxine [T_4], triiodothyronine [T_3]), by the anterior pituitary (thyroid-stimulating hormone [TSH]), and by the hypothalamus (thyrotropin-releasing hormone [TRH]). This plan includes care for these conditions and can be used in association with the THYROIDECTOMY care plan

NURSING DIAGNOSES

Altered nutrition: Less than body requirements related to biologic factor of increased metabolic rate resulting from hyperthyroidism causing weight loss as nutritional stores in the body are depleted

Altered nutrition: More than body requirements related to biologic factor of decreased metabolic rate resulting from hypothyroidism causing weight gain

EXPECTED OUTCOMES

Adequate nutritional status evidenced by gains or losses to regain and stabilize weight baseline or standard for height, age, sex, and frame

INTERVENTION	RATIONALE
I. Assess for:	
A. Weight changes, loss of muscle mass, weakness, appetite, activity level	A. Results from metabolic rate changes
B. Amount of food ingested and caloric content, dyspepsia, dysphagia, activity level	B. Provides data to plan for regulation of and well-balanced dietary intake to increase or decrease body weight
II. Monitor, describe, record:	
A. Weight daily or as appropriate, skinfold measurements	A. Determines gains or losses
III. Administer:	
A. Thyroid replacement PO	A. Promotes appetite and increases metabolism to normal levels in hypothyroidism
IV. Perform/provide:	
A. High-calorie (3000–4000), high-protein (1–2 g/kg), high-carbohydrate diet	A. Maintains or increases weight, prevents muscle mass tissue breakdown, provides energy and spares protein in both hypothyroidism, and as absorption is reduced by increased gastric motility/intestinal peristalsis in hyperthyroidism
B. Inclusion of vitamins and minerals, especially B complex and C	B. Supplements diet and assists in collagen synthesis in hyperthyroidism

INTERVENTION	RATIONALE
C. Low-calorie, high-protein diet, with inclusion of foods high in B_{12}, folic acid, iron, and vitamin C (citrus fruits, green leafy vegetables, whole grains, lean meats)	C. Reduces tendency for weight gain and promotes weight loss in hypothyroidism
D. Avoid cabbage, beans, and foods causing flatulence, highly seasoned and fibrous foods	D. Gas accumulation common and causes dyspepsia in hypothyroidism or increased peristalsis causing diarrhea in hyperthyroidism
E. Small, frequent meals spread over the daytime hours	E. Early satiety and decreased gastrointestinal motility common with decrease in metabolic rate in hypothyroidism
F. Obtain referral to nutritionist if appropriate	F. Assists with diet planning to ensure nutritional status and maintain optimal weight

NURSING DIAGNOSES

Activity intolerance related to generalized weakness resulting from decreased metabolic rate in hypothyroidism

Activity intolerance related to hyperactivity resulting from increased metabolic rate in hyperthyroidism causing fatigue

Sleep pattern disturbance related to internal factors of overactivity, agitation, and restlessness resulting from hyperthyroidism

EXPECTED OUTCOMES

Optimal activity tolerance and sleep and rest pattern evidenced by return of activity, energy, and endurance to normal parameters with full participation in ADL and uninterrupted sleep

INTERVENTION	RATIONALE
I. Assess for:	
A. Muscle and joint stiffness and cramping, slowing of movements and swelling	A. Mucinous deposits cause separation of fibers in muscle tissue and mucinous accumulation in joints in hypothyroidism
B. Weakness, loss of muscle mass and tone, fatigue, incoordination, tremors, change in strength and endurance	B. Result of overactivity and protein catabolism, increased metabolism leading to exhaustion or tissue hypoxia and decreased energy in hyperthyroidism
C. Restlessness, insomnia, irritability, wakefulness, difficulty falling asleep, listlessness	C. Increases in muscle tone and an elevated cerebral functioning interferes with sleep in hyperthyroidism
II. Monitor, describe, record:	
A. VS q4h or prior to and after activity to determine intolerance	A. Excessive activity indicated by P increases of 20 and BP increases of 40 mm Hg systolic and 20 mm Hg diastolic more than resting readings
B. Thyroid function tests (T_4, T_3 [RIA], [TAIU], TSH)	B. Indicates thyroid under- or overfunction affecting activity and implications for care
III. Administer:	
A. Thyroid hormone PO	A. Acts to replace hormone deficiency in hypothyroidism
B. Antithyroid PO	B. Acts to block synthesis of thyroid hormones in hyperthyroidism

INTERVENTION	RATIONALE
IV. Perform/provide:	
A. Quiet, calm environment and inform that sleep pattern returns when treatment to reduce thyroid secretion is implemented	A. Reduces stimuli that interferes with rest and sleep needed to prevent physical and mental fatigue
B. Alternate rest with activities within limitations	B. Conserves energy and prevents fatigue
C. Handle limbs gently and with support of hands and pillows when moving or repositioning	C. Prevents further discomfort in presence of muscle weakness or pain
D. Bed cradle, pads to limbs	D. Protects and reduces pressure to extremities if painful
E. Progressive program of exercises and participation in ADL within energy limits	E. Promotes activity and independence to increase endurance as these should improve with treatment

NURSING DIAGNOSES

Constipation related to less-than-adequate physical activity resulting from hypothyroidism causing activity intolerance, joint and muscle discomfort, lethargy, and reduced peristalsis

Diarrhea related to increased intestinal motility resulting from hyperthyroidism causing increased peristalsis and bowel motility

EXPECTED OUTCOMES

Bowel elimination patterns returned to baselines evidenced by absence of constipation or diarrhea with soft, formed brown feces daily or as determined from usual pattern

INTERVENTION	RATIONALE
I. Assess for: A. Bowel pattern and characteristics with presence of constipation or diarrhea, abdominal distention or fecal impaction, activity intolerance	A. Provides data to normalize adequate bowel elimination
III. Administer: A. Stool softener/laxative PO	A. Acts to soften feces for easier passage and to prevent constipation
IV. Perform/provide: A. Maintain activity within tolerance limitations and improvement in cardiac status	A. Promotes bowel peristalsis
B. Foods high in fiber and bulk (raw fruits and vegetables, whole grains)	B. Provides bulk to feces
C. Fluid intake of 2 to 3 L/day based on I&O ratio or fluid retention	C. Softens feces, replaces fluid loss from diarrhea
D. Avoid enemas if possible	D. Causes vagal stimulation that can alter VS

NURSING DIAGNOSES

Hyperthermia related to illness (hyperthyroidism) resulting in an increased metabolic rate causing heat production and increased oxygen consumption and increased cardiac output

Hypothermia related to illness (hypothyroidism) resulting in a decreased metabolic rate causing vasoconstriction and reduced cardiac output

EXPECTED OUTCOMES

Body temperature at optimal temperature evidenced by maintenance in the range of 98.6°F (37°C) oral temperature

INTERVENTION	RATIONALE
I. Assess for:	
A. Elevated temperature, heat intolerance, diaphoresis	A. Indicates increased heat production as metabolic rate increases in hyperthyroidism
B. Chilling, coldness, intolerance to cold	B. Indicates decreased heat production as metabolic rate decreases in hypothyroidism
IV. Perform/provide:	
A. Well-ventilated environment with temperature controlled to coolness or warmth depending on comfort level	A. Promotes comfort if experiencing intolerance to extremes in temperature
B. Extra blankets, warm clothing, warm fluid to drink	B. Provides additional warmth for feeling cold
C. Cool, loose-fitting, lightweight clothing	C. Promotes comfort and prevents overheating
D. Frequent bathing, change of linen/clothing, backrub	D. Promotes comfort if diaphoretic
E. Fluids of at least 3 L/day if allowed	E. Replaces fluid if diaphoretic

NURSING DIAGNOSES

Risk for impaired skin integrity related to internal factor of altered metabolic state resulting in edema, changes in texture and dryness/moisture/cold/warmth, changes in hair amount and integrity depending on hyper- or hypothyroidism

Fluid volume excess related to compromised regulatory mechanism resulting from thyroid dysfunction causing fluid retention and edema, change in cardiac output, bradycardia, possible increased blood pressure

EXPECTED OUTCOMES

I&O, VS within baseline determinations evidenced by absence of edema and urinary output of 30 mL/hr, skin intact and free of injury, return of hair and nails to normal state following treatment

INTERVENTION	RATIONALE
I. Assess for:	
A. Pressure points for redness, irritation, edema, disruption in skin surfaces, skin changes (dryness, leathery, scaly characteristics)	A. Indicates risk for skin breakdown from altered metabolic state, skin changes in texture and dryness occur in hypothyroidism, and changes of flushing and moisture in hyperthyroidism
B. Hair loss, changes in texture, nails that are thick, brittle, weak, and easily broken	B. Indicates effects of thyroid dysfunction on integumentary system
C. Edema of face and periorbital, pretibial areas	C. Indicates edema and potential for skin breakdown specific to hypothyroidism leading to myxedema
IV. Perform/provide:	
A. Position change q2h	A. Avoids prolonged pressure on skin that can lead to disruption

INTERVENTION	RATIONALE
B. Padding or protective device to vulnerable pressure points when in bed or in a chair, eggcrate mattress, sheepskin on bed	B. Protects skin from pressure that can lead to skin breakdown
C. Support edematous body parts, allow for privacy if face is puffy and area of eyes are edematous	C. Promotes comfort and body image until edema resolves
D. Skin and nail moisturizers, gentle hair care during personal hygiene activities	D. Preserves skin and appendages until hypothyroidism resolves
E. Cover head with a scarf, mark in eyebrows with pencil	E. Promotes positive body image until hair growth returns

NURSING DIAGNOSES

Sexual dysfunction related to altered body function resulting from reduction in thyroid hormone in hypothyroidism

Body image disturbance related to biophysical factor of change in appearance resulting from hyperthyroidism causing exophthalmos, anxiety, nervousness, mood swings, change in appearance resulting from hypothyroidism causing obesity, lethargy, apathy, depression, social isolation

EXPECTED OUTCOMES

Improved body image evidenced by return to level of social interaction, resolution of or adaptation to appearance changes and emotional responses, return to former sexual patterns following treatment

INTERVENTION	RATIONALE
I. Assess for:	
A. Decreased libido, impotence in men	A. Results of reduction in secretion and metabolism of androgens and progesterone in thyroid dysfunction
B. Irregular menses, menorrhagia, decreased libido, possible absence of ovulation in women	B. Results of hormonal imbalance in thyroid dysfunction
C. Exophthalmus, changes in vision, damage to sclera or cornea, night blindness	C. Results from hyperthyroidism causing protruding, dry eyes and decreased blinking or ability to close eyes
D. Thick speech, anxiety, apathy, depression, worry, paranoia	D. Responses from thyroid dysfunction resulting in social isolation
IV. Perform/provide:	
A. Inform that appearance, sexual patterns return with thyroid replacement therapy	A. Reduces anxiety and promotes ability to deal with temporary changes
B. Environment that is supportive and nonjudgmental during period of mental and emotional changes	B. Allows for behaviors that are temporary and caused by thyroid dysfunction
C. Elevate head of bed for sleep	C. Promotes fluid drainage from peri-orbital and facial areas

INTERVENTION	RATIONALE
D. Cool compress, isotonic eye drops, advise to turn eyes in complete ROM daily	D. Promotes comfort when eyes are irritated and exercises extraocular muscles
E. Suggest alternate sexual activities or sex therapist if not resolved	E. Sexual expression varies with individuals

NURSING DIAGNOSIS

Knowledge deficit related to follow-up care for long-term medication regimen, effect of condition on all systems, ongoing monitoring of disorder to prevent complications

EXPECTED OUTCOMES

Adequate knowledge and understanding of long-term care of thyroid dysfunction evidenced by compliance with medication regimen, nutritional requirements, and verbalization of signs and symptoms to report

INTERVENTION	RATIONALE
V. Teach patient/family:	
A. Anatomy and physiology of the thyroid gland, pathology present and effect on body systems	A. Information regarding the condition as a basis for rationale for treatment regimen enhances understanding
B. Importance for taking medication (hormone) for life and that compliance is imperative	B. Essential to avoid exacerbation of thyroid dysfunction

INTERVENTION	RATIONALE
C. Medication administration to include, dose, time, frequency, and side effects; report any change in temperature, weight loss or gain, fatigue, weakness, heat or cold intolerance, restlessness, constipation, nausea, vomiting, as well as increased pulse, palpitations, dyspnea, tremor, diarrhea	C. Prevents errors, over- or underdose of drug(s) and signs and symptoms of too much or too little thyroid medication to report
D. Dietary intake with inclusion of iodized salt and high-fiber foods, low- or high-calorie foods, increased protein intake	D. Provides nutritional requirements depending on hyper- or hypothyroidism
E. Maintain regular physician visits as scheduled	E. Monitors conditions and need to adjust replacement therapy

thyroidectomy

DEFINITION

Thyroidectomy is the total or subtotal (90%) surgical removal of the thyroid gland. The total thyroidectomy is done to treat cancer of the gland, the subtotal to treat hyperthyroidism as in Graves' disease, leaving a portion of the gland to supply the hormone and to avoid the need for replacement therapy. Preoperatively for subtotal thyroidectomy, antithyroid drugs and iodine preparations are administered to promote an euthyroid state and prevent a thyroid crisis postoperatively. Postoperatively for total thyroidectomy, internal radiation is administered with I-131 to ensure complete destruction of any residual thyroid tissue. This plan includes care specific to this procedure and can be used in association with the PREOPERATIVE CARE, POSTOPERATIVE CARE, HYPERTHYROIDISM/ HYPOTHYROIDISM, and NEOPLASM (CHEMOTHERAPY/EXTERNAL AND INTERNAL RADIATION) care plans

NURSING DIAGNOSIS

Pain related to physical injuring agent of edema, strain or stress of movement on the surgical incision

EXPECTED OUTCOMES

Pain reduced and controlled evidenced by verbalizations that pain relieved with analgesic and with neck supported and movement controlled

INTERVENTION	RATIONALE
I. Assess for: A. Neck pain, effect of movement or straining on neck, severity and type of pain postoperatively	A. Provides pain descriptors to determine need for incisional support and analgesic

INTERVENTION	RATIONALE
III. Administer: A. Analgesic IM	A. Acts on CNS to reduce pain by interfering with pain pathways
IV. Perform/provide: A. Head of bed elevation of 30 degrees with head aligned in position to avoid flexion or hyperextension	A. Reduces stress on incision
B. Support head with hands when moving patient, use pillows or sandbags to maintain head position	B. Reduces pressure on suture line when moving and maintains head support
C. Use small pillow under head at all times	C. Prevents excessive flexion of neck
D. Have articles within reach, suggest clasping hands behind neck for support when moving in bed or sitting up	D. Prevents need to strain or turn to reach articles
E. Advise to refrain from coughing when performing deep breathing	E. Creates additional stress on suture line

NURSING DIAGNOSES

Ineffective airway clearance related to tracheobronchial obstruction resulting from edema/bleeding at surgical site, pain resulting in the inability to cough and remove secretions

    Ineffective breathing pattern related to airway obstruction resulting from edema or hemorrhage at surgical site, laryngeal nerve damage causing spasms or vocal cord paralysis

EXPECTED OUTCOMES

Absence of respiratory distress and airway patency evidenced by respiratory rate, depth, and ease within baseline determinations, resolution of voice changes or distress, absence of pressure on trachea by bleeding or edema

INTERVENTION	RATIONALE
I. Assess for: A. Respiratory rate and characteristics, dyspnea, stridor, choking, dysphagia, voice changes with persistent hoarseness, whispery voice or absence of speech, deviation of trachea from midline	A. Indicates changes caused by edema that results in pressure against trachea or from nerve damage
B. Tachypnea, muscle retractions, cyanosis, restlessness, abnormal oxygen levels in ABGs or oximetry	B. Signs and symptoms of respiratory distress
III. Administer: A. Oxygen via nasal cannula	A. Supplements oxygen to tissues in presence of respiratory distress
B. Mucolytic, cool-mist INH	B. Acts to moisturize the air and liquefy secretions for easier removal
IV. Perform/provide: A. Place in semi- or low Fowler's position	A. Facilitates breathing effort and ventilation
B. Ice pack to neck	B. Reduces inflammation and edema causing pressure against trachea

INTERVENTION	RATIONALE
C. Loosen dressings on neck if respirations change or distress occur	C. Relieves pressure on trachea
D. Coughing and deep-breathing exercises, orotracheal suctioning when needed	D. Promotes removal of secretions to ensure clear airways
E. Encourage speech q30min, note voice weakness or hoarseness, which is temporary postoperatively	E. Identifies voice changes caused by laryngeal nerve damage
F. Offer pencil and paper, magic slate, hand gestures, facial gestures	F. Provides methods of communication and rests vocal cords
G. Anticipate needs, ask questions that require short or one-word answers	G. Prevents unnecessary talking
H. Answer light promptly, allow time for response depending on speech ability and effort	H. Prevents voice strain and reduces need to speak
I. Advise that hoarseness remains for 3 to 4 days and to refrain from talking when possible	I. Prevents anxiety about voice change caused by surgery
J. Have tracheostomy and emergency equipment and supplies on hand	J. Provides for respiratory distress emergency

NURSING DIAGNOSES
Risk for injury related to complications from surgery such as hypocalcemia resulting from accidental removal of parathyroid glands, excessive bleeding resulting from high level of vascularity at the surgical site

EXPECTED OUTCOMES
Uncomplicated postoperative course evidenced by absence of hypocalcemic tetany or hypovolemic shock from hemorrhage

INTERVENTION	RATIONALE
I. Assess for:	
A. Increased pressure at neck area with feelings of tightening of dressing, blood on dressing or at back of neck, increased respirations, change in VS (increased P and decreased BP)	A. Signs and symptoms of excessive bleeding that can lead to hemorrhage
B. Muscular twitching, spasms, irritability, numbness or tingling in digits or around mouth, positive Chvostek's and Trousseau's signs	B. Signs and symptoms of hypocalcemia
II. Monitor, describe, record:	
A. VS q2–4h, ECG if available	A. Monitors changes indicating hemorrhage or cardiac dysrhythmias
B. Serum Ca	B. Decreases indicate hypocalcemia and possible tetany
III. Administer:	
A. Calcium replacement IV or PO if appropriate	A. Acts to maintain Ca at normal levels

INTERVENTION	RATIONALE
B. Blood or blood products IV	B. Replaces blood loss

IV. Perform/provide:

A. Pressure dressing at surgical site or loosen if bleeding is present	A. Reduces risk of hemorrhage or promotes blood drainage from the wound
B. Elevate head of bed, advise to refrain from coughing or movement	B. Reduces pressure at the surgical site
C. Prepare for emergency tracheostomy, with oxygen administration and suctioning as appropriate, take precautions for seizure activity should this occur	C. Treats hypocalcemia
D. Prepare for drainage of bleeding or hematoma from the wound or ligation of vessels that are the origin of bleeding	D. Treats excessive bleeding or hemorrhage

NURSING DIAGNOSIS
Knowledge deficit related to postoperative follow-up care of medication regimen, wound care, neck exercises, signs and symptoms to report

EXPECTED OUTCOMES
Understanding of information and instructions for care evidenced by compliance with lifelong thyroid medication and verbalizations of postoperative plan for return to and maintenance of health status

INTERVENTION	RATIONALE
V. Teach patient/family:	
A. Anatomy and physiology of the thyroid gland, pathology present and surgical procedure performed	A. Information regarding the condition as a basis for rationale for treatment regimen, enhances understanding
B. Thyroid replacement regimen for life and importance of compliance, calcium replacement if appropriate, include dosage, time of day, frequency, and side effects	B. Essential if total thyroidectomy performed to avoid hypothyroidism and hypocalcemia that can lead to tetany
C. Neck ROM, exercises with head flexion forward and laterally, move head to each side, hyperextend the neck, instruct in hand placement in back of neck for support during these exercises	C. Promotes neck mobility and prevents contractures
D. Avoid wearing tight clothing or jewelry around neck	D. Promotes comfort at neck area
E. Eye and wound care using sterile technique in administering eye drops, cleansing surgical site and applying dressing if advised	E. Prevents eye irritation if exophthalmos or infection at the incision site present

INTERVENTION	RATIONALE
F. Report changes in temperature, weight loss or gain, fatigue, weakness, restlessness, heat or cold intolerances, constipation, nausea, vomiting, other unusual complaints	F. Indicates over- or underdose of thyroid replacement
G. Maintain regular physician visits as scheduled	G. Monitors conditions and need to adjust replacement therapy

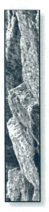

Gastrointestinal/ Hepatobiliary Systems Standards

gastrointestinal/hepatobiliary systems data base

anorectal disorders (fissure/fistula/hemorrhoids)

appendicitis/ruptured appendix/appendectomy

bowel resection/diversion (colostomy/ileostomy)

cholecystitis/cholelithiasis/cholecystectomy

cirrhosis of liver

diverticulosis/diverticulitis

esophagitis/achalasia

gastrectomy/gastroplasty

hepatitis

herniorrhaphy

inflammatory bowel disease (Crohn's disease/ulcerative colitis)

pancreatitis

peptic ulcer

gastrointestinal/hepatobiliary systems data base

HISTORICAL DATA REVIEW
Past events:
1. Acute and/or chronic gastrointestinal or hepatobiliary disease or disorders, presence of other diseases that affect these systems (diabetes, dental disorders, coagulation disorders, hiatal hernia, inflammatory disorders, eating disorders)
2. Chronic signs and symptoms related to oral (dryness, chewing or swallowing problems), esophageal (heartburn, dysphasia, reflux), stomach (dyspepsia, nausea, vomiting, pain, belching), intestine (pain, flatulence, constipation, diarrhea, color change of feces, rectal disorder), or hepatobiliary (jaundice, pruritis, edema, bleeding tendency, color change of feces and urine, anorexia)
3. Bowel tumor or inflammatory diseases, alcoholism, obesity of family members
4. Food allergies and effect on gastrointestinal and hepatobiliary function
5. Recent weight losses/gains, changes in food tolerance or eating pattern, dietary restrictions and/or inclusions
6. Anxiety, stressors, tobacco/alcohol/caffeine use, occupational/environmental hepatotoxins, water or food contamination
7. Treatments, hyperalimentation, rehabilitation associated with bowel incontinence, presence of bowel diversion or gastrostomy for feedings
8. Medications (prescription and over-the-counter) for gastrointestinal or hepatobiliary conditions and hepatotoxic drugs
9. Hospitalizations and feelings about care, surgery associated with organs of the gastrointestinal system (oral, esophageal, gastric, bowel, rectum), or hepatobiliary system (liver, gallbladder, pancreas)

Present events:
1. Medical diagnoses associated with or affecting gastrointestinal and hepatobiliary organ structures and function
2. Nutritional intake for 24 hours (food types, calories, likes and dislikes,

cultural influences), presence of partial or full dentures, over- or underweight for height, sex, and frame
3. Bowel elimination pattern (frequency, color amount, consistency, flatus), use of laxatives or enemas (frequency and type)
4. Bowel incontinence, abdominal distention, ascites
5. Presence of nasogastric tube for decompression or feedings
6. Jaundice, pruritis, bleeding (purpura), constipation, diarrhea (blood, mucus, pus), urine and fece color (dark urine, clay or fatty feces), fatigue, anorexia, nausea, vomiting, abdominal pain and severity, duration, pattern)
7. Activities of daily living and effect on self-care (feeding, toileting) and body image or self-esteem

PHYSICAL ASSESSMENT DATA REVIEW

1. Color, inflammation, lesions, odor, bleeding, pain in oral cavity, masses or tenderness of mouth lips, tongue palpated
2. Shape, size, of abdomen and umbilicus, skin color, bulging, tautness
3. Bowel sounds in all four quadrants for frequency, loudness, hyper- or hypo-activity (swishing, rushing sounds) auscultated, bruits over renal arteries, friction rub over liver/spleen auscultated
4. Abdominal distention percussed for dull or tympanic sounds, level of bladder distention percussed for dull sounds
5. Masses, nodes, tenderness, rigidity in all four quadrants palpated, liver, spleen, kidneys by deep palpation

NURSING DIAGNOSES CONSIDERATIONS

1. Altered nutrition: Less than body requirements
2. Altered nutrition: More than body requirements
3. Altered oral mucous membrane
4. Body image disturbance
5. Constipation
6. Diarrhea
7. Risk for impaired skin integrity
8. Risk for infection
9. Impaired swallowing
10. Knowledge deficit
11. Pain
12. Self-care deficit (feeding)

GERIATRIC CONSIDERATIONS

Gastrointestinal changes in geriatric patients depend on the aging process and include alterations in secretions, nutritional intake, absorption, and transport or motility. Common complaints made by the elderly begin with the mouth and end with elimination. Digestive disorders involve obstructive processes, absorption problems, vascular abnormalities, and neurological changes. Gastrointestinal changes associated with aging that should be considered when assessing the geriatric patient include:

1. Thinning teeth enamel resulting in brittle teeth, wearing down of grinding surface resulting in decreased force in biting and chewing
2. Loss of bone in oral structures resulting in reduced tooth support and difficulty in chewing and fitting dentures, thinning and drying of oral epithelium predisposing to irritation and damage to mucous membrane
3. Increased body fat and decreased lean body mass, fat decreased in extremities and increased in abdomen and hips, gradual weight decreases, decreased subcutaneous tissue predisposing to difficulty in environmental temperature adjustments
4. Decreased liver size, atrophy of pancreas, alveolar degeneration and duct obstruction resulting in decreased enzyme production and blockage of secretions
5. Decreased surface of small intestine mucosa resulting in alteration in nutrient absorption, atrophy of muscle layers and delay in peripheral nerve transmission of colon resulting in constipation or fecal incontinence, weakness of abdominal and pelvic musculature predisposing to difficulty in defecation
6. Decreased production of saliva and change of pH from acidic to alkalinic resulting in dry mouth and tendency for tooth decay, reduced number of taste buds resulting in reduced food intake, decreased gag reflex resulting in difficult swallowing
7. Decreased peristalsis and relaxation of lower esophagus muscle resulting in delayed emptying, dilatation, and reflux, decreased bowel motility, gastrocolic reflex, voluntary contraction of the sphincters, and amount of feces, all of which result in constipation or fecal incontinence
8. Decreased pepsin, hydrochloric acid secretion, intrinsic factor in stomach with a thinning and atrophy of mucosa resulting in reduced absorption of vitamins, decreased saliva/ptyalin in mouth and lipase/mucin in stomach resulting in slowing of digestion
9. Decreased hepatic enzyme concentration resulting in reduced drug

metabolism, decreased secretion of required enzyme resulting in increased time for digestion, reduced bacteria flora in large intestine
10. Decreased amylase, lipase, and trypsin secretions by pancreas resulting in reduced digestion of lipids and protein breakdown in the small intestine
11. Decreased absorption by small intestine, decreased efficiency of transport of nutrients
12. Increased cholesterol and thickness with a reduced volume of bile resulting in difficult gallbladder emptying and biliary tract disease, decreased absorption of fat-soluble vitamins by bile
13. Decreased metabolic rate resulting in weight gains, atherosclerosis resulting in reduced blood supply and transport of nutrients to the bowel for proper functioning in digestion and elimination

DIAGNOSTIC LABORATORY TESTS AND PROCEDURES

1. Abdominal flat plate (KUB), lower gastrointestinal series (LGI), upper gastrointestinal series (UGI), endoscopy (esophageal, gastric, duodenal), endoscopy (colon), proctosigmoidoscopy, peritoneoscopy, computerized tomography (CT), ultrasonography, magnetic resonance imaging (MRI), gastric analysis, esophageal manometry test, tissue, acid perfusion tests, oral or IV gallbladder series, cholangiography, angiography, nuclear scan, paracentesis and fluid analysis, abdominal laparoscopy, biopsy with laboratory examination, dental x rays
2. Complete blood count (CBC), electrolyte panel, carcinoembryonic antigen (CEA), feces analysis (fat, occult blood, toxins), d-xylose absorption, bilirubin (direct, indirect), urine and feces urobilinogen, amylase, lipase, lipid panel (cholesterol, triglycerides, lipid densities), albumin, globulin, protein, ammonia, aspartate aminotransferase (AST), alanine aminotransferase (ALT), alkaline phosphatase (ALP), gamma glutamyl transpeptidase (GGTP), alpha fetoprotein (AFP), prothrombin time (PT)

MEDICATIONS

1. Antacids: aluminum hydroxide/magnesium hydroxide/simethicone, aluminum hydroxide/magnesium carbonate, aluminum hydroxide, magnesium oxide
2. Anticholinergics/antispasmodics: propantheline bromide, dicyclomine hydrochloride, glycopyrrolate
3. Antidiarrheals: kaolin/pectate, bismuth subsalicylate, loperamide, diphenoxylate

4. Anti-emetics: metoclopramide, prochlorperaxzine, promethazine
5. Antimicrobials: sulfamethoxazole, sulfasalazine, trimethoprim, tinidazole, metronidazole, broad-spectrum antibiotics, acyclovir
6. Corticosteroids: prednisone, hydrocortisone
7. Histamine receptor antagonists: ranitidine hydrochloride, cimetidine, famotidine
8. Laxatives/cathartics: hydrophilic psyllium, docusate calcium, docusate sodium, mineral oil
9. Lipid-lowering agents: cholestyramine, colestipol, ursodeoxycholic acid
10. Mucosal protectants: sucralfate
11. Prostaglandins: misoprostol
12. Vitamins: multiple vitamins, vicon forte, fat-soluble vitamin replacement

anorectal disorders
(fissure/fistula/hemorrhoids)

DEFINITION

Hemorrhoids are external and/or internal varicose veins that result in dilated vessels that protrude down the anal canal and through the anus. It is a common condition caused by constipation and prolonged straining, pregnancy, heavy lifting, standing or sitting for prolonged periods of time, and at times portal hypertension associated with liver cirrhosis. The surgical excision of hemorrhoids is called a hemorrhoidectomy. Rectal fissure or fissure in ano is a tear, ulceration, or crack in the anal canal caused by trauma of straining and defecation of hard, enlarged feces. It can be excised surgically if chronic. A rectal fistula is a sinus tract that extends out of the anus or rectum or from an abscess. The only treatment for this is surgery (fistulectomy) in which the tract is excised and left open to heal by granulation. This plan includes care involved prior to (medical care) and following surgery and can be used in association with the PREOPERATIVE CARE and POSTOPERATIVE CARE plans if surgery is performed

NURSING DIAGNOSES

Pain related to physical injuring agent preoperatively resulting from thrombosed veins, prolapsed hemorrhoids, sphincter muscle spasms, and postoperatively resulting from inflammation, edema, defecation

Constipation preoperatively related to personal habits, pain on defecation, less-than-adequate dietary bulk and fluid intake resulting in dilation of hemorrhoidal veins, tear in the lining of the anal canal, and postoperatively resulting in recurrence of rectal disorder

EXPECTED OUTCOMES

Pain controlled or minimized and constipation avoided or relieved evidenced by verbalization that anorectal discomfort has subsided with preventive measures and/or treatment, and bowel elimination of soft formed feces daily or with regularly determined by baseline assessment

INTERVENTION	RATIONALE
I. Assess for:	
A. Severity of pain, itching, burning, sharp pain during defecation, draining or bleeding with defecation, edema and inflammation at anorectal area, prolapse of hemorrhoids	A. Information needed to implement measures to control pain, treat rectal condition, or determine thrombosis of hemorrhoids or other abnormalities
B. Feces characteristics, frequency and pattern of defecation and constipation pattern	B. Contributes to continuing pain or can result from avoiding defecation because of pain
III. Administer:	
A. Analgesic PO, SUP	A. Acts to control pain postoperatively
B. Stool softener PO	B. Acts to soften stool by increasing water content for easier removal
C. Bulk laxative PO	C. Acts to provide bulk to feces for easier defecation
D. Anesthetic, steroid cream TOP	D. Acts to reduce anal pain and itching
E. Astringent TOP	E. Acts to relieve pain and itching
IV. Perform/provide:	
A. Cleanse anorectal area after each defecation with warm water and mild soap, use baby wipes for wiping unless surgery performed	A. Promotes cleanliness and prevents irritation and itching of anorectal area

INTERVENTION	RATIONALE
B. Limit time to sit on toilet and avoid straining during defecation	B. Places pressure on anorectal vessels and constricts blood flow
C. Warm, moist packs to anorectal area for short time 12 hours postoperatively	C. Reduces inflammation by increasing blood supply to area, cleanses and promotes healing
D. Sitz bath TID 12 hours following surgery or after each bowel movement	D. Soothes and reduces pain by relieving spasms, cleanses and promotes healing of surgical area
E. Soft pillow or surface to sit on	E. Promotes comfort and reduces pressure to the operative site
F. Retention oil enema or mineral oil PO	F. Lubricates movement of feces following surgery to help control pain of first defecation
G. Sanitary napkin if drainage present	G. Useful as a dressing postoperatively
H. Diet containing fiber, fluid intake increased to 2 to 3 L/day if allowed	H. Promotes regular bowel elimination of soft formed feces, adequate urinary output

NURSING DIAGNOSES

Altered urinary elimination related to mechanical trauma resulting from the proximity of the bladder to the surgical site causing pain and urinary retention

Risk for injury related to surgery resulting in hemorrhage, possible infection

EXPECTED OUTCOMES
Urinary pattern reestablished and absence of surgical complications evidenced by no urinary or wound infection or hemorrhage

INTERVENTION	RATIONALE
I. Assess for:	
A. Prolapsed hemorrhoids with pain, edema, and inflammation	A. Indicates thrombosed or strangulated hemorrhoidal conditions preoperatively
B. Excessive or persistent bleeding, difficulty in defecation, hard feces	B. Signs and symptoms of postoperative hemorrhage caused by prolonged trauma during defecation
C. Dysuria, frequency, cloudy, foul-smelling urine	C. Indicates urinary tract infection
III. Administer:	
A. Antimicrobial PO	A. Acts to destroy infectious organisms by inhibiting cell wall synthesis
IV. Perform/provide:	
A. Cold compresses to anus TID for 20 minutes on and 20 minutes off	A. Reduces pain and edema
B. Place buttocks in an elevated position or carefully reinsert hemorrhoids with well-lubricated gloved finger	B. Assists to reduce prolapsed hemorrhoids
C. Catheterize for residual urine if voidings <50 mL of usual pattern	C. Prevents stasis of urine leading to infection

NURSING DIAGNOSIS

Knowledge deficit related to follow-up care, measures to prevent recurrence of anorectal disorders

EXPECTED OUTCOMES

Adequate knowledge of care of anorectal disorder and/or surgery evidenced by compliance with treatment protocol and progressive wound healing without complications

INTERVENTION	RATIONALE
V. Teach patient/family	
A. Pathophysiology of disorder, reason for procedure, importance of a regular bowel elimination pattern	A. Provides information as a basis for self-care and to prevent recurrence
B. Administration of medications to maintain bowel elimination, control pain, prevent infection to include name, action, dose, frequency, route, side effects to report; avoid laxatives and over-the-counter remedies for constipation	B. Prevents constipation and promotes urinary and bowel elimination
C. Fluid intake of 2 to 3 L/day, include fiber in daily diet	C. Promotes proper urinary and bowel elimination pattern
D. Avoid straining at defecation, prolonged standing, or sitting	D. Causes recurrence of hemorrhoids, possible prolapse and thrombosis, vessel strangulation
E. Dressing change using sterile technique if wound is left open to heal by granulation	E. Promotes wound cleanliness and healing following fistula surgery

INTERVENTION	RATIONALE
F. Cleansing of anorectal area with commercial wipes after each elimination, sitz bath for comfort if needed, avoid harsh wiping of anal area	F. Promotes cleanliness of area
G. Avoid anal intercourse following surgery	G. Prevents complications as healing takes place
H. Report bleeding, purulent drainage, inability to control constipation or to establish normal bowel pattern	H. Indicates possible complications

appendicitis/ruptured appendix/appendectomy

DEFINITION

Appendicitis is the inflammation of the appendix, which if left untreated leads to gangrene, rupture or perforation and spilling of the contents into the peritoneal cavity, causing peritonitis. Appendectomy is the surgical removal of the appendix with complete wound closure if the appendix is intact. It is also a procedure performed to remove the appendix with an open wound drainage of purulent fluids if contamination of the peritoneal cavity (peritonitis) has occurred from rupture of the organ. Appendicitis is usually caused by an occlusion of the appendix lumen by a fecal stone or of the bowel by adhesions, the kinking of the appendix, or changes in the bowel wall (edema or fibrosis). These can result in decreased circulation and bacterial invasion of the organ. This plan includes care of appendicitis preoperatively and the appendectomy procedures postoperatively. It can be used in association with the PREOPERATIVE CARE and POSTOPERATIVE CARE plans

NURSING DIAGNOSIS

Pain related to physical injuring agent of infectious process, ruptured appendix preoperatively, surgical trauma postoperatively

EXPECTED OUTCOMES

Pain relieved or controlled evidenced by verbalization that pain reduced by analgesic therapy following diagnosis

INTERVENTION	RATIONALE
I. Assess for:	
A. Pain severity and site, factors that increase or decrease pain, descriptors such as periumbilical (beginning stage) that is vague and becomes more generalized with shift to RLQ, abdominal rigidity and diminished bowel sounds (acute stage), becoming more severe with walking or coughing, increasing severity and more generalized with rebound tenderness (acute with rupture)	A. Provides data on intensity and locale of pain to identify appendicitis or appendix rupture
B. Abdominal guarding, grimacing, crying, restlessness	B. Nonverbal indications of pain when not able to reveal pain
II. Administer:	
A. Analgesic IM after diagnosis is made	A. Acts by inhibiting pain pathways in CNS and alters pain perception pre- and postoperatively
IV. Perform/provide:	
A. Place in semi-Fowler's or sidelying position with knees flexed	A. Reduces abdominal tension and increases comfort in appendicitis
B. Assist to deep-breathe and change position if needed	B. Relaxes muscles and reduces pain
C. Ice packs/compresses to area	C. Desensitizes nerves and decreases pain

INTERVENTION	RATIONALE
D. Assure that analgesic for pain will be administered when diagnosis is made	D. Prevents masking of symptoms
E. Place in sidelying position with knees flexed and pillow between them, alternate sides q2–3h	E. Position of comfort postoperatively

NURSING DIAGNOSES

Altered nutrition: Less than body requirements related to inability to ingest and digest food resulting from nausea, vomiting, abdominal distention, NPO status pre- and postoperatively (appendicitis, appendix rupture)

Risk for fluid volume deficit related to excessive losses through normal route (vomiting), abnormal route (nasogastric tube aspirate) during acute pre- and postoperative periods

EXPECTED OUTCOMES

Adequate nutritional and fluid intake during acute phase of illness evidenced by control of vomiting, IV infusion until oral intake permitted, I&O ratio within normal determinations

INTERVENTION	RATIONALE
I. Assess for:	
A. Nausea, vomiting, abdominal distention, and becoming more severe	A. Symptoms of appendicitis caused by irritation of vicera associated with inflammation of appendix and/or decreased gastrointestinal motility
B. NPO status, N/G tube and suctioning, fluid intake and output	B. Indicates causes for fluid imbalance with appendicitis with or without rupture pre- and postoperatively

INTERVENTION	RATIONALE
C. Skin and mucous membranes dryness, skin turgor, oliguria	C. Indicates risk for dehydration from fluid losses
II. Monitor, describe, record: A. I&O q4–8h including aspirate, vomitus	A. Determines fluid balance
B. Electrolytes	B. Reveals electrolyte imbalance with fluid losses (K, Na)
III. Administer: A. IV fluids/electrolyte replacement	A. Provides temporary fluids and nutrition until PO intake is resumed
B. Anti-emetic IM	B. Acts to reduce vomiting by depressing the chemoreceptor trigger zone
IV. Perform/provide: A. Assist to take deep breaths if patient is nauseated	A. Decreases urge to vomit
B. Place in semi-Fowler's position, and change position slowly	B. Movements can stimulate vomiting center
C. Oral care after each episode of vomiting	C. Promotes cleanliness and comfort of mouth
D. Environment that is odor free, quiet, and restful	D. Stimuli that can initiate vomiting
E. Maintain NPO status	E. Decreases peristalsis

INTERVENTION	RATIONALE
F. Insert N/G tube and attach to suction if ordered	F. Rests stomach and reduces vomiting, maintains gastrointestinal decompression in peritonitis postoperatively

NURSING DIAGNOSES

Risk for impaired skin integrity related to external factor of secretions/excretions resulting from drainage from open abdominal surgical site (ruptured appendix), mechanical factor of pressure resulting from N/G tube

    Risk for infection related to rupture of appendix resulting in peritonitis, sepsis

EXPECTED OUTCOMES

Reduced risk or absence of skin impairment and extension of inflammation/infection evidenced by nasal mucosa intact and free of irritation, wound site free of excoriation and breakdown, absence of intra-abdominal pain distenetion

INTERVENTION	RATIONALE
I. Assess for:	
A. Irritation, redness, drainage at wound site and characteristics	A. Leads to skin breakdown and infection, decreasing infectious process as drainage is reduced
B. Nasal mucosa for redness, dryness, irritation, breaks	B. Indicates risk for breakdown from N/G tube pressure
II. Monitor, describe, record:	
A. VS and temperature q2–4h	A. Decreased BP, increased P and temperature, rapid R indicates infection and ruptured appendix
B. CBC, WBC	B. Increases in WBC indicates infection

INTERVENTION	RATIONALE
III. Administer: A. Antimicrobial PO	A. Acts to inhibit synthesis of cell wall in prevention or treatment of infection pre- and postoperatively
B. Antipyretic PO	B. Acts to reduce temperature
IV. Perform/provide: A. Lubricate lips and nares, artificial saliva and mouth wash rinses q4h	A. Treats dryness and prevents breaks in oral mucosa
B. Encourage nasal breathing	B. Mouthbreathing increases dryness
C. Attach tubing to face in comfortable position	C. Prevents continued pressure or rubbing against nasal passages
D. Maintain dry, clean skin at closed wound site	D. Prevents skin irritation and breakdown
E. Change dressings as needed using sterile technique if drain is in place	E. Prevents saturation with drainage and further contamination from soaked dressings
F. Use caution not to disturb drains or pull on them or allow tubing to kink when changing dressings	F. Prevents accidental dislodgment
G. If wound drainage device in place, maintain suction, empty device as needed	G. Maintains patency of wound drainage to prevent pressure on wound

NURSING DIAGNOSIS

Knowledge deficit related to follow-up postoperative care to promote on-going wound healing and resumption of life-style activities

EXPECTED OUTCOMES

Knowledge and information provided evidenced by compliance with daily activities and restrictions for 2 to 4 weeks, wound care if appropriate postoperatively

INTERVENTION	RATIONALE
V. Teach patient/family:	
A. Pathophysiology and cause of appendicitis and overview of care	A. Provides information about surgery and rationale for care
B. Wound care, to cover with waterproof plastic when bathing if wound not completely healed	B. Protects wound and dressings from dampness
C. Dressing change using sterile or clean technique frequent as needed, inform that drain will be removed as healing takes place	C. Maintains clean, dry wound if drain is still in place
D. Fluid intake of 2 to 3 L/day, dietary intake of foods containing fiber, protein, stool softeners if prescribed	D. Promotes bowel elimination without straining and increasing intra-abdominal pressure following surgery
E. Advise refraining from returning to work or resume activities for 2 to 4 weeks, depending on physician's advice specific to activity	E. Prevents stress on wound site that may weaken area prior to complete healing

INTERVENTION

F. Report changes in wound appearance such as redness, swelling, pain, or increased drainage at the incisional site

RATIONALE

F. Indicates possible complication or wound infection

bowel resection/diversion
(colostomy/ileostomy)

DEFINITION
Bowel resection is the surgical removal of a portion of the small or large bowel or removal of the complete colon/rectum to treat ulcerative colitis, Crohn's disease (inflammatory disorders), tumors (colorectal, colon, small bowel cancer), bowel obstructions, abdominal perforation and trauma. A bowel diversion is a procedure performed in association with resection in which a portion of the ileum (ileostomy) or colon (colostomy) is brought to the surface of the abdomen to create a temporary or permanent diversion of fecal flow. Procedures for ileal diversion include a permanent ileostomy, continent ileostomy, or an ileorectal anastomosis, ileoanal reservoir. Procedures for colon diversion include a single (end ostomy and usually permanent) or double barreled (two ostomies and usually can be closed at a future time). This plan includes bowel diversion (ileostomy, colostomy, other procedures) care and can be used in association with the INFLAMMATORY BOWEL DISEASE (CROHN'S DISEASE/ULCERATIVE COLITIS), PREOPERATIVE CARE, and POSTOPERATIVE CARE plans

NURSING DIAGNOSES
Anxiety related to threat to or change in health status causing inability to manage feelings of uncertainty and apprehension regarding uncertain prognosis, disfigurement caused by the ostomy and ability to manage temporary or permanent bowel diversion

Ineffective individual coping related to inability to cope with change in control of bowel elimination, change in appearance (body image), and future life-style changes

Body image disturbance related to biophysical factor of change in structure and function of body part (change in bowel pattern with bowel diversion), and change in appearance (permanent ostomy on surface of abdomen), embarrassment of ostomy presence, affect on sexual function/pattern resulting from surgical diversion procedure

EXPECTED OUTCOMES

Anxiety and fear within manageable levels, development of coping and problem-solving skills, body image improved evidenced by verbalizations that anxiety is decreasing, fear reduced, participation in care activities and receptive to planning for ongoing ostomy care, change in bowel elimination and sexual pattern, and management of chronic anxiety

INTERVENTION	RATIONALE
I. Assess for:	
A. Level of anxiety, use of coping mechanisms, stated fears of uncertainty of disease outcome, life-style changes	A. Anxiety can range from mild to severe and high level associated with bowel diversion; assists in identifying inappropriate use of coping skills
B. Restlessness, diaphoresis, complaining, joking, withdrawal, talkativeness, increased P and R	B. Nonverbal expressions of anxiety when not able to communicate feelings
C. Personal resources to cope with stress, anxiety, and interest in learning to problem-solve, use of defense mechanisms	C. Support systems and personal strengths assist in developing coping skills
D. Feelings and response to change in appearance, permanent stoma, ability to carry out role and participate in care/social activities, fear of sexual inadequacy	D. Changes in body image and self-concept a common and serious problem with permanent changes in structure and function of a body organ
E. Looking or touching stoma, hiding stoma, feeling or preoccupation with the change, negative expressions about changes in life-style	E. Response to presence of stoma, negative or positive

INTERVENTION	RATIONALE
III. Administer: A. Anti-anxiety agent PO	A. Acts to reduce anxiety level and provides calming effect and rest, depresses subcortical levels of CNS, limbic system
IV. Perform/provide: A. Environment conducive to rest, time to express fears and anxiety, avoid anxiety-producing situations	A. Decreases stimuli that cause stress/anxiety, venting of feelings decreases anxiety
B. Suggest new methods to enhance coping skills and problem solving, allow to externalize and identify those that help	B. Offers alternative coping strategies that allow for release of anxiety and fear
C. Positive feedback regarding progress made, focus on abilities rather than inabilities	C. Provides support for adaptive behavior, promotes self-worth and responsibility
D. Avoid verbal or nonverbal reactions to stoma care or other procedures, display of distaste or alarm at surgical site	D. Promotes comfort with nurse–patient relationship
E. Privacy when dressings or appliance are changed, advise that feelings about the ostomy are normal	E. Reduces embarrassment caused by exposure to surgical procedure

INTERVENTION	RATIONALE
F. Diversional activities such as relaxation exercises, TV, radio, music, reading, tapes, guided imagery, encourage to continue usual interests	F. Reduces anxiety and promotes comfort
G. Allow to participate in planning of care to maintain usual activities when possible, allow to participate in ostomy care as soon as possible	G. Allows for some control over situations
H. Support grieving for loss of life-style and restrictions in activities, changes in physical appearance, and alternative bowel elimination	H. Provides assistance in adaptation to changes imposed by disease
I. Suggest visit from one who has had bowel diversion surgery and has made a successful recovery	I. Provides support and information from a reliable source

NURSING DIAGNOSES

Risk for infection related to inadequate primary defenses (surgical incision) resulting in pathogen invasion of wound, invasive procedures (ostomy irrigation, infusion of fluids/nutrients)

Risk for impaired skin integrity related to mechanical external factor of presence of collection appliance resulting in peristomal skin irritation, internal factor of secretions or wound drainage at incisional site or defecation at perianal site resulting in irritation and breakdown

EXPECTED OUTCOMES

Skin intact, healing, and free from breakdown at peristomal, perianal, and wound site, evidenced by absence of redness, irritation, excoriation at peristomal or perianal skin site, swelling, pain and exudate at incisional site, and redness, pain and swelling at IV site, WBC within normal levels

INTERVENTION	RATIONALE
I. Assess for:	
A. Irritation, excoriation, or redness at peristomal, perianal skin site, itching or burning under appliance or at anal site, type of drainage from stoma	A. Constant changing of temporary pouch, prolonged use of more permanent appliances, or excreta seepage around bag not properly applied can irritate skin from constant contact with effluent of ileostomy or fecal material of colostomy
B. Drainage on dressings with redness and swelling at incisional site	B. Indicates wound infection
C. Color of stoma changing from pink or red to bluish or purple	C. Indicates poor blood supply to stoma
D. Position of collection pouch and characteristics of drainage/feces	D. Prevents irritation of stoma by excretions, flow of drainage characteristics based on position of ostomy on colon (liquid to semisolid to solid from the ascending to descending portions of the large bowel), ileostomy drainage is fluid in nature
E. Patency of stoma	E. Indicates possible blockage of ostomy flow by constipation, obstruction
II. Monitor, describe, record:	
A. VS and temperature q4h	A. Temperature elevation indicates infection

INTERVENTION	RATIONALE
B. WBC, wound culture	B. Increased WBC of $>10,000/mm^3$ and positive wound cultures indicate infection and identifies the pathogen
III. Administer:	
A. Antibiotic PO, TOP	A. Acts to prevent or treat infection by inhibiting cell-wall synthesis
B. Antipyretic PO	B. Acts to reduce temperature
IV. Perform/provide:	
A. Proper handwash prior to any care or contact	A. Prevents transmission of pathogens
B. Use sterile technique and all sterile equipment, supplies, and dressings for wound and stoma care	B. Prevents contamination by pathogens
C. Dressing change q4–8h for 24 hours postoperatively or as needed (stoma and rectal)	C. Prevents contact of secretions with skin and promotes cleanliness, prevents infection
D. Cleanse peristomal or perianal skin with mild soap and warm water and gently pat dry	D. Promotes cleanliness and prevents irritation from intestinal secretions
E. If dressing worn instead of appliance, change and cleanse area after each exposure of skin to fecal material	E. Some colostomates do not use an appliance, only a dressing over stoma

INTERVENTION	RATIONALE
F. Colostomy irrigation daily at the same time (500–1000 mL), allow to assist using irrigating catheter and drainage bag without removing appliance	F. Cleanses bowel and begins training for regular bowel elimination pattern
G. Apply light to stoma covered with light dressing q4h, avoid use of soap, skin barrier, adhesive if skin irritated	G. Treatment for peristomal irritation
H. Apply skin barrier or skin sealant and then adhesive material when changing appliance, perform patch test prior to application (United Skin Prep and Hollister Skin Gel as sealants, Karaya and Stomahesive as skin barriers, antibiotic powder or ointment if ordered to peristomal skin)	H. Protects skin from contact with irritating substances and possible allergic reaction
I. Use a two-piece appliance if possible, change only when needed or ordered	I. Allows for changing of pouch without removing the skin adhesive plate, changes are more frequent early in postoperative period

INTERVENTION	RATIONALE
J. Remove and apply appliance and pouch as follows:	J. Ensures proper use of bowel collection system
a. Change appliance before meals or at night q4–5 days or longer if more permanent type used	a. Ostomy less likely to be active
b. Measure stoma for proper fit of appliance (opening should not extend more than $\frac{1}{4}$ inch from stoma)	b. Ensures proper fit to prevent leakage around stoma
c. Gently remove appliance in direction of hair growth and any substances with solvent prior to washing	c. Prevents skin damage when cleansing and changing appliance
d. Cover stoma with tampon or tissue when changing appliance	d. Absorbs drainage when changing appliance and prevents contact with peristomal skin
e. Fill in any irregular spaces around stoma with ostomy paste	e. Ensures seal to prevent leakage
f. Remove air pockets when applying pouch, empty q2–3h or when $\frac{1}{3}$ full, position pouch away from stoma	f. Prevents pull from skin caused by heavy bag and contents of pouch in contact with skin
g. Allow space of two fingers between skin and belt attached to appliance	g. Prevents pressure of belt or fasteners on belt to skin
K. Referral to enterostomal therapist if needed	K. Provides problem-solving assistance to prevent complications

NURSING DIAGNOSES

Altered nutrition: Less than body requirements related to inability to ingest (anorexia, nausea) or absorb (reduction in bowel surface following resection) nutrients resulting in malabsorption, weight loss, malnutrition, poor wound healing

Risk for fluid volume deficit related to excessive losses of fluids/electrolytes resulting from vomiting, diarrhea, ileostomy output causing possible imbalance (metabolic acidosis, alkalosis), constipation

EXPECTED OUTCOMES

Optimal nutritional and fluid level evidenced by stable weight pattern and protein, electrolyte levels, I&O within normal determinations, including intestinal output and absence of diarrhea and anorexia

INTERVENTION	RATIONALE
I. Assess for:	
A. Anorexia, nausea, vomiting, diarrhea, fatigue, ability to eat and drink and amounts/day	A. Affects oral intake of nutrients and fluid
B. Quantity and quality of ileostomy effluent (should decrease to 500–800 mL/day beginning in 1–2 weeks), changes in consistency of effluent	B. Provides output information to evaluate I&O ratio with as much as 2000 mL/day effluent from ileostomy postoperatively, consistency varies with foods eaten that are irritating
C. Volume, color, other characteristics of colostomy drainage based on segment of bowel with ostomy, passage of flatus	C. Provides data needed to plan care of colostomy and correct diarrhea or constipation, semiformed or formed feces with sigmoid or descending colon ostomy and semiliquid feces with ascending or transverse colon ostomy

INTERVENTION	RATIONALE
D. Nausea, vomiting, headache, disorientation, rapid respirations	D. Signs and symptoms of metabolic acidosis
E. Dry skin and mucous membranes, poor skin turgor, nausea, vomiting, muscle weakness	E. Signs and symptoms of fluid and electrolyte imbalance (K, Mg) caused by vomiting, N/G aspirate, inadequate fluid, electrolyte replacement

II. Monitor, describe, record:

A. Electrolytes, BUN, ABGs	A. Identifies abnormal levels indicating risk for or presence of deficiencies leading to metabolic acidosis/alkalosis
B. Weight daily or as needed on same scale, at same time, with same clothes	B. Indicates losses associated with fluid or nutritional inadequacy
C. I&O q4–8h (include effluent, vomitus, diarrhea, aspirate)	C. Provides data to determine imbalance in fluid status, decrease in output can indicate obstruction

III. Administer:

A. IV fluid and electrolyte replacement	A. Ensures adequate fluid and nutrition immediately postoperatively
B. Antidiarrheal PO, stool softener PO	B. Acts to control diarrhea and prevent constipation

INTERVENTION	RATIONALE
IV. Perform/provide:	
A. Patent N/G, gastrostomy, or jejunostomy tube attached to suction	A. Inserted postoperatively to remove gas and fluids that could cause intestinal distension, pressure on wound
B. Ice chips and small amounts of fluid PO if bowel sounds present, remove tube, and begin clear liquid diet in 24 hours	B. Begins oral intake of fluids
C. Progressive dietary inclusions to general diet, fluid intake to 2 to 3 L/day	C. Provides optimal nutrition and fluids for wound healing, maintain health status
D. Suggest to chew food well	D. Improves digestion and absorption
E. Avoid cheese, corn, celery, nuts, chocolate	E. Contributes to constipation
F. Avoid liver, spinach, raw or highly seasoned foods, hot or cold beverages, fried or fatty foods	F. Contributes to diarrhea
G. Avoid onions, cabbage, legumes, cucumbers	G. Contributes to gas formation
H. Include bananas, rice, potato, fruit juices, bouillon in diet	H. Prevents or corrects fluid and electrolyte imbalance if ileostomy effluent becomes watery
I. Referral to nutritionist	I. Assists to plan diet with foods that are best tolerated and avoid complications

NURSING DIAGNOSES
Knowledge deficit related to general post-operative care information, follow-up care including wound/ostomy procedures, nutrition/fluid needs, measures to prevent stoma or intestinal complications, signs and symptoms to report

EXPECTED OUTCOMES
Adequate information and teaching about follow-up care evidenced by performance of care required for proper ileostomy or colostomy function and absence of complications, expression of feelings about participation in care of ostomy, verbalization about monitoring of pattern related to elimination via bowel diversion

INTERVENTION	RATIONALE
V. Teach patient/family: A. Pathophysiology and bowel diversion anatomic changes, type of ostomy and consistency and characteristics of material eliminated	A. Provides information and rationale for functional pattern of bowel following surgery
B. Dressing change and wound/stoma protection during bathing	B. Maintains clean dry wound and stoma
C. Removal and application of appliance, pouch application and emptying with associated skin and stoma assessment and care (ileostomy and colostomy), allow to demonstrate and practice	C. Ensures proper and safe care and use of ostomy supplies and skin protection/barriers to prevent leakage and skin breakdown
D. Colostomy irrigation daily or q2days, allow to demonstrate and practice	D. Ensures bowel cleansing and trains for establishment of bowel elimination pattern

INTERVENTION	RATIONALE
E. Instruct in draining and irrigating of continent ileostomy, clamping of catheter if in the stoma, insertion of catheter into stoma to drain reservoir, allow to demonstrate and practice using catheter to drain into a toilet by gravity	E. Ensures correct method and schedule of emptying reservoir for progressive decrease in need for ileal draining, can begin in 3 to 4 days following surgery q2h for 2 weeks to prevent distention and pressure on suture line, then catheter removed and followed by catheter insertion to perform drainage
F. Application of pad, catheter placement in reservoir at night, and connection to drainage device	F. Provides care of ileoanal anastomosis postoperatively
G. Defecation prior to overdistention of rectum or to respond to urge to defecate to avoid incontinence while bowel adapts to change in pattern, include perianal cleansing and skin care	G. Ileorectal anastomosis and ileoanal reservoir bowel diversion procedures do not require stoma or appliance care as drainage is excreted via the colon
H. Proper cleansing of pouches/catheters, use of deodorant tablets in pouch, storage of reusable supplies, list of agencies that provide ostomy supplies	H. Minimizes embarrassing odors from the ostomy drainage and provides resources for supplies and equipment to care for various bowel diversions
I. Inform that stoma size will reach permanent status by 4 months	I. Prevents anxiety caused by changes in stoma

INTERVENTION	RATIONALE
J. Medication administration to include dose, frequency, time, how to take drug(s), condition being treated, expected effects, side effects and what to do if they occur, medications to avoid such as vitamins, enteric coated and time released, hormones as they are not absorbed in the small intestine	J. Protects or treats infection, skin irritation, diarrhea, or constipation
K. Avoid excessive exercises or lifting heavy objects, contact sports, or any trauma to the abdomen, plan for rest periods during convalescence	K. Activity restrictions following surgery to allow for healing and prevent trauma
L. Fluid intake of 2 to 3 L/day spread over 24 hours or amount based on ileostomy output or diarrhea associated with colostomy	L. Ensures adequate fluid intake to prevent fluid/electrolyte imbalance or constipation in bowel diversion surgery
M. Dietary modification of low-residue, high-protein, -carbohydrate, and -calorie intake; avoid raw foods, popcorn, greasy or spicy foods, hot or cold beverages, high-fiber foods	M. Promotes wound healing and prevents discomfort or elimination problems in ileostomy procedures (excessive output, diarrhea, constipation)
N. Exclude nuts, cabbage, legumes, broccoli, cauliflower, corn, carbonated beverages, seeds, others that affect elimination	N. Prevents gas formation, constipation, diarrhea, irritation of stoma with colostomy

INTERVENTION	RATIONALE
O. Suggest wearing loose or full clothing, use pads to cover stoma	O. Covers appliance, prevents soiling of clothing
P. Suggest alternative sexual activities, covering stoma during sexual activity, possibility of sexuality counseling	P. Assistive aids can enhance sexual satisfaction
Q. Report any redness, swelling, or pain at wound site, change in stoma and output characteristics, temperature elevation	Q. Signs and symptoms of possible complications of bowel diversion
R. Inform of planned chemotherapy or radiation therapy if appropriate	R. Postoperative therapy for malignancy
S. Importance of keeping appointments with physician as scheduled	S. Ensures that wound is healing and underlying disease is monitored
T. Suggest counseling if appropriate, community agencies such as American Cancer Society, Ostomy Club	T. Provides support and information that assists in adaptation to ostomy

cholecystitis/cholelithiasis/cholecystectomy

DEFINITION

Cholecystitis is the inflammation of the gallbladder involving the mucosa and wall that can eventually cause scarring, tissue fibrosis, and impaired function of the organ. It is usually associated with cholelithiasis, which is the presence of stones in the gallbladder that vary in size and commonly become lodged in the cystic or common bile duct resulting in biliary tract obstruction. Cholelithiasis is thought to be caused by the composition of the bile, bile stasis, or infection. Cholecystitis is usually a result of cholelithiasis or abnormality in the ductal system (kinks, twists) causing obstruction. Cholecystectomy is the most common surgical procedure performed to remove the gallbladder and stones and can include common bile duct exploration (choledocholithotomy) to treat inflammation or stones involved in the gallbladder system. Risk factors for these disorders are obesity, lack of exercise or active life-style, and underlying liver, pancreas, or ileal disorders. Procedures such as lithotripsy that can pulverize a small number of stones and remove them, or ingestion or instillation of an agent orally or by percutaneous cholecystolithotomy to dissolve the stones are also performed on selected patients. This plan includes the care of gallbladder disease and postoperative care specific to these diseases and can be used in association with the PREOPERATIVE CARE and POSTOPERATIVE CARE plans if surgery is performed

NURSING DIAGNOSIS

Pain related to physical injuring agent of inflammatory process, ductal spasms or obstruction resulting in irritation and distention of the gallbladder (choleycystitis, cholelithiasis), trauma of surgery postoperatively (cholecystectomy)

EXPECTED OUTCOMES

Pain relieved or controlled evidenced by verbalization that pain reduced by analgesic therapy, fewer requests for medication, ability to perform activities postoperatively

INTERVENTION	RATIONALE
I. Assess for:	
A. Pain severity and site, factors that increase or decrease pain (high-fat meal), descriptors such as biliary colic beginning in upper mid-abdomen that radiates to back and right scapula, flatulence	A. Provides data on intensity and locale of pain to identify gallbladder disease (acute and chronic)
B. Abdominal guarding, grimacing, crying, restlessness	B. Nonverbal indications of pain when not able to communicate pain
C. Incisional pain and characteristics (site, type, severity) and responses	C. Provides basis for postoperative analgesia to control pain
III. Administer:	
A. Analgesic IM	A. Acts by inhibiting pain pathways in CNS and alters pain perception pre- and postoperatively (morphine avoided as this increases spasms of sphincter of Oddi)
B. Anticholinergic PO	B. Acts to reduce spasms of ducts that cause pain
IV. Perform/provide:	
A. Quiet environment, backrub, relaxation exercises	A. Measures to reduce pain by decrease in stimuli
B. Place in low Fowler's or sidelying position, change position q2h	B. Reduces upper abdominal pressure, increases comfort in acute stages

INTERVENTION	RATIONALE
C. Assist to deep-breathe and to splint incisional area	C. Relaxes muscles and reduces pain
D. Assure that analgesic will be administered before pain becomes severe, advise to request analgesic as soon as pain appears and to report if medication does not relieve pain	D. Prevents extreme discomfort post-operatively

NURSING DIAGNOSES
Altered nutrition: Less than body requirements related to inability to ingest (nausea, vomiting, abdominal distention, NPO status, rejection of restrictive diet), digest food (lack of bile for fat digestion), and absorb nutrients (excretion of fats and fat-soluble vitamins with the lack of bile) pre- and postoperatively (cholecystitis, cholelithiasis, cholecystectomy)

Risk for fluid volume deficit related to excessive losses through normal route (vomiting), abnormal route (nasogastric tube aspirate) during acute pre- and postoperative periods

EXPECTED OUTCOMES
Adequate nutritional and fluid intake during acute phase of illness evidence by control of vomiting, effective replacement by IV infusion until oral intake permitted, I&O ratio and weight within normal determinations

INTERVENTION	RATIONALE
I. Assess for: A. Nausea, vomiting, abdominal distention or feeling of fullness, intolerance to fats in diet, regurgitation, dyspepsia	A. Symptoms of gallbladder inflammation or bile flow obstruction causing inadequate intake of nutrients

INTERVENTION	RATIONALE
B. NPO status, N/G tube and suctioning, restricted fluid intake	B. Indicates causes for fluid imbalance in inflammation with or without complications pre- and postoperatively
C. Weight loss, weakness, fatigue, anorexia, 24-hour intake of food groups and calories	C. Indicates reduced intake of protein, calories, and digestion and absorption of nutrients with reduced bile flow
D. Skin and mucous membranes dryness, skin turgor, oliguria	D. Indicates risk for dehydration from fluid losses
E. Muscle cramping, weakness, confusion, abdominal cramps, irregular pulse, muscle twitching, paresthesia	E. Symptoms of electrolyte deficits (K, Na, Cl)

II. Monitor, describe, record:

A. I&O q4–8h, including aspirate, vomitus	A. Determines fluid balance
B. Electrolytes	B. Reveals electrolyte imbalance with fluid losses (K, Na, Cl)
C. Weight daily or as needed on same scale, time, clothing, measurement of tricep skinfold	C. Determines weight loss or gain

III. Administer:

A. IV fluids/electrolyte replacement	A. Provides short-term fluids and nutrition until PO intake resumed

INTERVENTION	RATIONALE
B. Anti-emetic IM	B. Acts to reduce vomiting by depressing the chemore-ceptor trigger zone
C. Hydrocholeretics PO	C. Acts to stimulate bile pro-duction to assist with ab-sorption of fats/vitamins
D. Vitamins A, D, E, K	D. Acts to supplement vita-mins if not absorbed as a result of lack of bile salts

IV. Perform/provide:

A. Low-fat, -cholesterol diet, high protein and carbohy-drate intake	A. Prevents gallbladder at-tack by limiting fat in diet
B. Assist to take deep breathes if nauseated	B. Decreases urge to vomit
C. Place in semi-Fowler's po-sition, and change position slowly	C. Movements can stimulate vomiting center
D. Oral care after each episode of vomiting	D. Promotes cleanliness and comfort of mouth
E. Environment that is odor free, quiet, and restful	E. Stimuli that can initiate vomiting
F. Maintain NPO status, N/G tube and suction	F. Decompresses gastroin-testinal tract to rest stom-ach and prevent vomiting, distention
H. Clamp T-tube prior to and unclamp following meals as ordered	H. Allows for bile to flow into duodenum to assist in di-gestion and absorption of foods

INTERVENTION	RATIONALE
I. Progressive diet as tolerated with restriction in fatty foods such as cream, butter, cheese, milk, fried foods, ice cream	I. Fats are poorly digested with reduced bile
J. Increased fluid intake of 2500 mL/day PO as indicated	J. Provides adequate fluid intake
K. Referral to nutritionist	K. Provides information and instruction to ensure adequate nutritional intake with suggested inclusions and exclusions

NURSING DIAGNOSES

Risk for impaired skin integrity related to internal factor of altered pigmentation (jaundice) preoperatively resulting from duct obstruction causing bile salts accumulation under the skin, external factor of secretions/excretions postoperatively resulting from wound drainage at T-tube site causing skin irritation, mechanical factor of pressure to nasal mucosa resulting from N/G tube placement causing irritation and dryness

Risk for injury related to internal factors postoperatively of infection, inflammation resulting from leakage of bile into peritoneum, bile flow obstruction, trauma causing peritonitis, pancreatitis, abscess

EXPECTED OUTCOMES

Reduced risk or absence of skin impairment and surgical complications of inflammation/infection evidenced by wound site and mucous membranes intact and free of irritation, jaundice, excoriation, and breakdown, absence or resolution of increased abdominal pain, nausea, vomiting, elevated temperature, obstructed bile flow via T-tube, and WBC, VS within normal parameters.

INTERVENTION	RATIONALE
I. Assess for:	
A. Jaundice, pruritis, skin excoriation, scratching of areas causing redness and breaks	A. Results from bile flow obstruction causing bile salts to accumulate under skin
B. Irritation, redness, drainage around T-tube wound site and characteristics, dressings for bile drainage q2h, patency of T-tube for kinking or dislodgment	B. Indicates risk for skin breakdown and infection at wound site(s), T-tube patency determines leakage around site (bile) that irritates skin
C. Nasal mucosa for redness, dryness, irritation, breaks	C. Indicates risk for breakdown from N/G tube pressure and mouth breathing
D. Abdominal fullness when T-tube clamped, increased bile flow, clay colored feces, dark urine, jaundice	D. Signs and symptoms of continuing obstruction of bile flow caused by the trauma of surgery or inflammation
E. Abdominal pain, tachycardia, tachypnea, absent bowel sounds, hypotension, fever, chills, lethargy, confusion, nausea, vomiting	E. Signs and symptoms of complications associated with gallbladder disease that can occur pre- or postoperatively
II. Monitor, describe, record:	
A. VS and temperature q2–4h	A. Decreased BP, increased P and temperature, rapid R indicates infection resulting from biliary system complications
B. T-tube drainage q4h	B. Indicates amount and color that should decrease in amount and become dark brown in color

INTERVENTION	RATIONALE
C. CBC, WBC, amylase, lipase	C. Increases in WBC indicates infection, and pancreatic enzyme changes
D. ALT, AST, bilirubin	D. Reveals increases indicating organ involvement (obstruction, inflammation)
E. Urine bilirubin, fecal urobilinogen	E. Abnormalities indicate obstruction as bilirubin not converted to urobilinogen in intestine
F. Ultrasonography, computerized tomography (CT), cholangiography (oral, IV), abdominal flat plate	F. Diagnostic procedures for gallbladder disease (stones, patent duct system)

III. Administer:

INTERVENTION	RATIONALE
A. Hyperlipidemic PO	A. Acts to bind with bile salts and assist with excretion to reduce accumulation under skin
B. Antimicrobial PO	B. Acts to inhibit synthesis of cell wall in prevention or treatment of infection pre- and postoperatively
C. Antipyretic PO	C. Acts to reduce temperature

IV. Perform/provide:

INTERVENTION	RATIONALE
A. Cool, humidified environment, loose gown to wear	A. Increases comfort and reduces dry skin and mucosa

INTERVENTION	RATIONALE
B. Cool, moist compresses to skin, emollient bath with mild soap and warm water, pat dry thoroughly	B. Allays itching and soothes skin
C. Apply pressure, massage to areas instead of scratching	C. Reduces itching and urge to scratch
D. Lubricate lips and nares, artificial saliva and mouth wash rinses q4h, encourage nasal breathing, offer hard candy, lozenges, ice chips if permitted	D. Treats dryness and prevents breaks in oral mucosa, mouth breathing increases dryness of oral mucosa
E. Attach tubing to face in comfortable position	E. Prevents continued pressure or rubbing against nasal passages
F. Maintain dry, clean skin at closed wound site	F. Prevents skin irritation and breakdown
G. Change dressings as needed using sterile technique if T-tube is in place, apply zinc oxide or petrolatum to skin around tube	G. Prevents saturation with drainage and further contamination or skin irritation from dressings
H. Use caution not to disturb drain, pull on it, or allow tubing to kink when changing dressings, empty bag when $\frac{1}{3}$ full, and measure to prevent pull on wound by weight of container, maintain level of bag below drainage site	H. Prevents accidental dislodgment or backup of drainage into ducts and possibly peritoneal cavity; drainage varies from 500 to 1000 mL/day initially with gradual reduction to 200 mL/day

INTERVENTION	RATIONALE
I. Maintain low Fowler's position, assist to turn and ambulate, fasten drainage bag to clothing when ambulating	I. Facilitates drainage by gravity and prevents dislodgment of drainage system
J. Prepare for diagnostic tests or procedures, surgery with preoperative care (N/G tube and suction, NPO status, bed rest with position of comfort)	J. Begins interventions to diagnose and treat complications

NURSING DIAGNOSIS

Knowledge deficit related to follow-up postoperative care to promote ongoing wound healing and resumption of life-style activities

EXPECTED OUTCOMES

Adequate knowledge and information provided evidenced by compliance with dietary/medication/daily activities and restrictions, wound care postoperatively

INTERVENTION	RATIONALE
V. Teach patient/family:	
A. Pathophysiology and cause of gallbladder disease and overview of surgical procedure and care	A. Provides information about surgery and rationale for care
B. Wound care, to cover with waterproof plastic when bathing if not completely healed	B. Protects wound and dressings from dampness

INTERVENTION	RATIONALE
C. Dressing change using sterile or clean technique as needed, inform that drain will be removed as healing takes place, allow to return demonstration of dressing change and cleansing around drain, emptying bag twice daily	C. Maintains clean, dry wound if drain is still in place
D. Medications names, dose, time, frequency, side effects to report	D. Ensures correct administration of medication regimen
E. Fluid intake of 2 to 3 L/day, dietary intake of low-fat foods, fiber, protein, inform that loose feces can follow surgery for several months	E. Promotes bowel elimination without straining and increasing intra-abdominal pressure, wound healing following surgery
F. Advise refraining from returning to work or resume activities for 6 weeks, depending on physician's advice specific to activity	F. Prevents stress on wound site that may weaken area prior to complete healing
G. Report changes in wound appearance such as redness, swelling, pain, or increased drainage at the incisional site, change in color of feces or appearance of fatty feces, abdominal pain, temperature, chills, bleeding tendencies of mucous membrane, skin petechiae, hematoma, blood in feces or urine	G. Indicates possible complications of infection, obstruction, inadequate vitamin K absorption

cirrhosis of liver

DEFINITION

Cirrhosis is a chronic process of liver cell death and scarring or fibrosis formation. Nodules develop and cause structural changes as the liver attempts to regenerate resulting in obstruction of portal blood flow, bile flow, and by-products of hepatic function. This then results in venous congestion and causes collateral blood flow in veins of the lower esophagus (esophageal varices), rectum, and the pre-umbilical abdominal area, as well as ascites and encephalopathy. Portal hypertension develops as a reduction in hepatic function becomes more severe. Types of cirrhosis include Laennec's (most common) caused by alcohol abuse, postnecrotic caused by viral hepatitis and chemical hepatotoxins, and biliary caused by chronic biliary inflammation and bile stasis in hepatic tissue ducts. These causes constitute the risk factors involved in cirrhosis. This plan includes the care of this condition and can be used in association with the ANORECTAL DISORDERS and HEPATITIS care plans

NURSING DIAGNOSES

Anxiety related to change in health status causing inability to manage feelings of uncertainty, apprehension regarding prognosis and threat of death resulting from liver failure/hepatic coma, change in self-concept resulting from ascites and jaundice, situational crisis of chronic illness

Ineffective individual coping related to inability to cope with change in life-style, personal vulnerability, and inadequate support systems

Body image disturbance related to biophysical factor of ascites, jaundice, and edema resulting in change in appearance, and cognitive perceptual factor of alteration in thought process, dependence on others for care

EXPECTED OUTCOMES

Anxiety within manageable levels, development of coping and problem-solving skills, progressive adaptation to body image and life-style changes evidenced by verbalizations that anxiety is decreasing, fear reduced, and receptive to planning and participating in personal care and activities

INTERVENTION	RATIONALE
I. Assess for:	
A. Apprehension, anxiety level, feelings about change in body appearance and personal adequacy	A. Provides data regarding perceptions and anxiety that can range from mild to severe and high level associated with changes in body image
B. Use of coping mechanisms, stated fears of uncertainty of disease outcome, lifestyle changes	B. Assists in identifying inappropriate and appropriate use of coping skills, ineffective coping leads to depression and other psychosocial disorders
C. Restlessness, diaphoresis, complaining, joking, withdrawal, talkativeness, increased P and R	C. Nonverbal expressions of anxiety when not able to communicate feelings
D. Personal resources to cope with stress, anxiety, and interest in learning to problem-solve, use of defense mechanisms	D. Support systems and personal strengths assist in developing coping skills
E. Feelings and response to change in role, ability to carry out role and participation in sexual/social activities, fear of stigmatization and rejection	E. Changes in body image and self-concept a common and serious problem with changes in structure and function of a body part
III. Administer:	
A. Anti-anxiety agent PO (avoid hepatotoxic drugs)	A. Acts to reduce anxiety level and provides calming effect and rest, depresses subcortical levels of CNS, limbic system

INTERVENTION	RATIONALE
IV. Perform/provide:	
A. Environment conducive to expression of feelings about changes in body image, avoid judgments and negative responses to illness and feelings	A. Provides opportunity to vent feelings and reduce fear and anxiety about illness and feelings of inadequacy
B. Allow time for expression of feelings in privacy, encourage communications with significant others, encourage to focus on abilities rather than inabilities	B. Identifies positive behaviors and time and willingness to adapt to change in appearance and life-style
C. Diversional activities such as relaxation exercises, TV, radio, music, reading, tapes, guided imagery, encourage to continue usual interests	C. Reduces anxiety and promotes comfort
D. Allow to participate in planning of care to maintain usual activities when possible, allow to participate in care when possible, and formulate realistic expectations	D. Allows for some control over situations, self-image can improve with involvement in self-care
E. Referral to counseling or support group	E. Assists in providing information and support for long-term care

NURSING DIAGNOSES

Altered nutrition: Less than body requirements related to inability to ingest (anorexia, nausea, vomiting, dyspepsia, ascites, rejection of restrictive diet), digest food (lack of bile for fat digestion), and absorb nutrients (excretion of fats and fat-soluble vitamins with the lack of bile) resulting from decreased liver function causing inability to metabolize fats, proteins, carbohydrates and to store nutrients

Risk for fluid volume deficit related to excessive losses through normal route (vomiting, diarrhea)

EXPECTED OUTCOMES
Adequate nutritional and fluid intake evidenced by control of vomiting, optimal daily intake of planned meals, I&O ratio and electrolytes, VS, laboratory test results, and weight within normal determinations

INTERVENTION	RATIONALE
I. Assess for:	
A. Nausea, vomiting, dyspepsia, gas accumulation, flatulence	A. Symptoms of cirrhosis causing anorexia and reduced food intake
B. Weight loss, weakness, fatigue, anorexia, skinfold thickness, stomatitis, 24-hour recall of food groups and calories	B. Indicates reduced intake of protein, calories, and digestion and absorption of nutrients with reduced bile flow that can lead to malnutrition
C. Fluid intake, skin and mucous membrane dryness, skin turgor, oliguria	C. Indicates risk for dehydration from fluid losses
D. Muscle cramping, weakness, confusion, abdominal cramps, irregular pulse, muscle twitching, paresthesia	D. Symptoms of electrolyte deficits (K, Na) associated with fluid imbalance
E. Bowel, urinary elimination pattern changes	E. Indicates presence of diarrhea or constipation associated with altered liver metabolism of food intake or dietary restrictions

INTERVENTION	RATIONALE
II. Monitor, describe, record:	
A. Weight daily or as needed on same scale, time, clothing, measurement of tricep skinfold	A. Determines weight loss or gain
B. I&O q4–8h	B. Determines fluid balance ratio
C. Electrolytes	C. Reveals electrolyte imbalance with fluid losses/excesses (K, Na)
D. Total proteins with albumin and globulin, cholesterol, transferrin, Hb, Hct	D. Levels indicating nutritional status with total proteins <8.4 g/dL, albumin <3.5 g/dL, globulin >3.5 g/dL as liver is able to synthesize albumin but not globulins, cholesterol <120 mg/dL as the result of impaired fat metabolism
E. Serum and urine bilirubin, AST, ALT, alkaline phosphatase	E. Indicates liver dysfunction caused by impairment with bilirubin as high as 15 mg/dL, AST >27 U/L, ALT >21 U/L
F. Liver nuclear scan, computerized tomography (CT), biopsy	F. Reveals enlarged liver, destruction and fibrosis of tissue
III. Administer:	
A. IV fluids/electrolyte replacement	A. Provides short-term fluids and nutrition until PO intake resumed

INTERVENTION	RATIONALE
B. Anti-emetic IM	B. Acts to reduce vomiting by depressing the chemore-ceptor trigger zone
C. Antidiarrheal, stool soft-ener PO	C. Acts to inhibit motility or coats and protects intesti-nal lining, softens feces for easier elimination
D. Vitamins A, D, E, K PO	D. Acts to supplement vita-mins if liver is unable to store these

IV. Perform/provide:

A. Quiet, pleasant environ-ment for meals, offer 6 small meals/day	A. Promotes appetite and food intake and prevents feeling of fullness, nausea and dyspepsia
B. Encourage to take deep breaths if patient is nause-ated	B. Decreases urge to vomit
C. Place in semi Fowler's po-sition or higher for meals	C. Movements can stimulate vomiting center, elevated head of bed decreases dys-pepsia
D. Allow for time to eat slowly, to chew foods well and avoid drinking with meals, and rest following meals	D. Promotes nutritional in-take while reducing ten-dency for nausea and vom-iting
E. Oral care after each episode of vomiting and prior to meals	E. Promotes cleanliness and comfort of mouth

INTERVENTION	RATIONALE
F. Progressive diet as tolerated, high-calorie (3000/day) -protein and -carbohydrate and restriction in fatty foods such as cream, butter, cheese, milk, fried foods, ice cream	F. Maintains nutritional status while restricting fat intake with impaired liver function that limits flow of bile
G. Increased fluid intake of 2500 mL/day PO as indicated, include fruit juices, bouillon, Gatorade	G. Provides adequate fluid and electrolyte replacement
H. Offer hard candy, ginger ale	H. Provides fluids and reduces thirst and nausea
I. Referral to nutritionist	I. Provides information and instruction to ensure adequate nutritional and fluid intake with suggested inclusions and exclusions

NURSING DIAGNOSES

Fluid volume excess related to compromised regulatory mechanism of increased ADH secretion and aldosterone resulting from decreasing hormone metabolism by impaired liver, increased hydrostatic pressure, and decreased colloid osmotic pressure causing decreased water excretion and increased water and sodium retention, increased pressure in portal blood flow system, and third-spacing (ascites)

Ineffective breathing pattern related to decreased lung expansion resulting from increased intra-abdominal pressure of ascites

Pain related to physical injury agent of pressure and stretching resulting from distention of liver capsule and peritoneum, spasm of biliary ducts and vascular system of liver

EXPECTED OUTCOMES

Pain reduced or controlled, breathing maintained with optimal ease, and edema/ascites resolved evidenced by respiration rate, depth, I&O, and weight within baseline determinations, verbalizations that pain relieved and patient is able to participate in ADL

INTERVENTION	RATIONALE
I. Assess for:	
A. Abdominal pain with severity, locale (RUQ), type (dull, heavy feeling), enlarged liver palpable	A. Symptoms of liver dysfunction and disease
B. Dyspnea, changes in breath sounds, respiratory depth as fluid accumulation increases	B. Indicates compromised breathing pattern
C. Peripheral edema, neck vein distention, weight gain, increased abdominal girth, abnormal breath sounds (crackles, diminished)	C. Indicates fluid retention (ascites, pulmonary) as regulation of hormones are compromised with portal hypertension
II. Monitor, describe, record:	
A. VS q2–4h	A. P and BP increases as fluid is retained
B. I&O q4–8h	B. Indicates fluid balance with output decreasing as fluid retention increases
C. ABGs, pulse oximetry	C. Indicates hypoxemia and need for oxygen supplement
D. Weight daily same scale, same time, same clothing	D. Indicates fluid retention as weight increases

INTERVENTION	RATIONALE
E. Electrolytes	E. Decreases in K and increases in Na if ADH increased and diuretic therapy administered
F. Chest x ray	F. Reveals pulmonary edema or pleural effusion

III. Administer:

A. Analgesic PO with evaluation of those that are metabolized by the liver	A. Acts to relieve pain, narcotic analgesics and acetaminophen dosages are reduced if impairment severe
B. Diuretic PO, IV	B. Acts to promote fluid excretion or inhibit ADH secretion
C. Plasma, colloids IV	C. Acts to maintain albumin and protein levels that can be lost into peritoneal cavity
D. Salt-poor albumin IV	D. Acts to replace albumin to enhance movement of fluids from abdominal cavity for elimination
E. Oxygen via nasal cannula	E. Supplements oxygen based on ABGs or oximetry

IV. Perform/provide:

A. Place in semi- or high Fowler's position, and change position q2h, support arms and chest with pillows	A. Promotes ease in breathing pattern

INTERVENTION	RATIONALE
B. Assist with deep breathing exercises, incentive spirometry, IPPB if ordered	B. Improves breathing pattern
C. Elevate edematous areas, use eggcrate mattress on bed	C. Provides comfort and prevents pressure to susceptible areas
D. Restrict fluid intake to 1000 to 1500 mL/day, Na intake restriction of 200 to 500 mg/day	D. Maintains fluid balance by reducing fluid excess and prevent further fluid retention
E. Prepare for and assist with paracentesis and monitor for shock response to procedure q1h (VS)	E. Removes fluid accumulation from abdomen

NURSING DIAGNOSES

Risk for impaired skin integrity related to internal factor of altered pigmentation (jaundice) resulting from bile salts accumulation under the skin, external factor of skin irritation (scratching), mechanical factor of pressure to edematous areas

Risk for infection related to inadequate primary defenses (stasis of body fluids of lungs, urine), inadequate secondary defenses (leukopenia, loss of Kupffer cells in the liver) resulting from splenomegaly, and malnutrition resulting from chronic illness

Altered protection related to abnormal blood profile (leukopenia, coagulation) resulting from decreased absorption of vitamin K and production of coagulation factors causing bleeding tendency

EXPECTED OUTCOMES

Reduced risk or absence of skin impairment, bleeding abnormalities, and complication of inflammation/infection evidenced by skin intact and free of irritation, jaundice and breakdown, absence or resolution of elevated temperature, cloudy foul-smelling urine, abnormal breath sounds, bleeding from skin, mucous membranes, or other areas, and WBC, VS within normal ranges

INTERVENTION	RATIONALE
I. Assess for:	
A. Jaundice of skin and sclera, pruritis, irritation, scratching of areas causing redness and breaks	A. Results from bile flow obstruction causing bile salts to accumulate under skin, high bilirubin levels that diffuse into tissues
B. Redness, pressure on edematous parts	B. Indicates risk for skin breakdown
C. Ecchymosis, purpura, bleeding gums and mucous membranes, joints for pain, swelling, blood in urine, vomitus, feces	C. Indicates bleeding and possible hemorrhage
II. Monitor, describe, record:	
A. VS and temperature q2–4h	A. Decreased BP, increased P and temperature, rapid R indicates infection
B. CBC, WBC, Hct, Hb, coagulation factors	B. Increases in WBC >10,000/mm^3 indicates infection, an anemic condition can result from bleeding and decreased Hct <37% and Hb <10 g/dL, prothrombin, fibrinogen, VII, IX, X decreased as liver unable to produce factors
C. Urine, sputum culture	C. Identifies infectious agent
D. Urine, feces for occult blood	D. Indicates presence of bleeding

INTERVENTION	RATIONALE
III. Administer	
A. Hyperlipidemic PO	A. Acts to bind with bile salts and assists with excretion to reduce accumulation under skin
B. Antihistamine PO	B. Acts to allay itching if jaundice present
C. Antimicrobial PO	C. Acts to inhibit synthesis of cell wall in prevention or treatment of infection
D. Antipyretic PO	D. Acts to reduce temperature
E. Vitamin K PO, cryoprecipitate IV	E. Acts to provide vitamin needed for clotting as liver unable to absorb K, replaces clotting factors in more severe bleeding problems
IV. Perform/provide:	
A. Cool, humidified environment, loose gown to wear	A. Increases comfort and reduces dry skin and pruritis
B. Cool, moist compresses to skin, emollient bath with mild soap and warm water, pat dry thoroughly	B. Allays itching and soothes skin
C. Apply pressure, massage to areas instead of scratching	C. Reduces itching and urge to scratch
D. Maintain dry, clean skin at areas with edema present	D. Prevents skin irritation and breakdown

INTERVENTION	RATIONALE
E. Trim nails as needed	E. Prevents breaks in skin if scratching
F. Support for edematous areas and change position q2h	F. Relieves pressure that can lead to skin breakdown
G. Avoid shaving with razor, blowing nose with force, straining at defecation, using rough toothbrush or dental floss	G. Results in excessive bleeding when coagulation factors are low
H. Fluid intake of 2000 mL/day if allowed	H. Dilutes urine to prevent infection
I. Handwash, use of sterile supplies for treatments	I. Prevents transmission of pathogens

NURSING DIAGNOSES

Activity intolerance related to generalized weakness, presence of respiratory problems, fatigue resulting from sleep deprivation, anemia, bed rest status causing inability to perform self-care activities

Altered thought processes related to physiological changes (hepatic encephalopathy) resulting from inability of impaired liver to convert ammonia to urea causing its concentration in the brain

Social isolation related to alteration in physical appearance, mental status, and unaccepted social behavior (alcohol ingestion) resulting in feelings of rejection and hostility

EXPECTED OUTCOMES

Activity and mental status at optimal level evidenced by progressive participation in ADL, improved memory, orientation, and attention span, successful social interactions observed with verbalization of increased comfort in ability to participate in social situations

INTERVENTION	RATIONALE
I. Assess for:	
A. Fatigue, weakness, effect of bed rest on conditioning, amount of activity capable of performing, effect of illness on sleep pattern	A. Provides information about level of activity during various phases of illness
B. Memory, attention span, confusion, disorientation, personality changes, lethargy, speech changes	B. Indicates buildup of NH_3 as the liver is unable to convert it to urea for excretion
C. Social interactions, hostility, preference to limit interactions, family or peer acceptance, expressed feelings of insecurity, rejection, indifference	C. Indicates a discomfort with others or a desire to be alone
II. Monitor, describe, record:	
A. Ammonia	A. Reveals increases of >110 mcg/dL affecting thought processes
III. Administer:	
A. Sedative PO, unless respirations <12/minute	A. Acts on limbic and subcortical levels of CNS and increases sleep time
B. Oxygen via nasal cannula	B. Supplements oxygen during daily activities or sleep as needed if respiratory status compromised by ascites
IV. Perform/provide:	
A. Bed rest in a position of comfort with body parts supported with pillows	A. Conserves energy and provides needed rest

INTERVENTION	RATIONALE
B. Perform or assist in ADL and other activities as needed, place all articles and call light within reach to use as desired, utilize self-care aids as appropriate	B. Conserves energy while preserving as much control and independence as possible
C. Increase activities gradually from sitting up in bed, in chair, walking in room, to bathroom, and in hall with daily increase in distance and ADL activities	C. Progressive change in activities increases with endurance and energy level and prevents symptoms of activity intolerance
D. Organize activities around rest periods in a quiet, calm, dimly lit. environment free of stimuli and respiratory irritants	D. Permits rest without interruptions
E. Restrict or encourage visitors as appropriate for level of tolerance or need for socialization, encourage family and friends to visit	E. Prevents additional stimuli that interfere with rest, causes fatigue, but interaction with visitors can be a positive activity to prevent isolation
F. Compare mental capabilities daily such as writing samples, reorient to time, place, person, place a clock, radio, newspaper, TV in room	F. Identifies changes in neurological status if thinking and memory affected
G. Set aside time to interact, answer questions in simple terms and repeat when needed	G. Provide stimulation and socialization

INTERVENTION	RATIONALE

H. Reduce protein intake when NH_3 levels are high to 20 to 40 g/day, and increase of 10 to 20 g/day q2–3 days as tolerated (Lipomol-Oral can be administered if on tube feedings)

H. Provides restrictions to reduce buildup of ammonia in brain

NURSING DIAGNOSIS

Knowledge deficit related to ongoing long-term care and prevention of complications and further dysfunction associated with the disease with resumption of life-style activities

EXPECTED OUTCOMES

Adequate knowledge and information provided evidenced by compliance with dietary/medication/daily activities and restrictions, modification of social habits

INTERVENTION | RATIONALE

V. Teach patient/family:

A. Pathophysiology and cause of hepatic disease and overview of treatments and care

A. Provides information about disease and rationale for care

B. Medication names, dose, time, frequency, side effects to report, list of medication to avoid that depend on liver for metabolism such as sedatives, analgesics, and anti-anxiety agents, acetaminophen among others

B. Ensures correct administration of medication regimen without causing toxic condition

INTERVENTION	RATIONALE
C. Fluid intake of 2 to 3 L/day, dietary intake of low-fat foods, fiber, protein, low sodium intake and a list of foods to include and avoid (sample menus excluding fats and Na in particular)	C. Provides nutritional/fluid intake related to hepatic dysfunction
D. Advise refraining from any alcohol intake, and suggest support group that can assist to abstain, avoid making judgments about decision	D. Prevents further hepatic damage and metabolization of alcohol by impaired function
E. Avoid activities that are traumatizing such as safety razor, floss or hard brush for teeth cleansing, blowing nose hard, or straining at defecation, and strenuous contact sports	E. Prevents bleeding if tendency exists
F. Avoid intimate contact with large groups of people, those with hepatitis, perform handwash frequently	F. Prevents transmission of pathogens
G. Schedule daily routine activities to include rest and avoid fatigue	G. Adequate rest is important to maintain liver function

INTERVENTION	RATIONALE
H. Report changes in skin and mucous membrane such as redness, swelling, pain, temperature, chills, bleeding tendencies of mucous membrane, skin petechiae, hematoma, blood in feces or urine, weight gain, changes in mentation	H. Indicates possible complications of infection, inadequate vitamin K absorption, impending comatose state
I. Referral to counseling, nutritionist, sex therapist, smoking and alcohol rehabilitation	I. Provides support and information to modify life-style with long-term regimen
J. Importance of follow-up appointments with physician, referrals	J. Reinforces medical regimen to restore and maintain health status

diverticulosis/diverticulitis

DEFINITION

Diverticulosis is the pouching of areas of the large intestine's muscular wall, mostly in the sigmoid portion. Weakness in this wall develops as a result of increased intraluminal pressure caused by chronic constipation, pressure exerted to move feces into the rectum, or obesity. Diverticulitis, which can be acute or chronic, is the inflammation of these pouches caused by undigested material lodged in them that prevents adequate circulation and allows bacterial invasion of the area. Risk factors include the aging adult, presence of chronic overweight and constipation, and dietary ingestion of indigestible seeds or other substances. In more severe cases of inflammation, obstruction, or development of abscess or perforation, surgery is performed (colon resection with or without temporary colostomy). This plan includes the care of these conditions and can be used in association with the BOWEL RESECTION/DIVERSION (COLOSTOMY/ILEOSTOMY), PREOPERATIVE CARE, and POSTOPERATIVE CARE plans if surgery is performed

NURSING DIAGNOSES

Constipation related to less-than-adequate dietary intake of bulk resulting in hard formed feces and straining at defecation causing diverticulosis, narrowed colon resulting from chronic diverticulitis causing constipation and possible obstruction

Altered nutrition: Less than body requirements related to inability to ingest food to maintain normal daily bowel elimination pattern or because of nausea, anorexia resulting from inflammation in diverticulitis

EXPECTED OUTCOMES

Adequate bowel elimination pattern and nutritional intake evidenced by soft formed feces eliminated, progressive return to dietary intake with fiber inclusion following treatment for diverticulitis

INTERVENTION	RATIONALE
I. Assess for:	
A. Pattern of elimination, ribbonlike feces, constipation and characteristics (blood, mucus) constipation alternating with diarrhea, flatus, obstipation	A. Information regarding bowel elimination to determine disease status
B. Dietary habits, intake of foods containing fiber, undigestible roughage, foods containing seeds	B. Prevents constipation and treats diverticulosis by creating bulk and preventing material from blocking diverticula
III. Administer:	
A. Stool softener PO	A. Acts to soften feces by increasing fluid content for easier passage
B. Bulk laxative PO	B. Acts to provide bulk to feces to prevent constipation
IV. Perform/provide:	
A. NPO status during acute phase of diverticulitis	A. Rests colon until inflammation subsides
B. Soft diet including bulk such as bran, cereals, avoid high-bulk foods such as raw fruits, vegetables, seeds in foods such as strawberries, cucumbers, tomatoes, popcorn	B. Increases bulk in feces to prevent feces occluding diverticula leading to inflammation (diverticulitis)
C. Fluids to 2 to 3 L/day, especially if taking bulk laxative	C. Provides daily fluid needs and prevents constipation

INTERVENTION	RATIONALE
D. Fluids and nutrients IV, slowly progress to oral fluids and general high-residue diet plan	D. Provides hydration and nutrition until oral intake is allowed as pain, temperature, and inflammation are present
E. N/G tube care and patency	E. Maintains decompression and rests bowel during inflammation

NURSING DIAGNOSIS

Pain related to physical injuring agent of inflammation (diverticulitis) resulting from bacterial invasion causing edema, spasm, and irritability of colon

EXPECTED OUTCOMES

Relief or control of pain evidenced by verbalization that pain reduced or absent, decreased request for analgesic

INTERVENTION	RATIONALE
I. Assess for: A. Intermittent or continuous lower left quadrant abdominal pain, cramping	A. Indicates diverticulosis
B. Pain severity, type, referred back pain, abdominal guarding, flexed knees, mass in LLQ, temperature elevation	B. Indicates possible diverticulitis
II. Monitor, describe, record: A. Temperature q4h	A. Elevation indicates inflammation

INTERVENTION	RATIONALE
III. Administer:	
A. Analgesic PO	A. Acts to reduce pain by interrupting CNS pain pathways
B. Anticholinergic PO	B. Acts to control muscle spasms
C. Antibiotic PO	C. Acts to control inflammation causing the pain by interfering with cell wall synthesis
D. Antipyretic PO	D. Acts to reduce temperature in presence of inflammation
IV. Perform/provide:	
A. Bed rest in quiet, stimuli-free environment	A. Reduces pain perception
B. Place in position of comfort with hot dry application to painful area	B. Promotes comfort and reduces inflammatory process and pain by increasing circulation to the area

NURSING DIAGNOSIS

Knowledge deficit related to care regimen to prevent or treat diverticular disease

EXPECTED OUTCOMES

Compliance with dietary, activity restrictions and fluid, medication administration evidenced by absence of diverticulitis

INTERVENTION	RATIONALE
V. Teach patient/family:	
A. Medication administration, including name, action, dose, frequency, side effects; avoid over-the-counter laxatives unless advised by physician	A. Ensures correct medications to prevent constipation
B. Diet inclusions of fiber and restrictions of nuts, raw fruits and vegetables, alcohol, spicy foods, foods that contain seeds	B. Promotes regular bowel elimination while avoiding foods that can obstruct the diverticula or irritate the colon
C. Low-calorie diet with lists of foods to eat and avoid and sample menus	C. Promotes weight loss if obesity is a problem
D. Fluid intake of 2 to 3 L/day	D. Ensures adequate fluid intake and prevents constipation
E. Avoid activities such as lifting, stooping, coughing, straining	E. Increases intra-abdominal pressure that contributes to diverticula formation
F. Report fever, abdominal pain, diarrhea, persistent constipation, blood or mucus in feces	F. Signs and symptoms of diverticulitis for early treatment to control infection

esophagitis/achalasia

DEFINITION
Esophagitis is the inflammation of the esophagus caused by physical or chemical trauma. Reflux esophagitis is the reflux of gastric contents into the esophagus (gastroesophageal reflux disease) resulting from an incompetent lower esophageal sphincter or a sliding hiatal hernia. It can eventually lead to a breakdown of the esophageal mucosa from the constant exposure to gastric juices. Achalasia (cardiospasm) is the dilatation of the lower esophagus caused by a decrease in motility in the lower two-thirds of the esophagus and ineffective peristalsis. This results in a sphincter that does not relax in response to swallowing, causing an obstruction as food and fluid accumulate in the lower esophagus. It is a chronic progressive disease that causes esophageal inflammation, ulceration, and aspiration of material (respiratory infections, atelectasis). Risk factors for the disease are smoking, caffeine beverages, increased hormonal levels (estrogens, progesterone), drugs such as theophylline, and a high-fat diet. This plan includes care of these conditions with a focus on prevention or relief of the associated symptoms

NURSING DIAGNOSES
Pain related to physical injuring agent of esophageal spasms in achalasia and irritation of esophageal mucosa in gastric reflux

Chronic pain related to chronic physical condition resulting in progressive, continuous, or intermittent esophageal discomfort and dysphagia for at least 6 months

EXPECTED OUTCOMES
Pain controlled or minimized evidenced by verbalization that discomfort reduced or absent following meals or with medication

INTERVENTION	RATIONALE
I. Assess for:	
A. Retrosternal pain, severity and frequency, following swallowing, halitosis, inability to belch, regurgitation of food and/or mucus	A. Indicates achalasia associated with dysphagia with symptoms gradually becoming more severe and frequent
B. Substernal pain, heartburn moving up and down esophagus, pain that radiates to the back or neck, bloating or full feeling, regurgitation of sour-tasting material, dysphagia, factors that precipitate pain (supine position, abdominal distention, following meals)	B. Indicates esophagitis associated with gastroesophageal reflux that usually occurs after meals and can be frequent and intermittent or prolonged over time
II. Monitor, describe, record:	
A. Esophagogastroscopy with manometry	A. Determines degree of lower esophageal sphincter status, dilation and food retention
B. Gastric analysis, acid perfusion tests	B. Confirms diagnosis of reflux disease
C. Barium swallow	C. Determines diagnosis of achalasia and demonstrates the presence of reflux
III. Administer:	
A. Analgesic (non-narcotic) PO	A. Acts to relieve pain by interfering with CNS pain pathways

INTERVENTION	RATIONALE
B. Antacid PO	B. Acts to reduce acid concentration in the stomach and increase lower esophageal sphincter tone, relieves pain when taken prior to and following meals
C. Anticholinergic PO	C. Acts to lower esophageal pressure to treat achalasia by relaxing smooth muscle to prevent spasms, improves strength of esophageal sphincter
D. Cholinergic PO	D. Acts to increase lower esophageal pressure to prevent reflux if given with an antacid and histamine antagonist prior to meals for reflux disorder
E. Gastrointestinal stimulant PO	E. Acts to stimulate smooth muscle and motility to accelerate gastric emptying in reflux disease

IV. Perform/provide:

A. Place in position of comfort, preferably sitting for meals and avoid lying position for 2 to 3 hours after meals	A. Prevents regurgitation and reflux of gastric contents into esophagus, relieves pain following meals
B. Oral care prior to and after meals and as needed	B. Prevents halitosis

INTERVENTION	RATIONALE
C. Sleep with head elevated	C. Prevents gastric reflux that irritates esophagus mucosa and causes pain, promotes gastric emptying
D. Encourage standing or walking after meals	D. Relieves discomfort

NURSING DIAGNOSES

Altered nutrition: Less than body requirements related to inability to ingest foods and fluids because of dysphagia, reflux of gastric reflux resulting in irritation of mucosa and pain

Impaired swallowing related to obstruction resulting from edema or spasm, esophageal lumen that is narrowed from long-term inflammation causing dysphagia, possible aspiration

EXPECTED OUTCOMES

Adequate nutritional intake with minimal reflux and dysphagia evidenced by ingestion of six small meals/day without discomfort

INTERVENTION	RATIONALE
I. Assess for:	
A. Food and fluid intake/24 hr and preferences, cultural factors affecting eating pattern, weight loss or gain	A. Provides information needed for meal planning
B. Dysphagia, times and frequency, precipitating factors, effect on appetite and nutritional intake	B. Identifies severity and extent of swallowing impairment
II. Monitor, describe, record:	
A. Weight daily or as appropriate same clothes, scale, time of day	A. Reveals gains or losses and need to revise dietary plan

INTERVENTION	RATIONALE
B. Respiratory pattern q4h	B. Reveals pulmonary complications associated with aspiration
IV. Perform/provide:	
A. Small frequent meals (4 to 6/day) instead of 3 meals/day, bland diet to reduce irritation to mucosa	A. Prevents overdistention of lower esophagus and obstruction
B. Eat slowly and take fluids with food, chew foods well prior to swallowing	B. Assists to swallow food and prevents dysphagia
C. Fluids following meals	C. Cleanses esophagus to prevent irritation in esophagitis
D. Elevate head of bed to semi-Fowler's or higher during and following meals	D. Prevents reflux and minimizes dysphagia and regurgitation
E. Referral to nutritionist	E. Plans and supports dietary intake to provide adequate nutrition, weight loss or gain caloric diets

NURSING DIAGNOSIS

Knowledge deficit related to follow-up care to prevent or treat recurrent episodes of reflux and achalasia

EXPECTED OUTCOMES

Adequate understanding of care measures evidenced by compliance with instructions and absence of signs and symptoms associated with esophageal disorder

INTERVENTION	RATIONALE
V. Teach patient/family:	
A. Preparation and ingestion of semi-soft, warm foods rather than cold, rough foods	A. Provides ease of food passage through esophagus without further irritation to the mucosa
B. Avoid foods such as spicy, hot, iced foods, alcohol, fruit juices, caffeine or carbonated beverages	B. Irritates esophagus
C. Avoid sucking on candy, chewing gum, smoking, using a straw for fluids	C. Reduces chances of swallowing air
D. Inform to avoid coughing, straining at defecation, bending at waist, wearing tight clothing at the waist	D. Prevents gastric reflux
E. Administration of medications including name, action, dose, time, frequency, side effects to report	E. Ensures correct and effective medication regimen
F. Report pain that cannot be relieved with conservative measures, hematemesis, excessive bloating, persistent weight loss, changes in breathing pattern and sputum color, temperature elevation	F. Allows for early intervention to prevent complications

gastrectomy/gastroplasty

DEFINITION

Gastrectomy is the total or partial (up to 75%) surgical removal of the stomach. The choice of procedure depends on the reason for surgery (peptic ulcer or gastric malignancy) and location of the pathology. Other reasons for gastric surgery include repair of perforation, hemorrhage, or obstruction. A gastroenterostomy is a palliative procedure to connect the stomach to the duodenum done in place of gastrectomy to treat an obstruction caused by tumor size. Gastrojejunostomy is another procedure performed that involves a large portion of the stomach and connection of the stomach to the jejunum and preserving the section of the duodenum that collects the flow of digestive bile and other juices. A total gastrectomy involves the complete removal of the stomach and duodenum with an esophagus to jejunostomy anastomosis to treat late stage gastric malignancy. Gastroplasty (gastric partitioning) is the surgical reduction of the stomach size by dividing the stomach by transection or stapling that creates a gastric pouch capable of holding a limited amount of intake. It is done for extreme obesity that has resulted from excessive caloric intake over a long time that has not responded to weight reduction by other means. This plan includes care of these procedures and can be used in association with the PEPTIC ULCER, PREOPERATIVE CARE, and POST-OPERATIVE CARE plans

NURSING DIAGNOSIS

Anxiety related to threat to or change in health status causing inability to manage feelings of uncertainty and apprehension regarding prognosis (cancer), and ability to comply with lifelong dietary regimen

Ineffective individual coping related to inability to cope with illness and control of future life-style changes

Body image disturbance related to biophysical factor of change in appearance (obesity)

EXPECTED OUTCOMES

Anxiety and fear within manageable levels, development of coping and problem-solving skills, body image improved evidenced by verbalizations that anxiety is decreasing, fear reduced, participation in care activities and receptive to planning for ongoing care, progressive management of dietary regimen

INTERVENTION

I. Assess for:

A. Level of anxiety, use of coping mechanisms, stated fears of uncertainty of disease outcome, life-style changes

B. Restlessness, diaphoresis, complaining, joking, withdrawal, talkativeness, increased P and R

C. Personal resources to cope with stress, anxiety, and interest in learning to problem-solve, use of defense mechanisms

D. Feelings and response to appearance, role adequacy, embarrassment in social activities, feelings of stigma, negative expressions about appearance and need to change life-style

RATIONALE

A. Anxiety can range from mild to severe and high level associated with surgery for cancer, assists in identifying inappropriate use of coping skills

B. Nonverbal expressions of anxiety when not able to communicate feelings

C. Support systems and personal strengths assist in developing coping skills

D. Body image and self-concept can be a serious problem in overweight individuals

INTERVENTION	RATIONALE
III. Administer: 　　A. Anti-anxiety agent PO	A. Acts to reduce anxiety level and provides calming effect and rest, depresses subcortical levels of CNS, limbic system
IV. Perform/provide: 　　A. Environment conducive to rest, time to express fears and anxiety, avoid anxiety-producing situations	A. Decreases stimuli that cause stress/anxiety, venting of feelings decreases anxiety
B. Suggest new methods to enhance coping skills and problem solving, allow to externalize and identify those that help	B. Offers alternative coping strategies that allow for release of anxiety and fear
C. Positive feedback regarding progress made, focus on abilities rather than inabilities	C. Provides support for adaptive behavior, promotes self-worth and responsibility
D. Diversional activities such as relaxation exercises, TV, radio, music, reading, tapes, guided imagery, encourage to continue usual interests	D. Reduces anxiety and promotes comfort
E. Allow to participate in planning of care to maintain usual activities when possible, allow to participate in dietary planning as soon as possible	E. Allows for some control over situations

INTERVENTION	RATIONALE
F. Suggest visit from one who has lost weight by dieting or following gastroplasty	F. Promotes support and encouragement to achieve goal of weight loss

NURSING DIAGNOSES

Altered nutrition: less than body requirements post-operatively related to inability to ingest (anorexia, nausea, early satiety, dietary restrictions) or absorb (dumping syndrome, decreased digestive secretions) nutrients resulting in malabsorption, weight loss, malnutrition, poor wound healing

Altered nutrition: more than body requirements preoperatively related to excessive intake in relation to metabolic need, dysfunctional eating patterns resulting in persistent or recurrent weight gain and obesity

EXPECTED OUTCOMES

Optimal nutritional intake pre- and postoperatively evidenced by stable weight pattern within acceptable range for height, sex, and age, albumin, transferrin, Hb within normal levels, progressive weight loss of 1 to 2 lb/week and absence of unexpected weight gain (gastroplasty)

INTERVENTION	RATIONALE
I. Assess for:	
A. Appetite, cultural factors, amount and type of foods eaten daily, psychological factors, underlying medical problem, amount of weight over the ideal weight, weight reduction programs attempted, adherence to dietary/exercise regimens	A. Provides nutritional information regarding long-term obesity, dysfunctional eating patterns are often the result of internal or external cues other than hunger such as pairing food with activities, continued weight gain indicates noncompliance with dietary/activity regimen
B. Anorexia, nausea, vomiting, diarrhea, fatigue, ability to eat and accept dietary modifications in types, amounts, caloric value of foods when PO intake allowed	B. Indicates problem areas affecting nutritional intake postoperatively

INTERVENTION	RATIONALE
C. Reduction in PO intake, early satiety, diarrhea, abdominal cramping, diaphoresis, increased bowel weakness, dizziness within 1 hour following meals	C. Temporary postoperative symptoms resulting from reduced size of stomach or pouch size, early dumping syndrome in gastrectomy resulting from increased intestinal peristalsis and rapid movement of food into the jejunum
D. Nausea, vomiting, epigastric fullness	D. Indicates overdistention of gastric pouch
II. Monitor, describe, record: A. Weight daily or as needed on same scale, at same time, with same clothes	A. Indicates gains or losses associated with nutritional inadequacy, weight loss common in total gastrectomy and desired in gastroplasty (1–2 lb/week)
B. I&O q4–8h (include vomitus, diarrhea, aspirate)	B. Provides data to determine imbalance in fluid status, decrease in output can indicate obstruction
C. BUN, albumin, transferrin, CBC	C. Reveals changes that indicate malnutrition
III. Administer: A. IV fluid and nutritional replacement	A. Ensures adequate fluid and nutrition immediately postoperatively
B. Antidiarrheal PO	B. Acts to control diarrhea and prevent loss of fluid and nutrients postoperatively

INTERVENTION	RATIONALE
C. Anti-emetic PO, IM	C. Acts to reduce or control vomiting postoperatively
D. Vitamin/mineral supplement PO	D. Acts to ensure that necessary substances in intake pre- and postoperatively if on restrictive diet
E. Anticholinergic PO	E. Acts to delay gastric emptying in the presence of dumping syndrome
F. Antacid/histamine receptor antagonist PO	F. Acts to prevent recurrence of ulcer in remaining portion of stomach

IV. Perform/provide:

A. Patent N/G tube attached to suction	A. Inserted postoperatively to remove gas and fluids that could cause gastric distension, pressure on wound, prevent overdistention of pouch
B. Begin oral intake with about 30 mL, aspirate in 1 hour to determine if fluid is retained	B. Oral intake in small amounts while N/G tube in place and removed when bowel sounds return and water retained
C. Progressive diet with soft foods six times/day in small amounts PO when N/G tube is removed, feedings via jejunostomy when bowel sounds return	C. Diet plan until general diet tolerated to prevent too much food eaten at a time that can cause discomfort, about 3 months are needed to resume normal eating pattern

INTERVENTION	RATIONALE
D. Encourage to chew food well and eat slowly	D. Maintains adequate intake in a form that is easily digestible
E. Maintain fluid nutritional intake with protein supplement and progress to solid foods beginning with progressive feedings q1h to six/day with 60 mL water between meals within 2 months	E. Nutritional regimen following a gastrostomy to promote intake and prevent fullness, nausea, or vomiting
F. Oral care prior to meals/feedings, pleasant environment during meals	F. Promotes comfort and appetite
G. Referral to nutritionist for dietary inclusions and restrictions based on surgical procedure	G. Assists to plan diet with foods that are best tolerated and avoid complications

NURSING DIAGNOSIS
Knowledge deficit related to general postoperative care information, follow-up and maintenance care, including wound procedures, nutrition/fluid needs, signs and symptoms to report

EXPECTED OUTCOMES
Adequate information and teaching about follow-up care evidenced by compliance of dietary regimen and absence of complications associated with surgery (wound infection, late dumping syndrome, obstruction)

INTERVENTION	RATIONALE
V. Teach patient/family	
A. Pathophysiology and anatomic changes, type of surgery, possible recurrence of peptic ulcer	A. Provides information and rationale for functional pattern of gastrointestinal tract following surgery
B. Dressing change and wound protection during bathing, report pain, swelling, purulent drainage, temperature	B. Maintains clean dry wound
C. Medication administration to include dose, frequency, time, how to take drug(s), condition being treated, expected effects, side effects and what to do if they occur, medications to avoid such as aspirin, steroids or administer with antacid	C. Protects or treats infection, diarrhea, nausea, nutritional inadequacy
D. Avoid excessive exercises or lifting heavy objects, contact sports, or any trauma to the abdomen, plan for rest periods during convalescence	D. Activity restrictions following surgery to allow for healing and prevent trauma
E. Importance of dietary modification and importance of preventing weight gain	E. Improves compliance in weight control
F. Behavior modification in eating schedule, pattern, environment	F. Promotes compliance while integrating changes into life-style
G. Eat in sitting position, rest for 30 minutes after meals	G. Enhances digestion

INTERVENTION	RATIONALE
H. Dietary modification of adequate protein, carbohydrate, and caloric intake, six regularly scheduled meals/day plus snacks of calculated amounts based on size of remaining stomach, avoid skipping meals, drink fluids between meals in small amounts	H. Promotes wound healing and prevents discomfort and malnutrition following gastrectomy
I. Dietary modification of liquid or blenderized food, chew solid foods well when allowed and limit amounts/calories as ordered, eat/drink slowly, divide daily intake into six meals, fluids between meals to 1500 mL/day	I. Prevents overdistention of pouch or pressure on suture/staple line and prevents intake of excessive amounts and calories following gastroplasty
J. Avoid caffeine-containing beverages, foods irritating to gastric mucosa (spicy, raw, hot or cold, greasy), smoking, and stressful situations	J. Promotes dietary restrictions and activities to prevent recurrence of peptic ulcer
K. Report nausea, vomiting, diarrhea, epigastric fullness or discomfort, black tarry feces, weight loss or gain, weakness	K. Signs and symptoms of complications
L. Inform of planned chemotherapy or radiation therapy if appropriate	L. Postoperative therapy for malignancy

INTERVENTION	RATIONALE
M. Importance of keeping appointments with physician as scheduled	M. Ensures that wound is healing and nutritional/general health status is monitored
N. Suggest counseling if appropriate, community agencies such as American Cancer Society, weight loss group, smoking cessation group	N. Provides support and information that assists in adaptation to changes in lifestyle and nutritional patterns

hepatitis

DEFINITION

Hepatitis is an inflammatory condition of the liver. It can be caused by a virus, bacterium, or substance toxic to the liver. It results in damage in liver cells leading to impairment depending on the loss of the cellular function. Viral hepatitis conditions include hepatitis A (HAV) transmitted via food, water or milk, hepatitis B (HBV) transmitted via body fluids of an infected person, hepatitis C (HCV) transmitted via personal contact or blood transfusion, and hepatitis D (HDV) transmitted via contact with blood or blood products. Incubation periods vary with the different types of hepatitis. Immunization is available for hepatitis B prior to or during the disease, hepatitis A is prevented by good personal hygiene practices, monitoring water and public eating places, and an immunoglobin can be administered prior to a suspected exposure. Those at risk for the disease include health personnel, those who receive dialysis or multiple transfusions, homosexual males, and parenteral drug users. This plan provides general care for the various types of the disease and can be used in association with the ANEMIA, ACQUIRED IMMUNODEFICIENCY DISEASE, HEMOPHILIA, and CIRRHOSIS OF LIVER care plans

NURSING DIAGNOSES

Anxiety related to change in health status and interpersonal transmission of disease causing inability to manage feelings of uncertainty of the consequences of the disease, apprehension regarding change in life-style and personal vulnerability

Body image disturbance related to biophysical factor of jaundice resulting from diffusion of bilirubin in tissues causing change in appearance

EXPECTED OUTCOMES

Anxiety within manageable levels, development of coping with temporary change in appearance evidenced by verbalizations that anxiety is decreasing and receptive to planning and participating in personal care and activities, preventive measures

INTERVENTION	RATIONALE
I. Assess for:	
A. Apprehension, anxiety level, feelings about change in body appearance	A. Provides data regarding perceptions and anxiety that can range from mild to severe and high level associated with changes in body image
B. Use of coping mechanisms, stated fears of uncertainty about life-style changes	B. Assists in identifying inappropriate and appropriate use of coping skills, ineffective coping leads to depression and other psychosocial disorders
C. Personal resources to cope with anxiety and interest in learning to problem-solve	C. Support systems and personal strengths assist in coping with life-style changes
D. Feelings and response to ability to carry out role and participation in sexual/social activities	D. Changes in body image and self-concept a common problem with disease that affects appearance or life-style
III. Administer:	
A. Anti-anxiety agent PO (avoid hepatotoxic drugs)	A. Acts to reduce anxiety level and provides calming effect and rest, depresses subcortical levels of CNS, limbic system

INTERVENTION	RATIONALE
IV. Perform/provide:	
A. Environment conducive to expression of feelings about changes in body image, avoid judgments and negative responses to illness and feelings about cause	A. Provides opportunity to vent feelings and reduce fear and anxiety about illness
B. Allow time for expression of feelings in privacy, focus on abilities rather than inabilities	B. Identifies positive behaviors and time and willingness to adapt to change in life-style
C. Diversional activities such as relaxation exercises, TV, radio, music, reading, tapes, guided imagery, encourage to continue usual interests	C. Reduces anxiety and promotes comfort and social interaction
D. Allow to participate in planning of care to maintain usual activities when possible, allow to participate in care when possible	D. Allows for some control over situations, self-image can improve with involvement in self-care

NURSING DIAGNOSES

Altered nutrition: Less than body requirements related to inability to ingest (anorexia, nausea, vomiting, dyspepsia), digest food (lack of bile for fat digestion), and absorb nutrients (excretion of fats and fat-soluble vitamins with the lack of bile) resulting from decreased liver function causing inability to metabolize fats, proteins, carbohydrates and to store nutrients

Risk for fluid volume deficit and electrolytes related to excessive losses through normal route (vomiting) and reduced fluid intake

EXPECTED OUTCOMES

Adequate nutritional and fluid intake evidenced by control of vomiting, optimal daily intake of planned meals, I&O ratio, VS, laboratory test results, and weight within normal determinations

INTERVENTION	RATIONALE
I. Assess for:	
A. Nausea, vomiting, dyspepsia, gas accumulation	A. Symptoms of hepatitis causing anorexia and reduced food intake
B. Weight loss, weakness, fatigue, anorexia, skinfold thickness, 24-hour recall of food groups and calories, presence of diarrhea	B. Indicates reduced intake of protein, calories, and digestion and absorption of nutrients with reduced bile flow that can lead to malnutrition
C. Fluid intake, skin and mucous membrane dryness, skin turgor, oliguria	C. Indicates risk for dehydration from fluid losses
D. Muscle cramping, weakness, confusion, abdominal cramps, irregular pulse, muscle twitching, paresthesia, dizziness	D. Symptoms of electrolyte deficits (K, Cl) associated with fluid imbalance
II. Monitor, describe, record:	
A. Weight daily or as needed on same scale, time, clothing, measurement of tricep skinfold	A. Determines weight loss or gain
B. I&O q4–8h	B. Determines fluid balance ratio

INTERVENTION	RATIONALE
C. Electrolytes	C. Reveals electrolyte imbalance with fluid losses/excesses (K, Cl, Na)
D. Total proteins with albumin and globulin, cholesterol, transferrin, Hb, Hct	D. Levels indicating nutritional status with total proteins <8.4 g/dL, albumin <3.5 g/dL, globulin >3.5 g/dL as liver is able to synthesize albumin but not globulins, cholesterol <120 mg/dL as the result of impaired fat metabolism
E. Serum and urine bilirubin, AST, ALT, alkaline phosphatase	E. Indicates liver dysfunction caused by impairment with bilirubin as high as 15 mg/dL, AST >27 U/L, ALT >21 U/L

III. Administer:

A. IV fluids/electrolyte replacement	A. Provides short-term fluids and nutrition until PO intake resumed
B. Anti-emetic IM	B. Acts to reduce vomiting by depressing the chemoreceptor trigger zone
C. Vitamins A, D, E, K PO	C. Acts to supplement vitamins if liver is unable to store these

IV. Perform/provide

A. Quiet, pleasant environment for meals, offer six small meals/day	A. Promotes appetite and food intake and prevents feeling of fullness, nausea and dyspepsia

INTERVENTION	RATIONALE
B. Assist to take deep breaths if nauseated	B. Decreases urge to vomit
C. Place in semi-Fowler's position or higher for meals	C. Movements can stimulate vomiting center, elevated head decreases dyspepsia
D. Allow for time to eat slowly, to chew foods well and avoid drinking with meals, rest following meals	D. Promotes nutritional intake while reducing tendency for nausea and vomiting
E. Oral care after each episode of vomiting and prior to meals	E. Promotes cleanliness and comfort of mouth
F. Progressive diet as tolerated, high-calorie (3000/day), -protein, and -carbohydrate and restriction in fatty foods such as cream, butter, cheese, milk, fried foods, ice cream, and spicy, acidy foods that are irritating	F. Maintains nutritional status while restricting fat intake with impaired liver function that limits flow of bile, dietary plan should include 75 to 100 g/protein, 300 to 400 g/carbohydrate, 75 to 100 g/fat to enhance recovery of impaired liver
G. Increased fluid intake of 2500 mL/day PO as indicated, include fruit juices, bouillon, Gatorade, avoid caffeine-containing beverages	G. Provides adequate fluid and electrolyte replacement
H. Offer hard candy, ginger ale	H. Provides fluids and reduces thirst and nausea

INTERVENTION	RATIONALE
I. Referral to nutritionist	I. Provides information and instruction to ensure adequate nutritional and fluid intake with suggested inclusions and exclusions

NURSING DIAGNOSES

Risk for impaired skin integrity related to internal factor of altered pigmentation (jaundice) resulting from bile duct obstruction causing bile salts accumulation under the skin and pruritis

Altered protection related to abnormal blood profile (leukopenia, coagulation) resulting from decreased absorption of vitamin K and production of coagulation factors causing bleeding tendency

EXPECTED OUTCOMES

Reduced risk or absence of skin impairment, bleeding abnormalities evidenced by skin intact and free of irritation, jaundice and breakdown, absence or resolution of skin, mucous membrane, or other source of bleeding

INTERVENTION	RATIONALE
I. Assess for:	
A. Jaundice of skin and sclera, pruritis, irritation, scratching of areas causing redness and breaks	A. Results from bile flow obstruction causing bile salts to accumulate under skin, high bilirubin levels that diffuse into tissues
B. Ecchymosis, purpura, bleeding gums and mucous membranes, joints for pain and swelling, blood in urine, vomitus, feces	B. Indicates bleeding and possible hemorrhage

INTERVENTION	RATIONALE
II. Monitor, describe, record:	
A. CBC, Hct, Hb, coagulation factors	A. Abnormal levels in CBC indicates an anemic condition from bleeding and decreased Hct <37% and Hb <10 g/dL, prothrombin, fibrinogen, VII, IX, X decreased as liver unable to produce factors
B. Urine, feces for occult blood	B. Indicates presence of bleeding
C. HB_sAg, HB_cAg, HB_eAG (hepatitis B), and IgM, IgG (hepatitis A)	C. Diagnostic tests for positive results indicating hepatitis A or B
III. Administer:	
A. Hyperlipidemic PO	A. Acts to bind with bile salts and assist with excretion to reduce accumulation under skin
B. Antihistamine PO	B. Acts to allay itching if jaundice present
C. Vitamin K PO	C. Acts to provide vitamin needed for clotting as liver unable to absorb K
IV. Perform/provide:	
A. Cool, humidified environment, loose gown to wear	A. Increases comfort and reduces dry skin and pruritis
B. Cool, moist compresses to skin, emollient bath with mild soap and warm water, pat dry thoroughly	B. Allays itching and soothes skin

INTERVENTION	RATIONALE
C. Apply pressure, massage to areas instead of scratching	C. Reduces itching and urge to scratch
D. Maintain dry, clean skin at areas with edema present	D. Prevents skin irritation and breakdown
E. Trim nails as needed	E. Prevents breaks in skin if scratching
F. Avoid shaving with razor, blowing nose with force, straining at defecation, using rough toothbrush or dental floss	F. Results in excessive bleeding when coagulation factors are low
G. Relaxation techniques	G. Provides diversion from pruritis and desire to scratch

NURSING DIAGNOSES

Activity intolerance related to generalized weakness, fatigue resulting from sleep deprivation, anemia, bed rest status and immobility causing inability to perform self-care activities

Social isolation related to alteration in physical appearance, therapeutic isolation or limitations in personal contact with others resulting in restrictions in social/sexual activities and loneliness

EXPECTED OUTCOMES

Activity at optimal level evidenced by progressive participation in ADL, successful social interactions observed with verbalization of increased interest and comfort in social situations and reduced fear of transmitting the disease

INTERVENTION	RATIONALE
I. Assess for:	
A. Fatigue, weakness, effect of bed rest on conditioning, amount of activity capable of performing, effect of illness on sleep pattern	A. Provides information about level of activity during various phases of illness
B. Pain in upper abdomen (RUQ), joints, severity, and other characteristics	B. Results from liver inflammation that requires bed rest
C. Social interactions, interests, hobbies, desire for activity or visitors	C. Indicates a need for selective activities to relieve boredom if isolation precautions are in effect
D. Feelings regarding isolation procedures and effect (negative statements about self)	D. Prevents transmission of disease to others
III. Administer:	
A. Analgesic PO (evaluate those that are metabolized by liver)	A. Acts to reduce pain by interfering with CNS pathways
B. Anti-inflammatory agent PO	B. Acts to reduce inflammation
IV. Perform/provide:	
A. Bed rest in a position of comfort	A. Conserves energy and provides needed rest to prevent relapse

INTERVENTION	RATIONALE
B. Perform or assist in ADL and other activities as needed, place all articles and call light within reach to use as desired, utilize self-care aids as appropriate	B. Conserves energy while preserving as much control and independence as possible
C. Increase activities gradually from sitting up in bed, in chair, walking in room, to bathroom, and in hall with daily increase in distance and ADL activities	C. Progressive change in activities increases with endurance and energy level and prevents symptoms of activity intolerance
D. Organize activities around rest periods in a quiet, calm, dimly lit, environment free of stimuli	D. Permits rest without interruptions
E. Restrict or encourage visitors as appropriate for level of tolerance or need for socialization, encourage family and friends to visit	E. Prevents additional stimuli that interfere with rest, causes fatigue, but interaction with visitors can be a positive activity to prevent loneliness or depression
F. Set aside time to interact q2–3h, answer questions about isolation as needed	F. Provide stimulation and socialization

INTERVENTION	RATIONALE

G. Perform appropriate precautionary level of isolation as follows:
  a. For type A: careful handwash, handling of feces, disinfection of dishes, toilet, clothing, wearing gloves
  b. For type B and non-A, non-B: careful handwash, wear gloves for handling body fluids, needles, syringes, drawing blood, wear mask if necessary, autoclave articles not disposable and dispose of others according to universal standards (hazardous waste)
	G. Prevents transmission of disease to others

H. Suggest games, hobbies, or interests that can be done in the hospital	H. Provides stimulation and interest in environment

NURSING DIAGNOSIS

Knowledge deficit related to ongoing long-term care and prevention of complications and further dysfunction associated with the disease and allows for resumption of life-style activities

EXPECTED OUTCOMES

Adequate knowledge and information provided evidenced by compliance with dietary/medication/daily activities and restrictions, modification of social habits

INTERVENTION	RATIONALE
V. Teach patient/family:	
A. Pathophysiology and cause of hepatic disease, type and mode of transmission, overview of treatment and care	A. Provides information about disease and rationale for care
B. Jaundice is temporary and disappears with improvement	B. Provides positive feeling that skin will return to normal
C. Medications' names, dose, time, frequency, side effects to report; list of medication to avoid that depend on liver for metabolism such as sedatives, analgesics, and anti-anxiety agents, acetaminophen among others	C. Ensures correct administration of medication regimen without causing toxic condition
D. Fluid intake of 2 to 3 L/day, dietary intake of low-fat foods, fiber, protein, low sodium intake, and list of foods to include and avoid (sample menus excluding fats and Na in particular)	D. Provides nutritional/fluid intake related to hepatic dysfunction
E. Advise refraining from any alcohol intake and suggest support group that can assist to abstain, avoid making judgments about decision	E. Prevents further hepatic damage and metabolism of alcohol by impaired function
F. Advise to wear colors other than neutral or light shades	F. Accentuates yellow color of skin

INTERVENTION	RATIONALE
G. Avoid activities that are traumatizing such as using safety razor, floss or hard brush for teeth cleansing, blowing nose hard or straining at defecation, strenuous contact sports	G. Prevents bleeding if tendency exists
H. Schedule daily routine activities to include rest and avoid fatigue	H. Adequate rest is important to maintain liver function
I. Precautions to take such as handwash prior to eating and after bathroom use, use disposable utensils, wash with hot water or dishwasher, avoid sharing food, wash clothing and bed linens separately with disinfectant (chlorine bleach), dispose of tissues, needles and syringes, and other used articles according to universal precautions, avoid kissing and sexual intercourse until no transmission possible, do not donate blood	I. Measures to prevent transmission of disease to others
J. Report changes in skin and mucous membrane such as redness, swelling, pain, temperature, chills, bleeding tendencies of mucous membrane, skin petechiae, hematoma, blood in feces or urine, weight gain	J. Indicates possible complications of infection, inadequate vitamin K absorption

INTERVENTION	RATIONALE
K. Refer all contacts for evaluation of possible transmission	K. Contacts can be immunized against disease (immunoglobulin)
L. Referral to counseling, nutritionist, sex therapist, alcohol rehabilitation	L. Provides support and information to modify life-style
M. Importance of follow-up appointments with physician, referrals	M. Reinforces medical regimen to restore and maintain health status

herniorrhaphy

DEFINITION

Herniorrhaphy is the repair of a defect in the wall of a cavity that allows the protrusion of abdominal contents through a defect in the abdominal wall, the diaphragm, or through a structure within the cavity from its normal position. Hernias are thought to occur from a weakness in the abdominal muscles (acquired or congenital) and increased intra-abdominal pressure. They can be direct or indirect and occur at the femoral, inguinal, umbilical, or incisional sites. Most common is the indirect inguinal hernia occurring in men. The defect can be repaired and the contents of the sac replaced, sac closed and reinforced to prevent recurrence. A hernioplasty is the reinforcement of the weak area with fascia or mesh. Risk factors include obesity, sedentary life-style, and aging. Hernias can be repaired surgically for permanent reduction or as an emergency procedure to correct strangulation (circulation cut off from a portion of the bowel) or incarceration (irreducible) of a portion of the bowel associated with a hernia. This plan includes care of the various surgical procedures for hernias and can be used in association with the PREOPERATIVE CARE and POSTOPERATIVE CARE plans

NURSING DIAGNOSES

Pain related to physical injuring agent of surgical repair trauma resulting in tension of the incisional site

   Altered urinary elimination related to mechanical trauma of surgery, especially in men with inguinal repair resulting in urinary retention

EXPECTED OUTCOMES

Relief or absence of pain and resumption of urinary pattern postoperatively evidenced by verbalization that pain reduced, voiding with complete emptying of the bladder

INTERVENTION	RATIONALE
I. Assess for:	
A. Pain descriptors, tension or pull on incision, swelling at incisional site	A. Identifies pain characteristics, increases pain
B. Urinary pattern, bladder distention, inability to void postoperatively	B. Creates pressure and tension on incision caused by urinary retention
III. Administer:	
A. Analgesic PO, IM	A. Acts to relieve pain based on severity by interfering with CNS pathways
B. Antibiotic PO	B. Acts as a prophylactic postoperatively in more extensive surgical repairs
IV. Perform/provide:	
A. Place in semi Fowler's position with knees slightly flexed	A. Prevents tension on incision
B. Ice pack to surgical site, scrotal site if applicable	B. Provides vasoconstriction to reduce edema and pain
C. Apply scrotal support, and elevate scrotum in men with inguinal repair	C. Reduces tension on incisional site and reduces edema
D. Splinting with pillow during coughing or movement	D. Reduces stress and pain at incisional and prevents weakening of repair and possible recurrence of hernia
E. Urinary catheterization if unable to void in 6 to 8 hours postoperatively	E. Prevents stress on incision resulting from distention

NURSING DIAGNOSIS

Knowledge deficit related to follow-up care to prevent recurrence of hernia

EXPECTED OUTCOMES

Knowledge and information provided evidenced by compliance with daily activities and restrictions 4 to 6 weeks postoperatively

INTERVENTION	RATIONALE
V. Teach patient/family:	
A. Pathophysiology and cause of hernia and overview of care	A. Provides information about hernia formation and risk for recurrence
B. Application of truss daily in the morning	B. Reduces the hernia and maintains its position preoperatively or used postoperatively to prevent recurrence
C. Application of scrotal support	C. Provides support when up walking
D. Fluid intake of 2 to 3 L/day, dietary intake of foods containing fiber, stool softeners as prescribed	D. Promotes bowel elimination without straining and increasing intra-abdominal pressure
E. Advise refraining from returning to work or resume activities such as sexual activity	E. Prevents stress on repair site that may weaken area prior to complete healing
F. Walk for exercise until other activities allowed, avoid lifting heavy objects, straining, pushing, stretching, coughing hard, sneezing for 6 weeks	F. Provides exercises without stress on the incision by increasing intra-abdominal pressure

INTERVENTION	RATIONALE
G. Report changes in wound appearance such as redness, swelling, or drainage at the incisional site	G. Indicates possible complication or recurrence of hernia

inflammatory bowel disease
(Crohn's disease/ulcerative colitis)

DEFINITION

Inflammatory bowel disease (IBD) is a chronic condition that includes ulcerative colitis and Crohn's disease. The diseases are characterized by remissions and exacerbations. Crohn's disease affects any area of the alimentary tract, most commonly the ileum and involves deeper levels of the mucosa while ulcerative colitis affects the colon and involves more superficial levels of the mucosa. Causes have not been definitely established, but Crohn's disease is believed to be of an autoimmune or inherited nature and ulcerative colitis of an allergic or bacterial nature. This plan includes acute and ongoing care of these conditions and can be used in association with the ANORECTAL DISORDERS (FISSURE/FISTULA), BOWEL RESECTION/DIVERSION (COLOSTOMY/ILEOSTOMY), PREOPERATIVE CARE, and POSTOPERATIVE CARE plans if surgery is performed

NURSING DIAGNOSES

Anxiety related to change in health status causing inability to manage feelings of uncertainty and apprehension regarding uncertain prognosis of chronic disease

Ineffective individual coping related to inability to cope with change in bowel elimination (chronic diarrhea), and future life-style changes if surgery is planned (bowel diversion)

EXPECTED OUTCOMES

Chronic anxiety and fear within manageable levels, development of coping and problem-solving skills evidenced by verbalizations that anxiety is decreasing, fear reduced, participation in care activities and receptive to planning for long-term care of bowel elimination changes

INTERVENTION	RATIONALE
I. Assess for:	
A. Level of anxiety, use of coping mechanisms, stated fears of uncertainty of disease outcome, life-style changes	A. Anxiety can range from mild to severe and high level associated with chronic illness, assists to identify inappropriate use of coping skills
B. Restlessness, diaphoresis, complaining, joking, withdrawal, talkativeness, increased P and R	B. Nonverbal expressions of anxiety when not able to communicate feelings
C. Personal resources to cope with stress, anxiety, and interest in learning to problem-solve, use of defense mechanisms	C. Support systems and personal strengths assist to develop coping skills
D. Feelings or preoccupation with elimination pattern change, negative expressions about changes in life-style and effects of bowel disease	D. Responses to chronic illness, negative or positive
III. Administer:	
A. Anti-anxiety agent PO	A. Acts to reduce anxiety level and provides calming effect and rest, depresses subcortical levels of CNS, limbic system
IV. Perform/provide:	
A. Environment conducive to rest, time to express fears and anxiety, avoid anxiety-producing situations	A. Decreases stimuli that cause stress/anxiety, venting of feelings decreases anxiety

B. Suggest new methods to enhance coping skills and problem solving, allow to externalize and identify those that help

B. Offers alternative coping strategies that allow for release of anxiety and fear

C. Positive feedback regarding progress made, focus on abilities rather than inabilities

C. Provides support for adaptive behavior, promotes self-worth and responsibility

D. Avoid verbal or nonverbal reactions to bowel dysfunction or other procedures

D. Promotes comfort with nurse–patient relationship

E. Privacy when using bathroom, advise that feelings about the bowel pattern are normal

E. Reduces embarrassment caused by persistent and urgency in bowel elimination

F. Allow to participate in planning of care to maintain usual activities when possible, allow to participate in care as soon as possible

F. Allows for some control over situations

G. Relaxation techniques/exercises

G. Reduces stress and anxiety

NURSING DIAGNOSIS
Pain related to physical injuring agent of ulceration/erosion of intestinal wall resulting from inflammation

EXPECTED OUTCOMES
Pain episodes reduced or relieved evidenced by verbalization that pain is controlled or less severe and need for less frequent analgesic

INTERVENTION	RATIONALE
I. Assess for: A. Pain, cramping, locale (abdominal, joint, perianal), severity, type, and duration, flatulence, distension	A. Pain severity ranges from mild to severe and if not controlled, pain in LRQ with cramping and flatulence is associated with Crohn's disease and pain in LLQ, cramping with diarrhea is associated with ulcerative colitis
B. Factors that precipitate pain such as foods, stress, what relieves pain	B. Provides causative factors associated with exacerbations
II. Monitor, describe, record: A. Barium enema, colonoscopy	A. Differentiates between ulcerative colitis and Crohn's disease
III. Administer: A. Analgesic PO	A. Acts as agonist to decrease neurotransmitter release altering pain perception
B. Anticholinergic PO	B. Acts to relieve bowel spasms and cramping
C. Anti-inflammatory PO	C. Acts to reduce inflammatory process in bowel administered with antacid to prevent gastric irritation
IV. Perform/provide: A. Quiet, restful, nonstressful environment	A. Decreases stimuli that cause stress and pain

INTERVENTION	RATIONALE
B. Distractions, relaxation techniques	B. Diversional measures to relieve pain
C. Avoid fatigue and stress	C. Aggravates and precipitates condition causing pain
D. Administer analgesic prior to activities	D. Reduces or prevents pain
E. Protective ointment to anus	E. Reduces pain in areas affected by disease

NURSING DIAGNOSES

Altered nutrition: Less than body requirements related to inability to ingest (anorexia, pain, rejection of prescribed diet) or absorb (inflammation/damaged bowel mucosa, diarrhea) nutrients resulting in malabsorption, weight loss, malnutrition

Risk for fluid volume deficit related to excessive losses of fluids/electrolytes from normal routes (diarrhea), altered intake resulting from anorexia, nausea, causing possible imbalance (metabolic acidosis)

EXPECTED OUTCOMES

Optimal nutritional and fluid level within prescribed inclusions/exclusions evidenced by stable weight pattern and protein, electrolyte levels (K, Na, Cl, Ca, Mg), I&O within normal determinations, and absence of diarrhea, anorexia, nausea

INTERVENTION	RATIONALE
I. Assess for:	
A. Anorexia, nausea, diarrhea, fatigue, ability to eat and drink and amounts/day	A. Affects oral intake of nutrients and fluids
B. Eating pattern, likes and dislikes, cultural factors, food and fluid intake for 24–72 hours	B. Establishes baseline data for care and teaching needs

INTERVENTION	RATIONALE
C. Dry skin and mucous membranes, thirst, poor skin turgor, oliguria	C. Signs and symptoms of dehydration
D. Muscle weakness and cramping, nausea, vomiting, abdominal cramping, twitching, drowsiness	D. Signs and symptoms of electrolyte imbalance (decreased K, Na, Cl, lost with diarrhea and impaired absorption in the colon)
E. Numbness and tingling of digits, muscle cramps, positive Chvostek's and Trousseau's signs, neuromuscular irritability	E. Indicates decreased Ca, Mg, lost as excess fats bind with them and prevents their absorption
F. Nausea, vomiting, headache, disorientation, rapid respirations	F. Signs and symptoms of metabolic acidosis

II. Monitor, describe, record:

A. Weight daily or as needed on same scale, at same time, same clothes	A. Indicates losses associated with fluid or nutritional inadequacy and need for dietary changes
B. Electrolytes	B. Identifies abnormal levels indicating risk for or presence of deficiencies leading to metabolic acidosis
C. BUN, albumin, Hct, Hb, transferrin, cholesterol	C. Indicates lack of essential nutritional intake and possible anemia
D. I&O q4–8h (include diarrhea)	D. Provides data to determine imbalance in fluid status

INTERVENTION	RATIONALE
III. Administer:	
A. IV fluid and electrolyte replacement	A. Ensures adequate fluid and nutritional intake until oral intake is resumed
B. Vitamins (fat-soluble A, D, E, K) and (water-soluble C), and B_{12} (cyanocobalamin), folic acid	B. Fat absorption reduced and ascorbic acid (C) to enhance iron absorption, increase absorption of calcium (D), replacement for loss caused by reduced absorption in ileum (B_{12})
C. Iron preparation IM	C. Supplements to prevent anemia given by injection as iron is poorly absorbed in the inflamed intestines
IV. Perform/provide	
A. Quiet, clean, nonstressful environment	A. Promotes nutritional intake
B. Elemental formulae high in protein/calories/minerals, fat free	B. Provides complete nutritional intake in easily digestible form absorbed in upper part of small intestine allowing bowel to rest, fat is poorly absorbed by intestines, high protein needed for tissue repair and weight
C. Total parenteral nutrition (TPN) if ordered in Crohn's disease	C. Provides nutritional requirements while resting the bowel, decreases fecal bulk

INTERVENTION	RATIONALE
D. Bland, low residue diet in small feedings of six/day when allowed	D. Provides foods that are easy to digest and allow for absorption for time present in bowel
E. Allow time to rest prior to eating and time to eat slowly	E. Prevents fatigue during meals
F. Avoid inclusions of nuts, seeds, popcorn, alcohol, carbonated, and citrus beverages, chocolate, spicy, and gas-producing foods	F. Causes mechanical irritation of bowel mucosa and contributes to inflammation
G. Fluid intake of 2500 mL/day if allowed	G. Ensures adequate fluid balance in presence of losses from diarrhea
H. Referral to nutritionist	H. Assists in planning diet with foods that are best tolerated and avoid complications

NURSING DIAGNOSES

Diarrhea related to inflammation, irritation, or malabsorption of bowel resulting in increased peristalsis/hyperactivity of bowel causing frequent loose or liquid feces

Risk for infection related to inadequate secondary defense of immunosuppression resulting from steroid therapy and chronic illness (bowel inflammation)

Risk for impaired skin integrity related to internal factor of excretions (diarrhea) resulting in irritation or breakdown of perianal area

EXPECTED OUTCOMES

Skin intact and free from breakdown at perianal area evidenced by absence of redness, irritation, excoriation at perianal site, absence of infection in any body area evidenced by VS, WBC, cultures within normal parameters, reduced frequency of diarrheal episodes evidenced by soft, formed feces daily

INTERVENTION	RATIONALE
I. Assess for:	
A. Irritation, excoriation, or redness at perianal skin site, itching or burning at anal site	A. Indicates risk for skin breakdown resulting from persistent diarrhea
B. Pattern of diarrhea including frequency, amount, characteristics (blood, mucus, pus), bowel sounds for change in pitch or frequency, factors that precipitate diarrhea	B. Provides data base for plan of treatment and medication modifications
C. Changes in breath sounds and color of sputum, cloudy foul-smelling urine, temperature and chills	C. Indicates infectious process
II. Monitor, describe, record:	
A. VS and temperature q4h (avoid use of rectal thermometer)	A. Temperature elevation indicates infection
B. WBC, sputum, urine culture	B. Increased WBC of $>10,000/mm^3$ and positive cultures indicate infection and identify pathogen
III. Administer:	
A. Antidiarrheal PO	A. Acts to reduce peristaltic activity
B. Anti-inflammatory PO	B. Acts as an immunosuppressive in acute episodes
C. Bulk laxative PO	C. Increases feces' firmness without irritating mucosa

INTERVENTION	RATIONALE
D. Kaolin/pectin mixture PO	D. Decrease fluid content in feces
E. Antimicrobial PO, TOP	E. Acts to prevent or treat infection by inhibiting cell-wall synthesis
F. Antipyretic PO	F. Acts to reduce temperature

IV. Perform/provide:

A. Proper handwash prior to any care or contact	A. Prevents transmission of pathogens
B. Use sterile technique and all sterile equipment, supplies during acute phase or care of TPN	B. Prevents contamination by pathogens
C. Cleanse perianal skin with mild soap and warm water, and gently pat dry after each episode of diarrhea	C. Promotes cleanliness and prevents irritation from persistent diarrhea
D. Application of protective or antimicrobial ointment to anal area	D. Protects skin from constant irritation of diarrheal episodes
E. Sitz bath or warm compress to perianal area	E. Promotes comfort by soothing irritated anal area
F. Heat lamp 12–18 inches to anal area for 20 minutes	F. Treatment for irritation by vasodilation increasing blood flow to area for healing

INTERVENTION	RATIONALE
G. Close proximity to bathroom or bedpan, use deodorizer	G. Avoids embarrassment if diarrhea is difficult to control and eliminates unpleasant odors
H. Avoid gas-producing foods and food high in fat and roughage, also avoid smoking and laxatives	H. Produces distention, irritation to mucosa, and exacerbation of diarrhea

NURSING DIAGNOSIS

Knowledge deficit related to general care information including nutrition/fluid needs, measures to prevent intestinal complications, signs and symptoms to report

EXPECTED OUTCOMES

Adequate information and teaching about follow-up care evidenced by compliance with medication and nutritional/fluid regimens with reduced exacerbations of disease symptoms

INTERVENTION	RATIONALE
V. Teach patient/family: A. Pathophysiology and type of bowel disease, medical and surgical treatments	A. Provides information and rationale for bowel function, pattern of bowel elimination

INTERVENTION	RATIONALE
B. Medication administration to include dose, frequency, time, how to take drug(s), condition being treated, expected effects, side effects and what to do if they occur, medications to avoid such as laxatives and medications not prescribed, provide a written schedule and instructions to follow	B. Protects or treats infection, skin irritation, and especially diarrhea
C. Fluid intake of 2 to 3 L/day spread over 24 hours or amount based on fluid loss from diarrhea	C. Ensures adequate fluid intake to prevent fluid/electrolyte imbalance
D. Dietary modification of low-residue, high-protein, carbohydrate, and caloric intake, low fat	D. Promotes bowel healing and nutritional requirements when oral intake is allowed
E. Avoid raw foods, popcorn, greasy or spicy foods, hot or cold beverages, high-fiber foods, gas-forming foods (cabbage, legumes, carbonated beverages), milk, seeds	E. Absorption is difficult by damaged mucosa, increases stimulation to the tract and produces distention and irritation
F. Include foods that provide needed electrolytes (Ca, K, Na) such as soups, cheese, bananas, juices, add green vegetables, whole-grain cereals and meats if iron and folate needed	F. Encourages intake of necessary electrolytes while eliminating foods not allowed on bland, low-residue diet

INTERVENTION	RATIONALE
G. Cleanse anal area with soft tissue and with warm water and mild soap	G. Prevents skin irritation caused by frequent episodes of diarrhea
H. Arrange for continued TPN management upon discharge to home	H. Ensures that continuous nutritional and fluid requirements are met
I. Report any redness, swelling, or pain at anal site, blood in feces, persistent abdominal pain, cramping, diarrhea, vomiting, temperature elevation, drainage from rectum	I. Signs and symptoms of possible complications of bowel disease
J. Importance of keeping appointments with physician as scheduled, compliance with medical regimen	J. Ensures that disease is monitored and complications diagnosed
K. Suggest counseling if appropriate, community agencies dealing with stress management, smoking and alcohol use	K. Provides support and information that assists in adaptation to chronic disease

pancreatitis

DEFINITION
Pancreatitis is the acute or chronic inflammation of the pancreas. It is caused by the activation of the enzymes in the pancreas resulting in autodigestion of the organ. It is believed that the activation is caused by obstruction of the pancreatic duct, reflux of bile into the duct, ischemia or trauma to the organ. The chronic type leads to progressive destruction of the pancreas brought about by repeated episodes of acute pancreatitis. Risk factors include alcoholism and gallbladder disease. This plan involves the care of this disease and can be used in association with the CHOLECYSTITIS/CHOLELITHIASIS care plan

NURSING DIAGNOSIS
Anxiety related to threat to or change in health status causing inability to manage feelings of uncertainty about diagnosis and possible surgery, apprehension regarding pain and ability to manage stress

EXPECTED OUTCOMES
Anxiety and fear within manageable levels evidenced by verbalizations that anxiety is decreasing, fear reduced, participation in planning for care

INTERVENTION	RATIONALE
I. Assess for: A. Level of anxiety, use of coping mechanisms, stated fears of uncertainty of disease outcome, life-style changes	A. Anxiety can range from mild to severe and high level associated with acute illness

INTERVENTION	RATIONALE
B. Personal resources to cope with stress, anxiety, and interest in learning to problem-solve, use of defense mechanisms	B. Support systems and personal strengths assist to deal with anxiety
C. Negative expression about any changes in life-style, willingness to participate in care	C. Identifies effect of illness on feelings of self-concept (negative or positive)

III. Administer:

A. Anti-anxiety agent PO	A. Acts to reduce anxiety level and provides calming effect and rest, depresses subcortical levels of CNS, limbic system

IV. Perform/provide:

A. Environment conducive to rest, time to express fears and anxiety, avoid anxiety-producing situations	A. Decreases stimuli that cause stress/anxiety, venting of feelings decreases anxiety
B. Suggest new methods to enhance coping skills and problem solving, allow to externalize and identify those that help	B. Offers alternative coping strategies that allow for release of anxiety and fear
C. Positive feedback regarding progress made, focus on abilities rather than inabilities	C. Provides support for adaptive behavior, promotes self-worth and responsibility

INTERVENTION

D. Diversional activities such as relaxation exercises, TV, radio, music, reading, tapes, guided imagery, encourage to continue usual interests

E. Allow to participate in planning of care to maintain usual activities when possible

RATIONALE

D. Reduces anxiety and promotes comfort

E. Allows for some control over situations

NURSING DIAGNOSIS

Pain related to physical injuring agent of inflammatory process, ductal obstruction, biliary duct disease resulting in pancreatic distention

EXPECTED OUTCOMES

Pain relieved or controlled evidenced by verbalization that pain reduced by analgesic therapy, fewer requests for medication, ability to perform activities or rest/sleep as applicable

INTERVENTION

I. Assess for:
   A. Pain severity and site, factors that increase or decrease pain (high-fat meal), abdominal distention, descriptors such as epigastric or abdominal pain that radiates to back

   B. Abdominal guarding, grimacing, crying, restlessness

RATIONALE

A. Provides data on intensity and locale of pain to identify pancreas disease or peritoneal irritation if enzymes in the abdominal cavity

B. Nonverbal indications of pain when not able to communicate pain

INTERVENTION	RATIONALE
III. Administer:	
A. Analgesic IM	A. Acts by inhibiting pain pathways in CNS and alters pain perception (avoid opiate as this increases ductal spasms)
B. Anticholinergic PO	B. Acts to reduce spasms of ducts that cause pain
C. Histamine$_2$ receptor antagonist, antacid PO	C. Acts to prevent gastric acid production or to neutralize acid to protect the duodenum from exposure
IV. Perform/provide:	
A. Quiet environment, backrub, relaxation exercises	A. Measures to reduce pain by decreases in stimuli
B. Place in low Fowler's or side-lying position with knees flexed, change position q2h	B. Reduces upper abdominal pressure, increases comfort in acute stages
C. Assure that analgesic will be administered before pain becomes severe, advise to request analgesic as soon as pain appears and to report if medication does not relieve pain	C. Prevents extreme discomfort and anxiety related to the return of pain
D. Withhold oral intake of food/fluid	D. Stimulates secretion of pancreatic enzymes that increases pain

NURSING DIAGNOSES

Altered nutrition: less than body requirements related to inability to ingest (nausea, vomiting, abdominal distension, NPO status, rejection of restrictive diet), digest protein, carbohydrate, fat (decreased flow of pancreatic enzymes)

Risk for fluid volume deficit related to excessive losses through normal route (vomiting, diaphoresis), abnormal route (nasogastric tube aspirate), NPO status

EXPECTED OUTCOMES

Adequate nutritional and fluid intake evidenced by control of vomiting, effective replacement by IV infusion until oral intake permitted, I&O ratio, and weight within normal determinations

INTERVENTION	RATIONALE
I. Assess for:	
A. Nausea, vomiting, abdominal distention or feeling of fullness, intolerance to fats in diet	A. Symptoms of pancreatic inflammation or bile flow obstruction causing inadequate intake or digestion of nutrients
B. NPO status, N/G tube and suctioning, restricted fluid intake	B. Indicates causes for fluid imbalance
C. Weight loss, weakness, fatigue, anorexia, 24-hour intake of food groups and calories	C. Indicates reduced intake of protein, calories, and digestion and absorption of nutrients with reduced pancreatic enzyme flow
D. Skin and mucous membranes dryness, skin turgor, oliguria	D. Indicates risk for dehydration from fluid losses

INTERVENTION	RATIONALE
E. Muscle cramping, weakness, confusion, abdominal cramps, irregular pulse, muscle twitching, paresthesia, nausea, vomiting, positive Chvostek's and Trousseau's signs, numbness or tingling of digits	E. Symptoms of electrolyte deficits (K, Na, Cl, Ca)

II. Monitor, describe, record

A. Weight daily or as needed on same scale, time, clothing, measurement of tricep skinfold	A. Determines weight loss or gain
B. I&O q4–8h, including aspirate, vomitus	B. Determines fluid balance
C. Electrolytes	C. Reveals electrolyte imbalance with fluid losses (K, Na, Cl, Ca)
D. BUN, albumin, transferrin, Hb, Hct, glucose, serum and urinary amylase	D. Reveals risk for malnutrition and abnormalities associated with pancreatic disease
E. Upper GI series, computerized tomography (CT)	E. Reveals pancreatic structural abnormalities or changes

III. Administer:

A. IV fluids/electrolyte replacement	A. Provides short-term fluids and nutrition until PO intake resumed
B. Antiemetic IM	B. Acts to reduce vomiting by depressing the chemoreceptor trigger zone

INTERVENTION	RATIONALE
C. Hydrocholeretic PO	C. Acts to stimulate bile production to assist with absorption of fats/vitamins
D. Enzymes (pancreatic) PO	D. Acts to assist in the digestion of proteins, carbohydrates, and fats
E. Antiflatulent PO	E. Acts to reduce accumulation of gas and abdominal distention
F. Vitamin/minerals PO	F. Acts to supplement or replace substances in restricted dietary intake

IV. Perform/provide:

A. Place in position of comfort and allow to ambulate if tolerated, change position slowly	A. Decreases gas accumulation and release of flatus, movements can stimulate vomiting center
B. Maintain patency of N/G tube and NPO status if present	B. Decreases nausea and vomiting by maintaining empty stomach
C. Assist to take deep breaths if nauseated	C. Decreases urge to vomit
D. Oral care after each episode of vomiting	D. Promotes cleanliness and comfort of mouth
E. Environment that is odor free, quiet, and restful	E. Stimuli that can initiate vomiting and decrease appetite

INTERVENTION	RATIONALE
F. Begin oral intake when tolerated and when pain and distention subsides with liquid diet and slowly progress to solid foods with restriction in fatty foods such as cream, butter, cheese, milk, fried foods, ice cream, and gas-forming foods	F. Prevents exacerbation of symptoms
G. Offer small frequent meals six times/day with time to eat slowly	G. Prevents early satiety and vomiting
H. Include oral intake of electrolytes in foods such as bananas, bouillon, milk products, potatoes, cantaloupe	H. Replaces lost electrolytes via vomiting (K, Na, Ca)
I. Increased fluid intake of 2500 mL/day PO as indicated	I. Provides adequate fluid intake
J. Referral to nutritionist	J. Provides information and instruction to ensure adequate nutritional intake with suggested inclusions and exclusions

NURSING DIAGNOSIS

Knowledge deficit related to follow-up care to promote or maintain resolution of pancreatitis and resumption of life-style activities

EXPECTED OUTCOMES

Adequate knowledge and information provided evidenced by compliance with dietary/medication/daily activities regimens, absence of exacerbation of the disease

INTERVENTION	RATIONALE
V. Teach patient/family:	
A. Pathophysiology and cause of pancreatic disease and overview of care, importance of following planned discharge care	A. Provides information about disease and rationale for care
B. Medications names, dose, time, frequency, side effects to report, special instruction in insulin administration and glucose monitoring, allow to return demonstration	B. Ensures correct administration of medication regimen
C. Fluid intake of 2 to 3 L/day if allowed	C. Ensures adequate daily fluid intake
D. Dietary regimen with lists of inclusions and exclusions to supply a balanced nutritional intake with electrolytes while avoiding gas-forming, fats, irritating foods, provide sample menus and information for food purchase selection	D. Modifies dietary intake based on stage of disease and tolerances to specific food types
E. Avoid alcohol, smoking, and stressful situations	E. Prevents stimulation of pancreatic secretions leading to organ damage
F. Advise to plan and follow a daily exercise and rest regimen as tolerated depending on physician's advice specific to activity	F. Prevents fatigue and enhances a balanced regimen

INTERVENTION	RATIONALE
G. Report pain in abdomen or back, changes in feces (fatty and foul smelling), return of nausea and vomiting with abdominal distention, weight loss, temperature, chills, changes in breathing pattern and behavior, symptoms of hyperglycemia	G. Indicates possible complications of infection, obstruction, inadequate fat digestion, and general pancreatic dysfunction
H. Comply with follow-up appointments with physician and laboratory testing	H. Ensures continuing progress to wellness and allows to modify treatments if needed

peptic ulcer

DEFINITION

Peptic ulcer is an acute or chronic ulceration of the mucosa and deeper structures of the stomach, duodenum, lower esophagus, or jejunum (following surgical gastro-enterostomy). These are areas that come in contact with gastric juices that contribute to the cause of the disease depending on the ability of the mucosa to protect itself from injury and the associated regulation of these secretions and blood flow to the mucosa. Duodenal ulcer is more common than gastric ulcer. The chronic type can cause erosion followed by fibrosis of tissue with symptoms present over a long time, and the acute type, although superficial and inflammatory, heals in a short time. Risk for developing the disease includes ingestion of steroids, alcohol, smoking, aspirin and aspirin products, and stress. Alcohol and stress are believed to increase acid (HCl) secretion. Those with a critical illness are prone to stress ulcer as a result of low gastric pH, changes in gastric mucosa caused by the stress and is usually associated with hemorrhage. This plan includes care of peptic ulcer disease and can be used in association with the GASTRECTOMY/GASTROPLASTY, PREOPERATIVE CARE, and POSTOPERATIVE CARE plans if surgery is performed

NURSING DIAGNOSES

Anxiety is related to threat to or change in health status causing inability to manage feelings of uncertainty about diagnosis and apprehension regarding pain and ability to manage stress

Ineffective individual coping related to situational crisis of illness and expected changes in life-style, risk for possible chronicity of disease

EXPECTED OUTCOMES

Anxiety and fear within manageable levels, development of coping and problem-solving skills evidenced by verbalizations that anxiety is decreasing, fear reduced, participation in care activities and receptive to planning for ongoing care

INTERVENTION	RATIONALE
I. Assess for:	
A. Level of anxiety, use of coping mechanisms, stated fears of uncertainty of disease outcome, life-style changes	A. Anxiety can range from mild to severe and high level associated with critical illness, assists in identifying inappropriate use of coping skills
B. Personal resources to cope with stress, anxiety, and interest in learning to problem-solve, use of defense mechanisms	B. Support systems and personal strengths assist to develop coping skills
C. Negative expressions about any changes in life-style, willingness to participate in care	C. Identifies effect of illness on feelings of self-concept (negative or positive)
III. Administer:	
A. Anti-anxiety agent PO	A. Acts to reduce anxiety level and provides calming effect and rest, depresses subcortical levels of CNS, limbic system
IV. Perform/provide:	
A. Environment conducive to rest, time to express fears and anxiety, avoid anxiety-producing situations	A. Decreases stimuli that cause stress/anxiety, venting of feelings decreases anxiety
B. Suggest new methods to enhance coping skills and problem solving, allow to externalize and identify those that help	B. Offers alternative coping strategies that allow for release of anxiety and fear

INTERVENTION	RATIONALE
C. Positive feedback regarding progress made, focus on abilities rather than inabilities	C. Provides support for adaptive behavior, promotes self-worth and responsibility
D. Diversional activities such as relaxation exercises, TV, radio, music, reading, tapes, guided imagery, encourage to continue usual interests	D. Reduces anxiety and promotes comfort
E. Allow to participate in planning of care to maintain usual activities when possible	E. Allows for some control over situations

NURSING DIAGNOSES

Pain related to physical injuring agent of secretions acting on mucosa resulting in ulceration, inflammation

Altered nutrition: Less than body requirements related to inability to ingest foods and fluids resulting from anorexia, nausea, aversion to prescribed diet, and pain caused by irritating foods

EXPECTED OUTCOMES

Pain reduced or controlled and adequate nutritional intake evidenced by verbalization that pain relieved and ingestion of recommended diet without discomfort, weight within baseline parameters for age, height, sex, and frame

INTERVENTION	RATIONALE
I. Assess for:	
A. Pain descriptors, site and characteristics, pain following ingestion of irritating foods, time of onset after eating, other factors that increase or decrease pain, bloated or gaseous feeling	A. Symptoms of ulcer depending on site, usually epigastric 1 to 2 hours after meals in gastric ulcer, 2 to 4 hours in duodenal ulcer
B. Nausea, anorexia, food and fluid intake/24 hours and preferences, cultural factors affecting eating pattern, weight loss or gain, expressed feeling about bland diet and restrictions	B. Provides information needed for meal planning
II. Monitor, describe, record:	
A. Weight daily or as appropriate with same clothes, scale, time of day	A. Reveals gains or losses and need to revise dietary plan
B. Esophagogastroduodenoscopy (EGD)	B. Reveals site and extent of ulcer by direct visualization
III. Administer:	
A. Vitamin/mineral supplement PO	A. Acts to replace or provide essential substances if dietary intake inadequate
B. Antacid PO	B. Acts to relieve pain and enhance healing by neutralizing acid that results in protection to mucosa

INTERVENTION	RATIONALE
C. Histamine receptor antagonist PO	C. Acts to inhibit gastric acid secretion by blocking the H_2 receptors found in the stomach's parietal cells
D. Anticholinergic PO	D. Acts to inhibit gastric acid secretion and decrease hypermotility
E. Mucosal protective agent PO	E. Acts to coat and protect mucosa and inhibit pepsin activity on mucosa
F. Gastric motility and emptying agent PO	F. Acts to prevent retention of contents in stomach that stimulates acid production

IV. Perform/provide:

A. Stress-free environment with rest following meals	A. Stress increases acid production and pain
B. Limit visitors and phone calls until condition improves	B. Promotes rest and relaxation during acute painful stages of disease
C. Small frequent meals (4–6/day) instead of three meals/day, bland diet to reduce irritation to mucosa	C. Prevents overdistention and feeling of fullness
D. Advise to eat slowly and chew foods well	D. Provides a better dilution of gastric acid
E. Suggest and assist with stress-reduction techniques	E. Reduces acid production when relaxed and prevents pain

INTERVENTION	RATIONALE
F. Referral to nutritionist	F. Plans and supports dietary intake to provide adequate nutrition with the appropriate inclusions and exclusions

NURSING DIAGNOSIS

Risk for injury related to internal factor of hemorrhage, peritonitis, or obstruction complications resulting from erosion, perforation, pyloric scarring, and constriction

EXPECTED OUTCOMES

Absence of complications of peptic ulcer disease evidenced by progressive healing, absence of abdominal pain or distention, vomiting, and VS, Hct, Hb, WBC within normal ranges

INTERVENTION	RATIONALE
I. Assess for: A. Hematemesis, drop in BP, rapid pulse, cool moist skin, pallor, restlessness, confusion	A. Signs and symptoms of hemorrhage with risk for hypovolemic shock state
B. Severe abdominal pain, rigid abdomen, nausea, vomiting, bowel sounds absent, increased pulse and respirations, temperature	B. Signs and symptoms of perforation with associated peritonitis
C. Vomiting of undigested food, abdominal or gastric distention with a fullness or bloated feeling	C. Signs and symptoms of obstruction
II. Monitor, describe, record: A. VS q2–4h or as needed	A. Changes indicate complication of peptic ulcer

INTERVENTION	RATIONALE
B. CBC with Hb, Hct, WBC	B. Indicates complication with increases and decreases dependent on condition
III. Administer: A. Whole blood, packed RBC, volume expanders IV	A. Replaces blood losses with hemorrhage
B. Fluids IV	B. Replaces losses from vomiting associated with complications
IV. Perform/provide: A. NPO status and bed rest in semi Fowler's position	A. Prevents accumulation of contents in stomach
B. Insert N/G tube, and attach to suction	B. Maintains gastrointestinal decompression
C. Prepare for surgical intervention if planned	C. Procedures such as gastrectomy, gastroplasty, perforation repair
D. Supportive environment if complications arise	D. Complications result in life-threatening situations causing severe anxiety for patient and family

NURSING DIAGNOSIS

Knowledge deficit related to follow-up care and life-style modifications to promote healing of ulcer and prevent recurrence of peptic ulcer disease

EXPECTED OUTCOMES

Adequate understanding of care measures evidenced by compliance with instructions (dietary, smoking, drinking, stress reduction) and absence of signs and symptoms associated with peptic ulcer

INTERVENTION	RATIONALE
V. Teach patient/family:	
A. Pathophysiology of ulcer formation, type/location of ulcer, risk factors involved in recurrence, time it takes for ulcer to heal (6–8 weeks)	A. Provides information and rationale for disease and plan of care
B. Life-style modifications such as regular eating schedule, stress reduction, smoking cessation, adhering to prescribed dietary regimen	B. Reduces risk factors for peptic ulcer
C. Preparation and ingestion of bland diet, avoid raw, spicy, cold, rough foods, alcoholic, fruit juices, and caffeine containing beverages	C. Provides appropriate diet and restrictions during healing of ulcer
D. Take time eating meals, chew foods well, avoid skipping meals	D. Reduces irritation to gastric mucosa
E. Moderate activities to allow for rest periods	E. Promotes rest needed for healing process
F. Administration of medications including name, action, dose, time, frequency, side effects to report for each medication, avoid over-the-counter drugs such as aspirin	F. Ensures correct and effective medication regimen

INTERVENTION	RATIONALE
G. Report pain that cannot be relieved or pain that returns, black tarry feces, hematemesis or coffee-ground emesis, persistent weight loss, bloating, nausea	G. Allows for early intervention to prevent complications
H. Referral to counseling for stress, smoking, dietary regimen	H. Provides support for change in life-style and management of therapeutic regimen

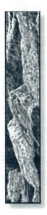

Musculoskeletal System Standards

musculoskeletal system data base

HISTORICAL DATA REVIEW
Past events:
1. Acute and/or chronic musculoskeletal disease or disorders, presence of disorders that affect the bones, joints, or muscles (trauma, congenital deformities, neuromuscular disorders, diabetes)
2. Chronic signs and symptoms related to musculoskeletal disorders (pain in bone or joint, back pain, stiffness of joint(s), edema, muscle weakness, burning, numbness, or tingling sensation in extremities, limited movements and range of motion, balance and coordination deficits, muscle cramping)
3. Musculoskeletal, neuromuscular diseases of family members
4. Childhood diseases affecting bones, joints, and muscles (poliomyelitis, osteomyelitis, hemophilia, infections), immunizations for polio, tetanus, and skin test for tuberculosis
5. Occupational/recreational/sports hazards for traumatic injury and safety gear used, proneness to accidents, presence of cast or splint, use of crutches, walker, or cane
6. Treatments, physical and occupational rehabilitation associated with this system, special dietary inclusions (calcium, vitamins, protein), restrictions (low caloric for obesity), exercise routine
7. Medications (prescription and over-the-counter) for musculoskeletal conditions
8. Hospitalization and feelings about care, surgery associated with bones, joints, or muscles, fractures and site(s), strains, dislocations, or sprains

Present events:
1. Medical diagnoses associated with or affecting musculoskeletal structure or function
2. Peripheral pulse and capillary refill in extremities
3. Presence of paralysis, contracture(s), amputation, reduction in mus-

cle mass and strength/endurance, muscle spasms, skeletal deformity, loss of mobility or weight-bearing ability, limited range of motion and joint site(s)
4. Cast, splint, traction application, limb prosthesis
5. Bone, joint pain and site(s), redness, swelling, warmth of affected site, sensory changes (burning, tingling, numbness)
6. Activities of daily living (self-care) and use of aids for personal care, meals, toileting, dressing and undressing, ambulation, ability to sit, stand, walk, use stairs with balance and coordination

PHYSICAL ASSESSMENT DATA REVIEW

1. Symmetry of extremities, shoulder's size and musculature and movements
2. Body alignment, posture, and contours, stance and gait
3. Deformities of spinal column, feet, toes, muscle strength, tone, and size
4. Crepitus, tenderness, bony irregularities or smoothness palpated
5. Presence or absence of reflexes

NURSING DIAGNOSES CONSIDERATIONS

1. Activity intolerance
2. Fatigue
3. Risk for impaired skin integrity
4. Risk for infection
5. Risk for peripheral neurovascular dysfunction
6. Risk for trauma
7. Impaired physical mobility
8. Knowledge deficit
9. Self-care deficits

GERIATRIC CONSIDERATIONS

Musculoskeletal changes in geriatric patients depend on the effect of the aging process on body movement, posture, stability, coordination and muscle agility, strength and endurance. Changes in neuromuscular function also contribute to alterations in movement. A common complaint includes difficulty in maintaining self-care activities of daily living causing changes in life-style. Musculoskeletal changes associated with aging that should be considered when assessing the geriatric patient include:

1. Decreased muscle fiber, mass, and muscle wasting resulting in reduced muscle weight, strength, endurance, and limited mobility and agility
2. Decreased bone minerals and resorption of bone faster than formation of new bone resulting in brittle bones and potential for fractures
3. Kyphosis and shortening of vertebral column resulting in reduced height and postural changes that affect balance and increase potential for falls
4. Stretched ligaments resulting in joint stiffness and decreased motion, increased synovial membrane and fluid thickness resulting in joint changes
5. Changed enzyme function resulting in muscle fatigue, decreased storage of muscle glycogen resulting in reduced energy needed for activities
6. Extrapyramidal system changes resulting in muscle stiffness, slowing, and resting tremor, decreased motor coordination and manual dexterity resulting in reduced reaction time
7. Increased muscle cramping and paresthesia of legs resulting in pain and sleep disturbance, long time weight bearing on feet resulting in foot changes and disabilities

DIAGNOSTIC LABORATORY TESTS AND PROCEDURES

1. X rays of specific bone(s), arthrography, nuclear scan (bone, Gallium or Indium), computerized tomography (CT), arthroscopy, arthrocentesis and fluid analysis, magnetic resonance imaging (MRI), electromyography (EMG), absorptiometry, biopsy with laboratory examination
2. Aspartate aminotransferase (AST), creatine phosphokinase (CPK), lactate dehydrogenase (LDH), aldolase, alkaline phosphatase (ALP), calcium (Ca), phosphorus (P), complete blood count (CBC), erythrocyte sedimentation rate (ESR), rheumatoid factors, antinuclear antibodies, C-reactive protein

MEDICATIONS

1. Analgesics/nonsteroidal anti-inflammatory agents: aspirin, acetaminophen, ibuprofen, naproxen sodium, sulindac, choline salicylate, ketoprofen, tolmetin
2. Antigout agents: allopurinol, colchicine, probenecid

3. Antimicrobials: penicillins
4. Calcium replacements: calcium lactate, calcium gluconate
5. Corticosteroids: prednisone, hydrocortisone, dexamethasone
6. Muscle relaxants: diazepam, baclofen, methocarbamol
7. Vitamins: vitamin D

amputation

DEFINITION
Amputation is the surgical removal of a limb at the joint, mid-upper, or lower arm or leg. Upper extremity amputations usually result from trauma, lower extremity amputations from peripheral vascular disease or occlusive disease (diabetes mellitus, atherosclerosis). Other causes include malignancy, thermal injuries, severe infection, and congenital conditions. Amputations can be open (guillotine) in which the wound is left open and draining, or closed (flap) in which a skin flap is fashioned by the surgeon and sutured over the stump with insertion of drains to enhance healing. This plan includes care of the amputation of a lower or upper limb and can be used in association with the DIABETES MELLITUS, DIMINISHED ARTERIAL CIRCULATION TO EXTREMITIES, PREOPERATIVE CARE, and POSTOPERATIVE CARE plans

NURSING DIAGNOSES
Anxiety related to change in health status causing inability to manage feelings of uncertainty, apprehension regarding prognosis (malignancy), change in role functioning and self-concept resulting from loss of extremity

Ineffective individual coping related to inability to cope with change in life-style, loss of independence, personal vulnerability resulting from loss of extremity

Body image disturbance related to biophysical factor of missing body part, resulting in change in appearance (mutilation) and function (loss of mobility or hand/arm use and dexterity) with use of a prosthesis

Dysfunctional grieving related to loss of physiopsychosocial well-being (actual loss of a limb) resulting in distress, sadness, denial, guilt, anger, depression

EXPECTED OUTCOMES

Anxiety and fear within manageable levels, development of coping and problem-solving skills, progressive adaptation to body image and life-style changes, initiation of grieving process evidenced by verbalizations that anxiety is decreasing, fear reduced, with willingness to participate in care and social activities, and receptive to planning for postoperative care and rehabilitation

INTERVENTION	RATIONALE
I. Assess for:	
A. Level of anxiety, use of coping mechanisms, stated fears of uncertainty of disease outcome, life-style changes	A. Anxiety can range from mild to severe and high level associated with loss of body part, assists in identifying inappropriate use of coping skills
B. Restlessness, diaphoresis, complaining, joking, withdrawal, talkativeness, increased P and R	B. Nonverbal expressions of anxiety when not able to communicate feelings
C. Personal resources to cope with stress, anxiety, and interest in learning to problem-solve, use of defense mechanisms	C. Support systems and personal strengths assist in developing coping skills
D. Feelings and response to change in role, ability to carry out role and participation in care/social activities, fear of stigmatization and rejection	D. Changes in body image and self-concept a common and serious problem with loss/changes in structure and function of a body part

INTERVENTION	RATIONALE
E. Looking or touching stump, feeling or preoccupation with changes, negative expressions about changes in life-style and use of prosthesis	E. Responses to presence of stump (negative or positive), adaptation to permanent loss and prosthesis use
F. Expression of grief (crying, withdrawal, anger, hostility, poor sleep and eating pattern, depression)	F. Grieving associated with any loss
III. Administer: A. Anti-anxiety agent PO	A. Acts to reduce anxiety level and provides calming effect and rest, depresses subcortical levels of CNS, limbic system
IV. Perform/provide: A. Environment conducive to rest, time to express fears and anxiety, avoid anxiety-producing situations	A. Decreases stimuli that cause stress/anxiety, venting of feelings decreases anxiety
B. Suggest new methods to enhance coping skills and problem solving, allow to externalize and identify those that help	B. Offers alternative coping strategies that allow for release of anxiety and fear
C. Positive feedback regarding progress made, focus on abilities rather than inabilities	C. Provides support for adaptive behavior, promotes self-worth and responsibility

INTERVENTION	RATIONALE
D. Avoid verbal or nonverbal reactions to stump care or other procedures, display of distaste or alarm of surgical site	D. Promotes comfort with nurse–patient relationship
E. Privacy when dressings are changed, advise that feelings about stump and prosthesis are normal	E. Reduces embarrassment caused by exposure of surgical site or prosthesis
F. Inform of phantom pain sensation or feeling that the limb has not been removed, activities to expect postoperatively	F. Reduces post-operative anxiety resulting from the unknown consequences of amputation
G. Diversional activities such as relaxation exercises, TV, radio, music, reading, tapes, guided imagery, encourage to continue usual interests	G. Reduces anxiety and promotes comfort
H. Allow to participate in planning of care to maintain usual activities when possible, allow to participate in stump care as soon as possible	H. Allows for some control over situations
I. Support grieving for loss of life-style and restrictions in activities, changes in physical appearance	I. Provides assistance in adaptation to changes imposed by amputated limb

INTERVENTION	RATIONALE
J. Suggest visit from one who has had an amputation and has made a successful recovery and rehabilitation	J. Provides support and information from a reliable source

NURSING DIAGNOSIS

Pain related to physical injury of underlying condition preoperatively, trauma from surgery postoperatively (incisional, phantom) resulting from amputation

EXPECTED OUTCOMES

Pain managed or controlled and skin at stump site intact evidenced by verbalization that pain reduced, skin free of redness, edema, irritation with progressive wound healing

INTERVENTION	RATIONALE
I. Assess for:	
A. Pain and severity, cause prior to surgery	A. Moderate to severe pain can exist from underlying conditions preoperatively from infections, ulcerations and necrosis, ischemia
B. Incisional pain and characteristics, presence of phantom pain	B. Results from surgical trauma, feeling that limb is still present postoperatively caused by intact peripheral nerves proximal to the amputation and feeling that limb is present and are normal responses that can exist for weeks or longer

INTERVENTION	RATIONALE
III. Administer:	
A. Analgesic PO, IM	A. Acts to control pain by interfering with CNS pathways pre- and postoperatively
B. Antimicrobial PO, wound infusion	B. Acts to destroy pathogens by interfering with cell-wall synthesis
IV. Perform/provide:	
A. Bed cradle preoperatively	A. Prevents pressure on painful extremities
B. Elevate stump slightly for 24 hours postoperatively	B. Reduces edema and pain
C. Application of heat to stump	C. Relieves phantom pain
D. Apply pressure to stump by pressing against a hard surface	D. Reduces phantom pain

NURSING DIAGNOSIS

Risk for impaired skin integrity related to external mechanical factor of pressure of improper weight bearing on stump or improper care of stump (dressings, cast, splint), secretions (drainage) from wound resulting in skin irritation, internal factor of altered circulation, nutritional state resulting in poor wound healing

EXPECTED OUTCOMES

Skin intact and progressive incisional healing evidenced by absence of redness, edema, irritation, breakdown, gradual reduction of drainage at stump site

INTERVENTION	RATIONALE
I. Assess for: A. Stump site for redness, tenderness, flabbiness, irritation, dryness at incisional site	A. Indicates potential for breakdown of skin exposed to drainage tube and drainage, tape on skin
B. Dressing, cast, or air splint position change or slippage, pressure by weight bearing on stump with prosthesis	B. Interferes with circulation and predisposes to breakdown and delayed healing
IV. Perform/provide: A. Reposition q2h, massage bony prominences	A. Prevents prolonged pressure on tissues and increases circulation
B. Eggcrate mattress or sheepskin, maintain dry, wrinkle-free linens	B. Protects skin from pressure
C. Application of lotion to skin, thin layer of powder to sheet, avoid use of lotions and powders on stump	C. Moisturizes the skin, absorbs any moisture on the sheets
D. Cleanse and gently dry and massage stump, allow exposure to the air for 20 minutes and reapply bandages firmly	D. Prevents breakdown at stump site
E. Application of sock provided by prosthetist, change daily	E. Prevents discomfort and pressure on stump

INTERVENTION	RATIONALE
F. Discontinue use of prosthesis if redness or skin irritation appears at stump site, have prosthesis fit checked	F. Prevents further irritation and skin breakdown, indicates improper fit or skin sensitivity to pressure

NURSING DIAGNOSES

Impaired physical mobility related to pain and discomfort, decreased strength and endurance (weakness) musculoskeletal impairment (loss of extremity, use of a prosthesis) resulting in inability to purposefully move within environment with or without prosthesis, impaired coordination and balance with loss of lower extremity

Risk for trauma related to internal factors of weakness, balancing difficulties resulting from control of prosthesis when ambulating or participating in ADL, and external factors of unsafe environment causing falls and injury

EXPECTED OUTCOMES

Optimal mobility and participation in activities evidenced by progressive self-care in ADL within imposed restrictions of movement, adaptation to prosthesis, absence of contractures, instability in ambulation, and accidental injury resulting from falls

INTERVENTION	RATIONALE
I. Assess for:	
A. Ability for movement, reluctance to attempt movement, limited ROM of residual limb, balancing, coordination	A. Provides data to determine mobility and potential for injury caused by use of prosthesis if immediate fitting is done

INTERVENTION	RATIONALE
B. Type of prosthesis, strength and endurance, psychological adaptation to prosthesis, ability to control prosthesis	B. Varies with type of amputation with a patellar tendon-bearing for below the knee, quadrilateral socket or ischial containment for above the knee, hook or hand with a harness and socket attachment for upper arm
IV. Perform/provide:	
A. Elevation of amputated limb on pillow for 12 to 24 hours, remove after 24 hours	A. Reduces edema and bleeding or drainage, removed to prevent knee or hip contracture
B. Prone position three to four times/day with hip in extension	B. Prevents hip flexion contracture
C. Application of compression bandage to stump snuggly, remove and reapply during and after bathing, physical therapy	C. Supports tissue and reduces edema, promotes stump shrinkage and healing while preventing residual stump edema if bandaging slips and does not maintain compression
D. If plaster mold or splint applied, check to be sure that it remains tight and snug	D. Ensures effective use of immobilization and compression, slippage allows for continued limb edema
E. Active and/or passive ROM to all joints	E. Maintains joint flexibility and prevents contractures

INTERVENTION	RATIONALE
F. Assist with exercises to shoulders, arms, legs, as appropriate, use of weights, pulleys, push-ups, knee bends, standing and walking with one foot	F. Prepares and strengthens muscles for crutch walking, trapeze use, standing and walking balance, transfer techniques
G. Assist to control weight bearing, ambulate for 5-minute periods, sitting and rising from chair	G. Promotes activity and participation in ADL, prevents falls
H. Accompany during ambulating and crutch walking until balance and gait achieved, transfer technique when needed	H. Prevents accidental falling and injury as center of gravity changes and the prosthesis is different in weight and movement from the amputated limb
I. Encourage and reinforce rehabilitation regimen (physical and occupational)	I. Rehabilitation and prosthesis training assists in achieving independence and adaptation to change in body image and life-style

NURSING DIAGNOSIS

Knowledge deficit related to follow-up care for stump and prosthesis and remaining limbs, prevention of complications (contracture, wound infection), safely manage independence in ADL and mobility

EXPECTED OUTCOMES

Adequate preparation and knowledge of ongoing care of amputated limb and consequences evidenced by progressive adaptation to life-style changes, compliance with rehabilitation program, demonstrated ability to resume mobility and care for stump and prosthesis

INTERVENTION	RATIONALE
V. Teach patient/family:	
A. Pathophysiology of underlying condition(s), reason for surgery and procedure performed	A. Provides information to assist in teaching and planning ongoing care
B. Stump bandaging and wrapping until prosthesis fitted, permanent prosthesis usually fitted in 3 to 4 weeks by a prosthetist	B. Promotes healing and shrinking and protects stump
C. Care of stump including daily inspection for redness, irritation, blisters, breaks, daily washing, rinsing, drying, application of special sock over stump and care of socks for reuse	C. Identifies abnormalities to report for early interventions/treatments, enhances independence in self-care
D. Inform that arm and hook or cosmetic hand available	D. Prostheses available for arm amputation
E. Care of prosthesis including daily cleansing of the socket with rinsing and drying, adjustments and maintenance, avoid moisture touching metal or leather parts of prosthesis, proper shoes, keep appointments with prosthetist	E. Promotes proper fit and ensures optimal use of prosthesis necessary for successful rehabilitation
F. Muscle strengthening exercises, crutch walking, ROM daily and as prescribed	F. Prevents contractures and allows for mobility with prosthesis

INTERVENTION	RATIONALE
G. Physical therapist visits and availability for support and adaptation to loss of limb and prosthesis	G. Provides management of mobility with prosthesis
H. Skin and nail care, protection from skin irritation and circulatory impairment in extremities, use a podiatrist for foot care	H. Maintains health status of remaining extremities
I. Report changes in stump and remaining extremities such as pain, color change, edema, changes in sensation, breaks, drainage	I. Allows for early interventions and prevents complications

arthritis
(gout/osteoarthritis/rheumatoid)

DEFINITION
Arthritis in a term used to identify disorders affecting joints, cartilage, and connective tissue resulting in limitations in mobility and activity. Included is rheumatoid arthritis, a chronic, systemic, inflammatory collagen disease affecting the synovial membrane (synovitis) initially, leading to extension of the membrane into the joint itself and invasion of the cartilage, and finally ankylosis that prevents joint movement. Osteoarthritis is a degenerative joint disease that is chronic, localized, and progressive leading to erosion of the cartilage. Gouty arthritis is a metabolic disease (purine metabolism) leading to deposits of uric acid crystals in joints and connective tissues. All can result in acute or chronic pain, reduced function, and deformity of the involved joints. Various surgical procedures are performed to treat arthritic conditions such as synovectomy or joint replacements (total hip, knee, elbow, finger, ankle). This plan includes the care of these conditions and can be used in association with the TOTAL HIP/KNEE REPLACEMENT, PREOPERATIVE CARE, and POSTOPERATIVE CARE plans if surgery is done

NURSING DIAGNOSES
Anxiety related to threat to or change in health status and outcome of illness causing inability to manage feelings of uncertainty and apprehension regarding situation crisis, change in breathing pattern and inability to sleep

Ineffective individual coping related to inability to cope with long-term chronic illness, change in appearance, and future life-style changes

Body image disturbance related to biophysical factor of change in structure and function of body parts (hip, knee, ankle, feet, elbow, wrist, hand) resulting in change in appearance (deformities of joint areas) and loss of mobility or hand/arm use and dexterity (pain, grasp, imposed immobility)

EXPECTED OUTCOMES

Anxiety within manageable levels, development of coping and problem-solving skills verbalizations that anxiety is decreasing and positive feelings about functional changes and social involvement, participation in care activities and receptive attitude to planning for ongoing care needed to manage disease and chronic anxiety

INTERVENTION	RATIONALE
I. Assess for:	
A. Level of anxiety, use of coping mechanisms, stated fears of uncertainty of disease outcome, life-style changes, possible future surgery	A. Anxiety can range from mild to severe and rest and disease maintenance will be affected accordingly, assists in identifying inappropriate use of coping skills
B. Restlessness, diaphoresis, complaining, joking, withdrawal, talkativeness, increased P and R	B. Nonverbal expressions of anxiety when not able to communicate feelings
C. Personal resources to cope with stress, anxiety, and interest in learning to problem-solve	C. Support systems and personal strengths assist in developing coping skills
D. Feelings and response to change in appearance (deformed joints), declining ability to carry out role and participate in activities	D. Changes in body image and self-concept common problems associated with long-term systemic and degenerative joint disorders
III. Administer:	
A. Anti-anxiety agent PO	A. Acts to reduce anxiety level and provides calming effect and rest, depresses subcortical levels of CNS, limbic system

INTERVENTION	RATIONALE
IV. Perform/provide:	
A. Environment conducive to rest, expression of fears and anxiety, avoid anxiety-producing situations	A. Decreases stimuli that cause stress/anxiety, venting of feelings decreases anxiety
B. Suggest new methods to enhance coping skills and problem solving, allow to externalize and identify those that help	B. Offers alternative coping strategies that allow for release of anxiety and fear
C. Positive feedback regarding progress made, focus on abilities rather than inabilities	C. Provides support for adaptive behavior, promotes self-worth and responsibility
D. Relaxation activities such as exercises, TV, radio, music, reading, tapes, guided imagery, biofeedback	D. Reduces anxiety and promotes comfort, releases muscle tension
E. Allow to participate in planning of care to maintain usual activities when possible	E. Allows for some control over situations
F. Support grieving for loss of life-style and restrictions in activities, changes in physical appearance	F. Provides assistance in adaptation to changes imposed by disease

NURSING DIAGNOSIS

Chronic pain related to physical/psychosocial disability resulting from inflammation and fibrosis of the joint capsule and supporting structures, irritation and pressure on nerves and bones causing joint destruction, deformities, and disability in performing daily routine activities

EXPECTED OUTCOMES

Pain controlled or minimized evidenced by verbalizations that able to manage daily life and continue activities and analgesic regimen effective in pain control

INTERVENTION	RATIONALE
I. Assess for:	
A. Severity of pain, joints and areas involved, type and duration, remission and exacerbations of pain, time of occurrence of pain as on arising in the morning, swelling and stiffness of joints in the morning, redness and heat at joint site	A. Characteristic symptoms of arthritic conditions caused by inflammatory process (rheumatoid), cartilage deterioration bringing bony surfaces together (rheumatoid and osteo), deposits of crystals in joints (gout)
B. Factors that precipitate pain such as movement, stress on joints	B. Accelerates osteoarthritic changes, increases joint pain during inflammatory phase in gout and rheumatoid arthritis
C. Grimacing, moaning, rubbing, and trying to protect painful joint or limb	C. Nonverbal symptoms associated with arthritic pain
D. Muscle aching, elevated temperature, chills, prostration, joint pain and swelling (usually the smaller joints)	D. Symptoms associated initially with rheumatoid arthritis
II. Monitor, describe, record:	
A. Synovial fluid analysis	A. Reveals WBC increased to $50,000/mm^3$

INTERVENTION	RATIONALE
B. X rays of affected joints	B. Reveals tissue swelling, cartilage changes (erosion), narrowed joint spaces, and progressive degeneration and deformity
III. Administer:	
A. Analgesic, nonsteroidal anti-inflammatory PO	A. Acts to reduce pain and inflammatory response caused by disease
B. Antirheumatic salicylate PO	B. Acts to reduce symptomatic arthritic conditions by its analgesic and anti-inflammatory action
C. Anti-inflammatory corticosteroid PO, intra-articular	C. Acts as anti-inflammatory agent to support body defenses
IV. Perform/provide:	
A. Bed rest in acute periods with affected joints supported and immobilized	A. Reduces movement that is painful to joints
B. Handle joints and limbs gently when moving them	B. Careless, rough handling causes pain
C. Bed cradle over painful limbs	C. Protects joints from weight of linens
D. Allow time for movement in bed, moving to chair, and during walking	D. Hurrying movements cause pain

INTERVENTION	RATIONALE
E. Warm-up movements such as flexing knees, sitting or standing in warm shower, soaking hands in warm water	E. Relieves stiffness common on arising in the morning
F. Plan activities and procedures around most painful time or delay until pain and stiffness reduced	F. Activity and movement will increase pain and discomfort
G. Application of heat such as moist or dry (whirlpool, ultrasound, diathermy), cold such as ice pack to painful area	G. Relieves inflammation and local pain
H. Careful massage of muscles if acute inflammation has subsided	H. Relieves joint pain and muscle aches
I. Relaxation techniques, diversional activities, biofeedback	I. Reduces anxiety and stress that increase or cause exacerbation of pain
J. Application of lightweight splint	J. Rests inflamed joint and reduces pain by immobilization in rheumatoid-type arthritis
K. Exercises and strengthening exercises (isometric), inform that pain can increase at beginning of exercises	K. Relieves pain rather than having continuous immobility that can cause increased pain

NURSING DIAGNOSES

Impaired physical mobility related to pain and discomfort and musculoskeletal impairment resulting from joint inflammatory and degenerative changes in joints and associated structures causing immobility, limited ROM (joint destruction), reluctance to attempt movement/exercises (pain), imposed restrictions of medical protocol (splint, bed rest), and possible risk for falls (weakness)

Activity intolerance related to generalized weakness and bed rest or immobility resulting from musculoskeletal impairment (inflammation and pain)

Bathing/hygiene, dressing/grooming self-care deficits related to musculoskeletal impairment (joint pain, deformity, immobility) and weakness/fatigue resulting in inability to perform ADL independently

EXPECTED OUTCOMES

Improved or optimal joint function, maintenance, and endurance within identified limitations for mobility (ambulation) and participation in ADL evidenced by ability to perform ADL with or without assistance or aids (washing, putting on and taking off clothing, combing hair, applying facial makeup, brushing teeth, shaving, others), walking with or without assistive aids with absence of falls or trauma

INTERVENTION	RATIONALE
I. Assess for:	
A. Pain on movement, ROM and limitations of any joint, ability to perform self-care activities, deformities in joints if present	A. Provides data regarding mobility, ability to maintain activities within limitations without injury to joints
B. Overall functional ability in daily routines, tolerance for treatments and activity, attitude about importance of self-care	B. Assists to determine need for assistance or assistive aids to encourage independence

INTERVENTION	RATIONALE
C. Presence of contractures and deformities (ulnar drift, swan neck, subcutaneous nodules, raised toes with lower metatarsal heads), tight, glossy skin near arthritic joint	C. Manifestations of arthritic disorders especially rheumatoid arthritis that can affect mobility and function
D. Ability to ambulate safely, muscle strength, coordination, fatigue	D. Predisposes to risk for falls

II. Monitor, describe, record:

INTERVENTION	RATIONALE
A. Rheumatoid factor (RF), erythrocyte sedimentation rate (ESR), C-reactive protein, antinuclear antibodies (ANA)	A. Reveals RE titers greater than 1:160, ESR and C-reactive protein increased, ANA present in rheumatoid arthritis
B. Uric acid	B. Reveals increases of >8 mg/dL in gouty arthritis

III. Administer:

INTERVENTION	RATIONALE
A. Immunosuppressive PO	A. Acts to block the inflammatory response of rheumatoid arthritis
B. Anti-inflammatory agent, gold IM	B. Acts to relieve inflammation and slow progression of disease in rheumatoid arthritis

IV. Perform/provide:

INTERVENTION	RATIONALE
A. Bed rest for limited time or depending on severity of disease and number of joints involved	A. Provides physical and emotional rest and reduces inflammation

INTERVENTION	RATIONALE
B. Proper positioning in body alignment and posture in bed and erect while sitting in straight chair or standing and walking	B. Reduces stress on joints
C. Bedboard or firm mattress, footboard, sandbags, small pillows under joints to maintain extension or positioning in bed	C. Maintains body alignment and prevents flexion contractures
D. Balance exercises and activities with rest, reinforce activities and exercises learned in physical and occupational therapy, modify if overactivity causes intolerance (fatigue, pain) or perform most important activities when tolerance and energy is at highest level	D. Enhances mobility and prevents fatigue and exacerbation of inflammation and pain
E. Clear pathways, night lights, hand rails in halls and bathroom, cane, walker, or other aid	E. Prevents stumbling, falls, support while walking
F. Assist with ADL activities as needed, assistive aids for specific activities (crutches, braces, supportive shoes for ambulation, special utensils for eating, personal hygiene)	F. Conserves energy and prevents stress on joints and deformity, aids are useful if ROM is compromised

INTERVENTION	RATIONALE
G. Isometric exercises with or without splint use, perform when analgesic at optimal effect, ROM at least daily if advised	G. Prevents immobilization and maintains muscle strength
H. Limit time in one position, encourage to move periodically	H. Prevents stiffness and prolonged stress on joints
I. Comply with physical and occupational therapy regimens and reinforce practice of activities	I. Promotes joint function and prevents complications caused by immobilization

NURSING DIAGNOSIS

Knowledge deficit related to ongoing care including medication, exercises/rehabilitation/dietary regimens, life-style modifications, follow-up monitoring of disease progression

Ineffective management of therapeutic regimen (individual) related to complexity of therapeutic regimen, powerlessness, excessive demands made on individual resulting in progression or acceleration in symptoms and debilitating effect of disease (damage to joints)

EXPECTED OUTCOMES

Adequate knowledge, understanding, and compliance of long-term medical regimen evidenced by effective results of medication administration with pain and inflammation controlled, reduced exacerbation of signs and symptoms, ability to maintain optimal mobility, and deformities/joint damage minimized

INTERVENTION	RATIONALE
V. Teach patient/family:	
A. Importance of continued physical and occupational therapy and perform ROM daily (hip and trunk extension, trunk flexion, hip abduction, knee extension, dorsiflexion and aversion of feet, shoulder and elbow exercises, shoulder external rotation, finger exercises)	A. Provides ongoing joint mobility and muscle strength maintenance
B. Allow for 8 hours of sleep at night, rest periods periodically during activities	B. Prevents fatigue, weakness, and exhaustion, possible damage to joints
C. Sit when possible and avoid prolonged standing, move around q2h	C. Reduces stress on hip and knee joints with increased energy needed to stand or walk
D. Application of splints, removal and skin assessment as advised	D. Prevents possible injury to joints by immobilizing them
E. Warm shower, jacuzzi on arising in the morning	E. Promotes comfort by providing heat to relax muscles and reduce pain

INTERVENTION	RATIONALE
F. Ways to perform tasks such as spreading over longer periods, organize to avoid stairs, use carts to carry objects, keep articles in easy-to-reach areas, use electrically run articles instead of hand-operated ones, slide instead of lifting objects, delegate activities to other family members, eliminate unnecessary tasks such as bending, stretching, gripping, reaching	F. Lessens fatigue and stress to joints
G. Correct and safe use of assistive devices such as built-up utensils and toilet seat or chair, buttonhooks, clothing with easy closures, lightweight dishes, modified handles, grooming aids with attachments	G. Provides means to maintain independence in ADL without adding stress to joints leading to deformity
H. Suggest positions for sexual closeness, altered timing for activity	H. Provides adaptation to sexual needs
I. Dietary avoidance of foods high in purine such as sardines, liver, kidneys, goose, crab, herring, ham, salmon, bacon, pork, meat soups, and limited intake of alcohol	I. Increases uric acid and exacerbates gout
J. Modification of home for long-term progressive restrictions/disabilities	J. Provides safe environment for life-style changes

INTERVENTION	RATIONALE
K. Correct medication administration including action, dose, time, frequency, expected response, side effects and to report bleeding, tarry feces, easy bruising	K. Controls inflammation, pain, and eventual loss of function and deformity, early intervention if gastric irritation results from anti-inflammatory medications
L. Identification in wallet or purse, bracelet if taking corticosteroids	L. Provides information in event of emergency
M. Importance of compliance with regimen even if feeling better	M. Exacerbation can occur if health and medications are not maintained
N. Referral to psychological counseling, social worker, interdisciplinary team to prepare for surgery if needed	N. Supports specific needs during long-term illness

fractures
(cast/traction)

DEFINITION

A fracture is a break in a bone usually accompanied by surrounding soft tissue injury caused by trauma or a disease process (pathogenic fracture). It can be a complete or incomplete fracture and classified as simple or compound. Fractures can involve bones of the vertebrae, ribs, clavicles, upper and lower leg, patella, foot, hand, upper or lower arm, or hip. Correction can be accomplished by a closed reduction, external fixation, or open reduction with internal fixation. Immobilization essential to healing is provided by cast, splint, or traction depending on the type and site of the fracture. Traction can be continuous or intermittent (a constant or periodic pull). Skeletal traction is performed by the insertion of wires or pins or metal tongs with the traction attached at the site of the insertion. Casts are immobilizing devices made of plaster or fiber glass applied to a body part, usually an extremity but also the torso area of the body. Bones heal in stages by regeneration (new bone tissue is formed) in approximately 6 weeks depending on the type of bone and fracture. Complications include deformity (malunion), delayed or nonunion of bone healing, fat embolism, infection, compartment syndrome, and arterial damage. This plan includes care of a fracture and immobilization device and can be used in association with the TOTAL HIP/KNEE REPLACEMENT, ARTHRITIS (OSTEOARTHRITIS), PREOPERATIVE CARE, and POSTOPERATIVE CARE plans if surgery is planned for open reduction procedures

NURSING DIAGNOSIS

Pain related to physical injuring agent of trauma or disease affecting a bone resulting in fracture causing spasms and inflammation, use of immobilizing device to treat fracture resulting in pressure and discomfort

EXPECTED OUTCOMES

Pain relieved or controlled evidenced by verbalization that pain reduced and fewer requests for analgesic

INTERVENTION	RATIONALE
I. Assess for: A. Pain descriptors, severity, site, muscle spasms, edema at injured site, site of pinning, need to bivalve cast to relieve pressure on injured part	A. Movement of bone fragments causes spasms and pain that usually subsides in 48 to 72 hours after application of traction or a cast, edema is the result of inflammatory response to injury or surgery
III. Administer: A. Analgesic PO, IM	A. Acts to reduce pain by interfering with CNS pathways with route depending on pre- and postoperative needs
B. Muscle relaxant PO	B. Acts to relieve muscle spasms by depressing nerve transmission through pathways in spinal cord and brain stem
IV. Perform/provide: A. Elevate limb above heart level, position on pillows	A. Relieves edema by promoting return circulation to heart
B. Position and move extremity with gentle smooth movements in proper alignment	B. Prevents spasms that cause pain
C. Change position q2h	C. Prevents pain and stiffness caused by immobility and continuous pressure of cast on one body part

INTERVENTION	RATIONALE
D. Ice pack to site of injury	D. Reduces inflammation and edema by vasoconstriction
E. Avoid heavy covers, bumping bed, pin, traction, or weights, removal of weights when moving in bed or giving care, use bed cradle over casted area if appropriate	E. Causes muscle spasms and pain

NURSING DIAGNOSES

Risk for impaired skin integrity related to the external factors of pressure on skin by cast, physical immobilization by traction or body cast resulting in skin irritation and disruption, internal factors of altered circulation and sensation resulting in impaired peripheral tissue perfusion and flow of oxygen and nutrients to the skin

Risk for infection related to inadequate primary defenses (broken skin resulting from open reduction, pinning, and/or traumatized tissue from injury/fracture)

Risk for peripheral neurovascular dysfunction related to mechanical compression (cast, brace, traction), immobilization resulting in interruption of arterial blood flow or neurological innervation to tissues that can lead to ischemia, paresthesia, or paresis

EXPECTED OUTCOMES

Skin integrity with adequate circulation and sensation in extremity maintained, absence of infection evidenced by no redness, swelling, purulent drainage, at incisional or pin site, no redness, irritation of skin under cast, color, temperature, and sensation at distal extremity sites within normal determinations with cast in place

INTERVENTION	RATIONALE
I. Assess for:	
A. Redness, edema, pain, purulent drainage around pin site, foul odor from under cast, drainage through the cast, heat felt on cast over injury or operative site	A. Indicates infection at surgical incision or pin site, tissue necrosis resulting from skin breakdown
B. Cyanosis, pallor, coldness, swelling, delayed capillary refill, diminished peripheral pulse, tightness of cast, pain and swelling peripheral to cast, skin irritation at cast edges	B. Indicates impaired circulation to the extremity, possible skin breakdown from pressure of cast edges
C. Numbness, tingling, burning, loss of motion of part distal to cast, persistent local pain, paralysis	C. Indicates neurological impairment resulting from nerve compression by cast
II. Monitor, describe, record:	
A. VS, temperature, capillary refill, peripheral pulses q2–4h	A. Elevated temperature associated with infection, diminished peripheral pulses, slow capillary refill indicate circulatory impairment
B. Bone x ray, CT scan	B. Reveals site and extent of fracture
C. CBC with WBC and differential	C. Elevated WBC indicates infection

INTERVENTION	RATIONALE
IV. Perform/provide:	
A. Place in position of comfort with casted extremity elevated, change position q2h and provide skin care and padding to body prominences q8h, assist with position change for those in traction	A. Prevents prolonged pressure on skin, bony prominences
B. Maintain bed free of wrinkles, crumbs, dampness	B. Prevents pressure and irritation to skin
C. Allow for cast to dry and change position to expose all areas to air, handle cast with palms of hands, place on a pillow protected by cover	C. Enhances cast to set and immobilize body part
D. Petal cast edges with tape or moleskin	D. Prevents irritation and excoriation of skin caused by rough edges
E. Cleanse pin site with peroxide, rinse with sterile normal saline (NS), gently dry and dress with sterile technique and supplies	E. Removes exudate and prevents infection
F. Cleanse outside of plaster cast with warm water, cleanse skin under cast edges, dry gently, massage with alcohol, avoid lotions to skin	F. Prevents skin irritation, creams and lotions soften and cause skin to stick to cast

INTERVENTION	RATIONALE
G. Split cast (bivalve) if warranted to allow for edema	G. Prevents permanent neurovascular damage from prolonged nerve pressure causing possible paralysis

NURSING DIAGNOSES

Impaired physical mobility related to musculoskeletal impairment (bone fracture) resulting in imposed restriction in movement by cast or traction application causing possible complications of immobility

Bathing/hygiene, dressing/grooming, toileting self-care deficits related to musculoskeletal impairment and impaired mobility status resulting from the imposed restrictions in movement by presence of cast and/or traction

EXPECTED OUTCOMES

Improved or optimal mobility and use of extremities for ambulation, maintenance, and participation in ADL evidenced by ability to move in and out of bed (walking), perform ADL with or without assistance or aids (washing, personal hygiene, grooming, dressing, toileting) with absence of falls or trauma, circulatory (thrombophlebitis), pulmonary (pneumonia), gastrointestinal (constipation), musculoskeletal (contracture) complications of immobility

INTERVENTION	RATIONALE
I. Assess for:	
A. Ability to move in bed, to ambulate with or without aids, ability to use overhead trapeze for movement in bed if traction applied	A. Provides data regarding mobility, ability to maintain activities within limitations of cast or traction
B. Ability to perform self-care daily routines and activities, attitude about importance of self-care	B. Assists to determine need for assistance or assistive aids to encourage independence

INTERVENTION	RATIONALE
C. Ability to ambulate with cast safely, muscle strength, ROM, coordination	C. Predisposes to risk for falls

IV. Perform/provide:

INTERVENTION	RATIONALE
A. Bed rest for limited time or depending on type of immobilization with proper alignment and positioning	A. Provides physical and emotional rest
B. Active or passive ROM of uncasted joints and those not involved in traction	B. Promotes joint mobility and prevents contractures
C. Restrictive exercises, isometric exercises to contract muscles of uninvolved areas first and then of casted muscles, include gluteal setting, abdominal contractions	C. Promotes muscle strength to prepare for crutches, walker use, stimulates circulation and facilitates healing
D. Balance exercises and activities with rest, reinforce activities and exercises learned in physical and occupational therapy, gradually increase activities	D. Enhances mobility and prevents fatigue
E. Splint casted foot or support in a 90-degree angle	E. Prevents footdrop
F. Assist with ADL activities as needed while traction in place	F. Conserves energy, allows for self-care, independence, and additional exercising of body parts

INTERVENTION	RATIONALE
G. Allow ambulation and weight bearing when walking cast is dry	G. Promotes early ambulation
H. Assistive aids for ADL such as covering cast during bathing, aids to reach articles, put on and take off clothing, suction cups for toothpaste, shaving cream, chair for shower, fracture pan if in traction	H. Reduces frustration associated with personal hygiene and other ADL activities

NURSING DIAGNOSES

Risk for trauma/injury related to internal factor of weakness resulting from prolonged immobility of imposed bed rest associated with traction, lack of safety precautions associated with use of crutches, other assistive aids during or following use of immobilization devices; and external factors of unsafe environment causing falls, incorrect traction maintenance causing ineffective healing of fracture and postponement in return to normal function

Diversional activity deficit related to long-term treatment of traction resulting in possible sensory deprivation

EXPECTED OUTCOMES

Provision of hazard-free environment, resolution of boredom evidenced by absence of injury resulting from falls or traction/cast maintenance, verbalization that participating in interactions and activities

INTERVENTION	RATIONALE
I. Assess for:	
A. Environmental hazards such as slippery floors, cluttered pathways, poor lighting, improper shoes; presence of hand rails, aids to assist safe ambulation (crutches, walker, cane)	A. Provides support and safety measures to prevent falls
B. Desire for leisure activity, boredom, people to visit with	B. Indicates lack of stimulation and need for diversion
C. Correct weights, knots, pulleys, ropes on traction apparatus	C. Ensures effective traction
IV. Perform/provide:	
A. Clear pathways, night lights, hand rails in halls and bathroom, cane, walker, or other aid	A. Prevents stumbling, falls, provides support while walking
B. Use safety straps when transferring or moving a patient	B. Provides secure assistance to those with casts applied
C. Progressive ambulation using belt around waist starting with 10 to 15 min, three times/day	C. Provides stabilization during early ambulation following removal of traction
D. Radio, TV, books, games, newspapers, telephone, clock and calendar within reach	D. Prevents sensory deprivation

INTERVENTION	RATIONALE
E. Adjust traction for weights that hang away from pulley, pulley does not interfere with rope, correct amount of weight removed or added if ordered, frayed rope, loose knots, or pulley clamps not fastened	E. Traction not effective if weights are not hanging, knots caught in pulleys, defective parts to traction

NURSING DIAGNOSIS

Knowledge deficit related to follow-up care of cast and care following traction/cast removal including skin, positioning, mobility and exercises, dietary, and rehabilitation regimen

EXPECTED OUTCOMES

Adequate knowledge to comply with follow-up care evidenced by progressive fracture healing and resumption of routine activities

INTERVENTION	RATIONALE
V. Teach patient/family:	
A. Avoid allowing cast to get wet or dirty, refrain from sticking anything into cast to scratch itchy areas to avoid removing any pads from cast	A. Dampness affects shape of cast, soiling or break in skin can predispose to infection
B. Transfer techniques to chair or commode, use of aids for personal care	B. Promotes independence in mobility and self-care
C. Continue muscle and joint exercises	C. Maintains muscle strength and prevents atrophy following traction

INTERVENTION	RATIONALE
D. Crutch walking, use of walking cast, gait training, weight bearing, use of walker	D. Allows for mobility, can be non-weight-bearing, partial- or full-weight-bearing
E. Proper shoe for uncasted foot, application of cast shoe	E. Protects cast and prevents falls
F. Soak, wash, and dry area following cast removal	F. Allows for skin to return to normal
G. Report cast that is cracked, soft, loose, or rubbing skin, skin that is dry, irritated, edematous, or change in color, sensation	G. Cast that does not fit must be replaced to continue effectiveness, skin changes can indicate risk for breakdown
H. Time for cast removal and to keep appointments for follow-up x rays as scheduled	H. Length of time for casts depends on the type and severity of fracture

laminectomy/spinal fusion

DEFINITION

Laminectomy is the most common type of spinal surgery performed to remove a tumor, correct a herniated intervertebral disc, or relieve pressure on the cord from bone fragments (trauma). It involves the removal of a portion of a vertebra (posterior arch) and possible spinal fusion that removes bone fragments from the iliac crest or tibia and implants them at the surgical site. This is done to provide stability to the spine when a disc is removed and in cases of trauma (fracture) or degenerative disease by fusing the vertebrae together. Metal rods or wires can also be used to provide stability to the spine in certain disorders (spinal curvature). The procedure can be performed via an anterior or posterior approach with the anterior usually reserved for cervical repair. Those at risk for spinal surgery include presence of a past back injury, occupation that involves strenuous physical labor, use of incorrect body mechanics, and activities (exercises) that produce continuous stress on the back muscles. This plan includes some considerations for the medical care of spinal disorders with a concentration on care following surgery and can be used in association with the LOW BACK SYNDROME, SPINAL CORD INJURY, PREOPERATIVE CARE, and POSTOPERATIVE CARE plans

NURSING DIAGNOSIS

Pain related to physical injury of underlying condition preoperatively (disc herniation), trauma from surgery postoperatively (graft and incisional sites) resulting in irritated spinal nerves, spasms, and edema

EXPECTED OUTCOMES

Neck or back pain managed or controlled by medication and activity regimen preoperatively and incisional pain postoperatively evidenced by verbalization that pain reduced or absent and progressive resumption of positioning and activities

INTERVENTION	RATIONALE
I. Assess for:	
A. Pain severity and location, spasm of muscles, stiff neck, shoulder pain, factors that precipitate pain such as straining, coughing, bending, lifting	A. Moderate to severe pain can exist from underlying conditions preoperatively from ruptured disc, trauma, deformities
B. Incisional pain and characteristics, pain in an extremity after anesthesia has worn off	B. Results from surgical trauma postoperatively caused by edema and spasms in back and thigh
II. Monitor, describe, record:	
A. Spinal x rays	A. Reveals degenerative changes and other disorders that are the source of pain
B. Myelography, computerized scan (CT)	B. Reveals narrowed disc space, spinal stenosis, degenerative disease, level of herniation
III. Administer:	
A. Analgesic PO, IM	A. Acts to control pain by interfering with CNS pathways pre- and postoperatively
B. Muscle relaxants PO	B. Acts to reduce muscle spasms
C. Anti-inflammatory PO	C. Acts to enhance body defenses and reduce inflammation caused by surgery

INTERVENTION	RATIONALE
IV. Perform/provide:	
A. Bed rest on a firm mattress during periods of pain or supine in low or semi-Fowler's position with knees slightly flexed or with pillows under the legs, or sidelying on unaffected side with pillow between knees and affected leg flexed	A. Relieves stress on back muscles and vertebrae and stress on the sciatic nerve to relieve pain preoperatively
B. Application of back brace or corset, intermittent cervical traction until pain is relieved	B. Provides support and relieves pain preoperatively and postoperatively
C. Proper alignment, spine and affected leg in comfortable position; avoid flexion, hyperextension of the lumbar or cervical spine, sitting for prolonged periods	C. Reduces pain and muscle spasms postoperatively
D. Logroll to turn and change position	D. Prevents stress on incisional and fusion sites
E. Massage near the operative site	E. Reduces pain by relaxing muscles

NURSING DIAGNOSES

Risk for peripheral neurovascular dysfunction related to trauma to nerves or vessels involved in sensation and blood flow associated with surgery, mechanical compression (corset, brace, collar), immobilization (bed rest) postoperatively resulting in interruption of arterial blood flow or innervation to tissues causing motor or sensory impairment

Risk for impaired skin integrity related to the external factors of pressure on skin by immobility devices, excretions from wound or tube drainage, resulting in skin irritation and disruption, internal factors of altered circulation and sensation resulting in impaired peripheral tissue perfusion and flow of oxygen and nutrients to the skin for wound healing

EXPECTED OUTCOMES

Skin integrity with adequate circulation and sensation maintained, evidenced by absence of redness, irritation of skin under device or burning, numbness, and tingling sensation in upper or lower extremities, no skin irritation or breakdown at surgical site evidenced by dry, progressive wound healing

INTERVENTION	RATIONALE
I. Assess for:	
A. Redness, edema, pain, irritation, drainage, excoriation around drain/surgical site	A. Indicates risk for skin breakdown or infection at surgical site, drain can be removed 2 days postoperatively
B. Skin under brace, collar or other device for irritation, fit of device	B. Excessive, continuous pressure on skin leads to impaired circulation and breakdown both pre- and postoperatively, cervical collar usually applied following cervical surgery, brace or corset following lumbar or thoracic surgery whether in or out of bed
C. Delayed capillary refill, diminish peripheral pulse, pain, pallor, coolness, cyanosis, numbness, tingling, burning in arms or legs, loss of motion in feet, hands, or digits q2h, compare to baseline determinations prior to surgery	C. Indicates impaired circulation and neurological function to the extremity that can be caused from cord edema or hemorrhage

INTERVENTION	RATIONALE
II. Monitor, describe, record:	
A. VS, temperature, capillary refill, peripheral pulses q2–4h	A. Elevated temperature associated with infection, diminished peripheral pulses, slow capillary refill indicate circulatory impairment
B. Neurological signs q4h	B. Indicates neurological dysfunction and possible spinal fluid leakage and infection at site
IV. Perform/provide:	
A. Correct application and positioning of device snuggly but not tightly	A. Prevents rubbing or pressure to skin
B. Wrinkle-free cotton shirt under device, apply powder on skin under device	B. Prevents pressure from creases on skin and maintains dryness without irritation
C. Avoid poking anything under device, pad edges and bony prominences under device	C. Can scratch or cause breaks in skin
D. Massage to back, neck, and head in areas away from surgical sites	D. Stimulates circulation to the area
E. Use sterile technique for all postoperative dressing change or other procedures	E. Prevents transmission of pathogens

INTERVENTION	RATIONALE
F. Maintain patency of wound drainage	F. Removes drainage that can accumulate and increase pressure on the vessels and nerves at the surgical site
G. Use gentle firm movements when changing positions and giving care	G. Reduces stress on surgical area that can dislocate bone chips in fusion

NURSING DIAGNOSES

Impaired physical mobility related to pain and discomfort, and musculo-skeletal impairment resulting from surgery, imposed restrictions of protocol (positioning, splint, brace), reluctance to attempt movement/exercises (pain)

Bathing/hygiene, dressing/grooming, toileting self-care deficits related to musculoskeletal impairment (imposed restrictions of protocol) resulting in temporary inability to perform ADL independently

EXPECTED OUTCOMES

Improved or optimal movement, maintenance, and endurance within identified limitations evidenced by progressive improvement for positioning, mobility (ambulation) and participation in ADL with or without assistance

INTERVENTION	RATIONALE
I. Assess for:	
A. Pain on movement, ability to perform self-care activities, fear or reluctance to move in bed, muscle strength and control	A. Provides data regarding movement status and potential for postoperative mobility
B. Ability to ambulate safely, fatigue, weakness	B. Predisposes to risk for falls

INTERVENTION	RATIONALE
IV. Perform/provide:	
A. Bed rest in flat position postoperatively for at least 1 hour, 10 days to 2 weeks if fusion done	A. Promotes hemostasis immediately following laminectomy to remove disc, promotes comfort and proper alignment until healing is achieved, raising the head of bed puts strain on or can dislodge bone graft
B. Proper positioning in body alignment and posture in bed by logrolling q2h	B. Reduces strain or flexion at the surgical site, prevents twisting of spine or hips while maintaining alignment
C. Bedboard or firm mattress	C. Maintains body alignment and prevents flexion of spine
D. Place in sidelying position with spine straight, flexing legs with a pillow between legs and a pillow to support upper arm	D. Positioning for lumbar and cervical surgery for comfort and support
E. Place all articles and call light within reach	E. Prevents reaching and pull on surgical site
F. Start ambulation in 2 to 3 days unless a fusion was performed, apply a cervical collar for cervical fusion to stabilize surgical site	F. Begins progressive activity program to promote circulation

G. Balance exercises and activities with rest, active or passive ROM only if permitted by order, modify if overactivity causes intolerance (fatigue, pain)

G. Enhances progressive movement without stress on back

H. Assist with ADL activities as needed

H. Conserves energy and prevents stress on surgical site

I. Sturdy shoes for walking

I. Provides support and alignment to reduce strain on back

NURSING DIAGNOSES

Constipation related to neuromuscular impairment (paralytic ileus) resulting in loss of parasympathetic function causing decreased peristalsis and bowel sounds

Urinary retention related to neuromuscular impairment resulting in loss of bladder function and an inability to urinate

EXPECTED OUTCOMES

Urinary and bowel elimination pattern resumed within 48 hours postoperatively evidenced by daily soft formed feces and urination in amounts and frequency compared to baseline determinations preoperatively

INTERVENTION   RATIONALE

I. Assess for:

A. Ability to urinate, urinary bladder distention with associated pain

A. Indicates urinary retention

B. Bowel sounds, abdominal distention, nausea, vomiting

B. Indicates paralytic ileus causing bowel elimination problems

INTERVENTION	RATIONALE

III. Administer:
  A. Stool softener, bulk laxa-
     tive, suppository
	A. Acts to promote bowel
	    elimination by providing
	    bulk and fluid to feces

IV. Perform/provide:
  A. Use fracture pan while in
     bed and able to void
	A. Allows voiding in an al-
	    most flat position

B. Allow to stand or sit up if
     unable to void or have
     bowel elimination
	B. A natural position for void-
	    ing or defecation

C. Clear liquid diet and pro-
     gression to general diet
     with fiber inclusions
	C. Provides fluid and nutri-
	    tional intake to promote
	    elimination without exer-
	    tion

D. Increased fluid intake	D. Promotes elimination

E. Catheterize intermittently
     for inability to void, resid-
     ual urine
	E. Bladder function should re-
	    turn in 48 hours but pa-
	    tient may not be able to
	    completely empty the blad-
	    der

NURSING DIAGNOSIS
Knowledge deficit related to ongoing care, including activities/dietary regimens, life-style modifications related to back care, follow-up monitoring of convalescence

EXPECTED OUTCOMES
Adequate knowledge and understanding of postoperative regimen evidenced by compliance with preventive care of back and successful resumption of life-style

INTERVENTION	RATIONALE
V. Teach patient/family:	
A. Importance of back care to include rolling out of bed near edge and pushing up to sitting position without twisting, use of proper body mechanics when lifting, stooping, bending with muscles of legs and arms	A. Promotes optimal back function with freedom from discomfort
B. Allow for 8 hours of sleep at night on firm mattress, rest when tired, bend a knee during periods of prolonged standing	B. Prevents fatigue and stress on low back
C. Dietary intake that includes fiber, increase fluid intake to 2 to 3 L/day, maintain as near-ideal weight as possible	C. Prevents constipation and need to strain that increases stress on back
D. Application of brace or collar to cervical or lumbar region, note condition of skin	D. Prevents possible injury to operative site postoperatively
E. Use straight-back chair for sitting and driving	E. Maintains back alignment
F. Avoid lifting heavy objects, climbing stairs, driving, sport activities, sexual activity until advised	F. Activities vary according to physician and type of surgery

INTERVENTION	RATIONALE
G. Report any change in incisional sites, drainage or pain, change in sensation or appearance in extremities, discomfort from use of device	G. Allows for early interventions if complications occur
H. Importance of keeping scheduled appointments with physician	H. Ensures smooth postoperative course

low back syndrome

DEFINITION

Low back syndrome is chronic pain in the low lumbar and lumbosacral areas caused by degeneration changes (osteoarthritis), strain on the muscular supporting structures (spasms), osteoporosis, rupture/herniation of the nucleus pulposus, infectious processes (osteomyelitis), inflammatory disorders (spondylitis), tumor, fractures (vertebral), or congenital deformities

NURSING DIAGNOSES

Chronic pain related to physical injuring agents resulting from disorders of the lumbar spine causing poor body mechanics, intermittent discomfort for 6 months or more

Impaired physical mobility related to pain and discomfort resulting from unstable lumbrosacral structures

EXPECTED OUTCOMES

Pain reduced or controlled for extended time with optimal activity and mobility evidenced by pain free ability to walk, work, and function within imposed or painful limitations

INTERVENTION	RATIONALE
I. Assess for: A. Location, severity and length of pain, posture, body mechanics (sitting, standing, stooping, walking), what relieves or precipitates back pain	A. Provides data base for prevention or control of pain

INTERVENTION	RATIONALE
B. Strain or fatigue with performance of ADL, stiffness, contractures, foot drop, loss of sensation in extremity	B. Provides data base regarding mobility and determinants of mobility
III. Administer: A. Non-narcotic analgesic PO	A. Acts to control pain by interference with CNS pain pathways
B. Muscle relaxant PO	B. Acts to reduce muscle spasms
C. Anti-inflammatory, epidural	C. Acts to reduce pain and edema
IV. Perform/provide: A. Bed rest with head elevated and knees slightly flexed	A. Promotes comfort and relieves tension on back
B. Cold or heat applications, massage to lower back q4h	B. Provides comfort and relaxation of muscles to ease pain
C. Pelvic traction continuously or intermittent in proper body alignment with head of bed slightly elevated and hips and knees flexed 30 degrees	C. Provides traction to lumbar spine to relieve pressure on nerves of lumbosacral area and muscle spasms
D. ROM, muscle strengthening exercises for low back and trunk	D. Maintains muscle and joint function, prevents stiffness and strengthens back structures

INTERVENTION	RATIONALE
E. Encourage progressive activity and ambulation using a correctly fitted lumbrosacral corset	E. Maintains mobility and enhances a positive self-concept, corset supports back structures

NURSING DIAGNOSIS

Knowledge deficit related to follow-up care to manage chronic back syndrome and prevent acute exacerbation of pain and immobilization

EXPECTED OUTCOMES

Adequate ongoing management of chronic low back condition evidenced by optimal pain-free activity, participation in exercises and practices to improve body mechanics and posture

INTERVENTION	RATIONALE
V. Teach patient/family:	
A. Pathophysiology involved in the symptomology, debilitating effect of chronic pain on life-style	A. Promotes understanding of disorder and rationale for treatments
B. Proper body mechanics for sitting, standing, stooping, walking, lifting, pushing, pulling	B. Prevents back strain/injury and exacerbation of pain
C. Avoid prolonged sitting or standing, extreme hip or knee extension, high heeled shoes, uncomfortable positions, bending or twisting from the waist	C. Prevents stiffness or strain to the back muscles

INTERVENTION	RATIONALE
D. Maintain erect posture when sitting or standing with frequent change in position, feet flat on floor or on footstool when sitting, stoop with back straight	D. Prevents unnecessary pressure on back muscles
E. Exercises or fitness regimen for back-conditioning and strengthening in lying, sitting, and standing positions for 15 minutes BID	E. Strengthens back muscles
F. Avoid weight gain/obesity, follow low-calorie diet if indicated	F. Prevents pressure on muscles and joints and ligaments of the spine
G. Correct application of corset	G. Provides support for lower back
H. Report extreme back pain or extremity pain, change in sensation	H. Indicates severe lumbrosacral intravertebral pressure

osteoporosis

DEFINITION

Osteoporosis is a condition characterized by a decrease in skeletal bone mass resulting from an increase in bone resorption. It causes a suscepti-bility to fractures especially in the hip and spinal column. It is associated with menopause (most common) or an underlying condition such as hy-perparathyroidism, Cushing's syndrome, or hepatic or renal disease. Those at risk include older female adults, thin small women, immobility, endocrine diseases, smoking, alcohol, and long-term use of medications such as antacids, laxatives, steroids, psychotropics, and others

NURSING DIAGNOSES

Pain related to biologic injuring agent resulting from fracture causing lim-ited mobility, change in life-style and reduced independence in ADL

Body image disturbance related to biophysical deformity of kyphosis of thoracic spine (dowager's hump), height reduction, changes in ap-pearance resulting from long-term effect of bone resorption

Risk for injury related to internal regulatory function of loss of bone mass resulting from bone resorption and causing spontaneous fractures, poorly fitting dentures or tooth loss, fractures from falls

EXPECTED OUTCOMES

Pain reduced or controlled, improved body image, and reduced risk for trauma evidenced by verbalization that pain is relieved, adaptation to changes in appearance with maintenance of bone mass without further deterioration or deformity, reduction of potential for fractures

INTERVENTION	RATIONALE
I. Assess for:	
A. Back pain and characteristics, effect on mobility, history of fractures, pain characteristics of a new fracture	A. Provides data as to extent of disorder or proneness to fracture
B. Menopausal status, changes in height, deformity or crippling effect, expressed feelings about changes	B. Affects body image and self-esteem
C. Dietary intake of calcium, vitamins, estrogen therapy	C. Prevents decrease in bone mass if requirements are met
II. Monitor, describe, record:	
A. Serum and urinary calcium, phosphorus, alkaline phosphatase	A. Confirms diagnosis of osteoporosis caused by underlying bone disease
B. Densitometry	B. Measures amount of bone tissue
C. Bone biopsy	C. Reveals pathology if therapy is ineffective
III. Administer:	
A. Calcium PO	A. Acts to provide mineral to treat or prevent further age-related bone loss and promote bone growth
B. Vitamin D PO	B. Acts to assist in absorption of calcium by intestines

INTERVENTION	RATIONALE
C. Analgesic PO	C. Acts to control pain by interfering with CNS pathways

IV. Perform/provide:

A. Environment free from hazards such as lighting, clear pathways, bed in low position, articles within reach	A. Prevents injury from falls
B. Daily exercises (weight bearing and strengthening), ambulation (distance and time determined by physician)	B. Decreases risk of osteoporosis by activating osteoblast formation
C. Assist with ADL as needed, use aids as appropriate	C. Promotes independence
D. Measure and apply corset	D. Provides support for spine and prevents vertebral collapse
E. Suggest clothing to cover deformity	E. Enhances self-image
F. Referral to nutritionist	F. Ensures dietary intake of calcium

NURSING DIAGNOSIS
Knowledge deficit related to measures to prevent or treat disorder and rehabilitative program following fracture

EXPECTED OUTCOMES
Adequate knowledge of follow-up care and preventive measures evidenced by compliance with exercise/dietary/medication regimens

INTERVENTION	RATIONALE
V. Teach patient/family:	
A. Home modifications with hand rails, safe pathways, assistive aids for ADL to prevent safety hazards	A. Allows posthospital return to home environment during rehabilitation
B. Dietary inclusion of milk, cheese, other dairy foods, soy beans, green leafy vegetables, seafood	B. Provides needed calcium and vitamin D
C. Avoid caffeine and alcohol	C. Increases bone resorption
D. Daily exercise regimen, importance of participating in rehabilitation program	D. Decreases risk for further osteoporosis or return to baseline mobility following a fracture
E. Medication regimen including drug, action, dose, frequency, side effects	E. Promotes correct administration to maintain desirable calcium levels and bone mass
F. Report pain, inability to maintain activity	F. May indicate fracture

total hip/knee replacement

DEFINITION
Total hip replacement is the surgical removal of the ball (femoral head) and socket (acetabulum) of the hip joint and the placement of a prosthesis. It is done to correct damage caused by arthritis, congenital hip disease, fractures, and failure of previous prosthesis placement. Hemiarthroplasty is the surgical removal and replacement of either the ball or socket and is usually done to correct arthritis. Total knee replacement is the surgical removal of the surfaces where the tibia and femur articulate and of the patella if necessary of the knee joint with the placement of a prosthesis. It is done to correct damage caused by rheumatoid or degenerative osteoarthritis. Prostheses available are varied and made of metal, cemented in the desired position or cementless that allows for bone growth to ensure fixation. Less common are joint replacement procedures for shoulder, elbow, ankle, and finger joints. Hip fracture (femoral neck, introtrochanteric) are surgically repaired with the use of pins, nails, compression screw as well as the total replacement or hemi-arthroplasty. This plan includes care of hip and knee arthroplasty and can be used in association with the ARTHRITIS (RHEUMATOID/OSTEOARTHRITIS), PREOPERATIVE CARE, and POSTOPERATIVE CARE plans

NURSING DIAGNOSIS
Pain related to physical injuring agent of disease (arthritis) or injury (hip fracture) affecting joint(s) preoperatively resulting in inflammation and destruction, trauma from surgical repair or joint replacement postoperatively resulting in spasms and inflammation

EXPECTED OUTCOMES
Pain relieved or controlled evidenced by verbalization that pain reduced, increased comfort, and fewer requests for analgesic

INTERVENTION	RATIONALE
I. Assess for: A. Pain descriptors, severity, site (hip, knee, other joints), muscle spasms, edema at site	A. Provides data regarding need for analgesia pre- and postoperatively, edema and spasms are the result of inflammatory response to injury, disease, or surgical trauma
B. Operative limb and factors that contribute to pain (anxiety, improper positioning of operative limb, prolonged immobilization)	B. Indicates tolerance for pain and activities that increase discomfort
III. Administer: A. Analgesic PO, IM	A. Acts to reduce pain by interfering with CNS pathways with route depending on pre- and postoperative needs
B. Muscle relaxant PO	B. Acts to relieve muscle spasms by depressing nerve transmission through pathways in spinal cord and brain stem
IV. Perform/provide: A. Extremity in abducted position by suspension or pillows between legs (hip surgery), extremity in proper alignment without flexion beyond recommended degree (knee surgery)	A. Relieves pain by correct positioning following hip or knee surgery

INTERVENTION	RATIONALE
B. Position and move extremity with gentle smooth movements and maintain body alignment	B. Prevents spasms or pressure on operative site that causes pain
C. Restrict hip flexion as ordered to 45–60 degrees for 3 days	C. Prevents pain postoperatively
D. Change position q2h, keep pillow between legs when moving	D. Prevents painful positioning and continuous pressure on one body part
E. Ice pack to surgical site for 24 to 48 hours	E. Reduces inflammation and edema by vasoconstriction
F. Application of TENS machine for total knee surgery	F. Reduces pain sensations by applying electrical nerve stimulation

NURSING DIAGNOSES

Risk for impaired skin integrity related to the external factors of pressure to skin resulting from physical immobilization, excretions of wound drainage resulting in irritation and possible breakdown; internal factors of altered circulation and sensation resulting in impaired peripheral tissue perfusion and flow of oxygen and nutrients to the skin and wound

Risk for infection related to inadequate primary defenses resulting from broken skin from surgical procedure, traumatized tissue from injury/fracture

Risk for peripheral neurovascular dysfunction of extremity related to orthopedic surgery resulting from trauma to vessels and/or nerves, incorrect positioning of the extremity, possible dislodgment of prosthesis

EXPECTED OUTCOMES

Skin integrity with adequate circulation and sensation in extremity maintained, absence of infection evidenced by no redness, swelling, purulent drainage at incisional site, color, temperature, and sensation at distal extremity sites within normal determinations postoperatively

INTERVENTION	RATIONALE
I. Assess for:	
A. Redness, irritation at pressure points	A. Indicates risk for skin breakdown from prolonged pressure to areas
B. Redness, edema, pain, purulent drainage at surgical site	B. Indicates infection at surgical incision, prosthesis is considered a foreign body and source of infection
C. Cyanosis, pallor, coldness, swelling, delayed capillary refill, diminished peripheral pulse, pain increased with movement	C. Indicates impaired circulation to the extremity with joint replacement
D. Numbness, tingling, burning, loss of motion	D. Indicates neurological impairment resulting from nerve damage
II. Monitor, describe, record:	
A. VS, temperature, capillary refill, peripheral pulses, neurological check q2–4h	A. Elevated temperature associated with infection, diminished peripheral pulses, slow capillary refill indicate circulatory impairment, neurological check associated with nerve trauma
B. Bone x ray, CT scan	B. Reveals joint pathology, prosthesis placement
C. CBC with WBC and differential	C. Elevated WBC indicates infection

INTERVENTION	RATIONALE
III. Administer:	
A. Antimicrobial PO	A. Acts to interfere with cell-wall synthesis to destroy pathogens given as a prophylactic and postoperatively
IV. Perform/provide:	
A. Place in position of comfort with extremity in limited flexion or abduction with immobilizing device in place, change position q2h	A. Prevents prolonged pressure on skin, bony prominences or uneven pressure of device
B. Maintain body alignment when changing position or performing care	B. Prevents unnecessary pressure on skin and possible contractures
C. Maintain proper tightness and placement of elastic bandage, device, trochanter roll, dressings at surgical site	C. Prevents undue pressure or restriction to knee, ankle, popliteal area that can cause neurovascular complication
D. Cleanse incision and change dressing with sterile technique and supplies as needed	D. Removes exudate and maintains dry wound that prevents infection, dressing changes usually occur by 3 days postoperatively
E. Maintain drainage system patency, avoid kinking of tubing, keep device below level of wound, ensure suctioning, empty collection bag as needed	E. Reduces accumulation of fluid at the wound site and prevents infection, average wound drainage is usually 600 mL/24 hours

INTERVENTION	RATIONALE
F. Maintain dry, wrinkle-free bed, remove elastic hose and cleanse and massage skin at pressure points and heels/elbows, use lotion to moisturize skin	F. Prevents skin irritation and breakdown

NURSING DIAGNOSES

Impaired physical mobility related to musculoskeletal impairment (surgical hip or knee replacement) resulting in pain, imposed restriction in movement, fear of falling or dislocating prosthesis causing possible loss of strength and endurance and complications of immobility

Risk of trauma related to internal factor of weakness, impaired weight bearing and movement of operative extremity resulting in inability to ambulate, transfer, perform ADL independently

Bathing/hygiene, dressing/grooming, toileting self-care deficits related to musculoskeletal impairment and impaired mobility status resulting from the surgical procedure

EXPECTED OUTCOMES

Improved or optimal mobility and use of extremities for ambulation, maintenance, and participation in ADL evidenced by ability to move in and out of bed (walking), perform ADL with or without assistance or aids with absence of falls or trauma, circulatory (thromboembolism), gastrointestinal (constipation), or musculoskeletal (prosthesis displacement) complications of immobility or surgery

INTERVENTION	RATIONALE
I. Assess for: A. Ability or reluctance to move in bed with or without aids, ability to use overhead trapeze for movement in bed	A. Provides data regarding mobility, ability to maintain activities within imposed limitations

INTERVENTION	RATIONALE
B. Ability to perform self-care daily routines and activities, attitude about importance of self-care	B. Assists to determine need for assistance or assistive aids to encourage independence
C. Ability to ambulate safely, muscle strength, ROM, coordination, attitude about beginning rehabilitation	C. Predisposes to risk for falls
D. Environmental hazards, awareness level affected by medications, weakness, fatigue	D. Leads to falls and injury
IV. Perform/provide:	
A. Bed rest for limited time or depending on type of surgery with proper positioning of extremity	A. Provides physical and emotional rest during healing
B. Active or passive ROM of areas not involved in surgery	B. Promotes joint mobility and prevents contractures
C. Restrictive exercises, isometric exercises to contract muscles of uninvolved areas first and then gluteal and quadriceps setting, knee flexion and extension about 3 days postoperatively	C. Promotes muscle strength to prepare for walking without dislocating prosthesis, promotes circulation and facilitates healing

INTERVENTION	RATIONALE
D. Balance exercises and activities with rest, reinforce activities and exercises learned in physical therapy; stand at bedside on second day, assist to chair without hip flexion of more than 90 degrees, progressive ambulation with bars, walker, and cane, transfer techniques	D. Enhances mobility and prevents fatigue, rehabilitation can begin as early as 5 days postoperatively
E. Careful active ROM to extremity daily following rehabilitation routine	E. Strengthens muscles
F. Assist with ADL activities as needed while device is in place, use aids for personal care and place articles within reach	F. Conserves energy, allows for self-care, independence, and additional exercising of body parts
G. Clear pathways, place furniture in stragetic positions, hand rails, in halls and bathroom, night lights	G. Prevents barriers to ambulating and falls

NURSING DIAGNOSIS
Knowledge deficit related to follow-up care including wound, positioning, mobility/exercises, and rehabilitation regimens

EXPECTED OUTCOMES
Adequate knowledge to comply with follow-up care evidenced by progressive resumption of routine activities

INTERVENTION	RATIONALE
V. Teach patient/family:	
A. Continue physical therapy and transfer techniques to chair or commode, use of aids for ambulation and personal care (raised toilet seat, walker, cane)	A. Provides for support and continued rehabilitative progress, independence in self-care
B. Continue muscle and joint exercises	B. Maintains muscle strength and promotes endurance
C. Crutch walking, use of walker and cane, gait training, weight bearing, use of proper shoes	C. Allows for mobility, can be non-weight-bearing, partial- or full-weight-bearing
D. Avoid leaning forward, reaching for articles on floor, use of pillow under knees, avoid any extremes related to internal rotation, flexion, or adduction of hip, use long-handled utensil for putting on shoes and hose	D. Prevents hip or knee flexion of more than 90 degrees that can dislocate the prosthesis
E. Avoid crossing legs, keep the knees parted, lifting heavy objects, jumping, running, prolonged sitting, sitting in low chairs with soft seats	E. Prevents strain on operative limb and possible injury
F. Avoid position during intercourse that cause hip to turn inward or any rotation of the knee, begin driving a car and climbing stairs as advised by physician	F. Prevents positioning that can cause injury or displacement of prosthesis

INTERVENTION	RATIONALE
G. Report skin that is dry, irritated, color or sensation changes in operative extremity, persistent pain, inability to move or bear weight on limb, wound drainage and pain	G. Indicates possible complications to allow for early intervention
H. Modify home environment to provide good lighting, clear pathways, holding bars in bathroom, elevated seats with arms	H. Prevents falls following discharge from hospital
I. To keep scheduled appointments for follow-up care, x rays, rehabilitation therapy as scheduled	I. Length of time for healing is 4 to 6 weeks, but rehabilitation can continue until ability to ambulate and perform other activities is regained

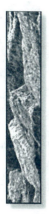

Reproductive System Standards

reproductive system data base

HISTORICAL DATA REVIEW
Past events:
1. Acute and/or chronic female (gynecologic) or male reproductive disease or disorders, presence of other disorders that affect the reproductive system (genitourinary tract disorders, sexually transmitted diseases, hormone over- or undersecretions, bleeding disorders, diabetes, cardiovascular disease)
2. Chronic signs and symptoms related to reproductive system (external genitalia irritation, pruritis, dysmenorrhea, amenorrhea, meatal/vaginal discharge, dyspareunia, urinary abnormalities)
3. Reproductive/breast disorders of family members
4. Allergies to tampons, personal hygienic products
5. Childhood diseases and immunizations (mumps, measles)
6. Menstrual date, menopause date, maternal history
7. Tobacco/alcohol/caffeine use, self-examination of breasts and/or testes, female/male contraceptive/birth control use
8. Medications (prescription and over-the-counter) and effect on libido, impotence, and fertility
9. Hospitalization and feelings about care, surgery associated with female or male reproductive organs or disorders

Present events:
1. Medical diagnoses associated with or affecting reproductive structures or functions
2. Known or suspected disorders of the reproductive system (tumor, sexually transmitted disease, infertility, sexual dysfunction, hypertrophy of prostate, prostatitis, menstrual disorders, endometriosis, uterine prolapse, vaginitis)
3. Abnormal vaginal or penile bleeding/discharge, genital pruritis, irritation, lesions, dyspareunia, impotence, urinary problems (hematuria, pyuria, urgency, incontinence), pain and site(s)

4. Presence of penile implant, breast augmentation, indwelling catheter
5. Cleanliness and personal hygiene practices, sexual orientation
6. Activities of daily living and effect of sexuality impairment on life-style and self-esteem or body image (intercourse frequency and satisfaction)

PHYSICAL ASSESSMENT DATA REVIEW
Female:

1. Symmetry of breasts' size, contour, presence of lesions, rash, discoloration, dimpling, edema, venous pattern, symmetry of nipples' size, contour, presence of inversion, rash, cracks, discharge
2. Axillary lymph nodes and site(s), breast and nipple tenderness, mobility, elasticity, fullness, masses palpated
3. Discharge, redness, swelling, lesions, infectious process of external genitalia; bulging, color, masses, irritation, discharge of vaginal wall; position, color, shape, ulceration, discharge of cervix; pubic hair distribution and infestation
4. Tenderness of vaginal wall; mobility, tenderness, smoothness, firmness of cervix; size, mobility, firmness, contour, position, tenderness of uterus; masses, size, of ovaries, all by palpation

Male:

1. Size and shape for age, rash, ulcer, and swelling of penis; position, discharge, inflammation of meatus; shape, swelling, of scrotum with testes in position; pubic hair distribution and infestation; circumcision present or absent
2. Symmetry, lesions, masses, tenderness, enlargement, discharge of breasts
3. Tenderness, masses, firmness, smoothness of penile shaft; size, shape, tenderness, masses of scrotum, all by palpation
4. Prostate tenderness, enlargement, softness by rectal palpation
5. Bulging at inguinal area during straining; mass or hernia by inguinal area palpation

NURSING DIAGNOSIS CONSIDERATIONS

1. Altered sexuality pattern
2. Altered urinary elimination
3. Anxiety
4. Body image disturbance

5. Risk for infection
6. Knowledge deficit
7. Sexual dysfunction
8. Stress incontinence
9. Urge incontinence

GERIATRIC CONSIDERATIONS

Reproductive tract changes in geriatric patients depend on the aging process and the physical health of the older adult. They can result in urinary and sexuality (impotency) problems. Sexual expression and drive continue throughout life and remain an important activity in the elderly unless there is a lack of privacy, illness, or problem with sexual organs that interfere with arousal, erection, vaginal lubrication, or libido. Reproductive changes associated with aging that should be considered when assessing the geriatric patient include:

1. Decreased size of uterus, cervix, ovaries, weakness of muscles resulting in uterine prolapse
2. Decreased subcutaneous fat resulting in reduced amount and sagging of breast tissue, flattening and folding of labia
3. Vagina shorter and narrower with thinning and atrophy of lining resulting in atrophic vaginitis, dyspareunia
4. Decreased size and firmness of testes and thickness of testicular tubules resulting in decreased sperm production, increased size of prostate gland
5. Decreased estrogen secretion resulting in "hot flashes" and other symptoms of climacteric, decreased Bartholin gland secretions resulting in reduced mucus to lubricate the vagina
6. Decreased testosterone secretion resulting in reduced sexual energy, decreased seminal fluid amount and viscosity resulting in reduced force of ejaculation, delayed erection resulting in delayed orgasm

DIAGNOSTIC LABORATORY TESTS AND PROCEDURES

1. Mammography, ultrasonography, thermography, transillumination, magnetic resonance imaging (MRI), computerized tomography (CT), colposcopy, culdoscopy, pelvic laparoscopy, cystoscopy, urodynamic tests, tissue biopsy
2. Papanicolaou smear and cytology, culture of secretions from reproductive tract, sperm antibodies, fertility tests, prolactin, follicle stim-

ulating hormone (FSH), luteinizing hormone (LH), testosterone, fluorescent treponemal antibody absorption (FTA), venereal disease research laboratory (VDRL), urinalysis (routine and culture)

MEDICATIONS

1. Alpha-adrenergic blockers: prozasin, phenoxybenzamine
2. Analgesics: aspirin, ibuprofen, mefenamic acid, naproxen sodium
3. Antiestrogens: tamoxifen
4. Antigonadotropins: danazol
5. Antimicrobials: specific to identified organism and sexually transmitted diseases (penicillin, tetracycline, ceftriaxone sodium, acyclovir, metronidazole)
6. Antitestosterone/Androgen agents: flutamide, cyproterone acetate, and gonadotropin-releasing hormones such as leuprolide, nafarelin acetate
7. Hormone replacement agents: estrogen, estrone sulfate, estradiol, progesterone
8. Male infertility agents: testosterone

colporrhaphy/vaginal hysterectomy

DEFINITION
Colporrhaphy is the surgical repair of a cystocele (anterior), rectocele (posterior), and enterocele or urethrocele. A cystocele is the protrusion or herniation of the bladder into the vagina and rectocele is the protrusion of the rectum into the vagina. Both are associated with a weakness in the pelvic and vaginal muscles and uterine prolapse, which pulls these structures out of position. Causes include multiple childbirths and aging. Anterior and/or posterior colporrhaphy tightens these weak muscles via a vaginal approach. An abdominal approach can also be performed to suspend the pelvic ligaments and fix the bladder to a higher position in the pelvis. Uterine prolapse is the descent of the uterus into the vagina and is corrected by the surgical removal of the uterus through the vagina (vaginal hysterectomy). Vaginal hysterectomy is also performed to treat abdominal conditions that lend themselves to this approach if salpingectomy or oophorectomy is not done. It can be done alone or in conjunction with colporrhaphy. This plan includes care specific to these procedures and can be used in association with the HYSTERECTOMY, PREOPERATIVE CARE, and POSTOPERATIVE CARE plans

NURSING DIAGNOSIS
Stress incontinence preoperatively related to weak pelvic muscles and structural supports, uterine prolapse resulting in urinary urgency, frequency, dribbling with increased abdominal pressure

EXPECTED OUTCOMES
Strengthened pelvic muscles evidenced by compliance with exercises and incontinence episodes minimized

INTERVENTION	RATIONALE
I. Assess for:	
A. Urgency, frequency, loss of urine with coughing, difficulty in entirely emptying bladder, frequent urinary tract infections	A. Indicates presence of cystocele
B. Feeling of heaviness, hemorrhoids that are painful, constipation	B. Indicates presence of rectocele
C. Stress incontinence, feeling of heaviness and pressure, backache, protrusion of cervix through the vaginal orifice	C. Indicates uterine prolapse with symptoms depending on degree of prolapse
III. Administer:	
A. Stool softener PO	A. Acts to promote bowel elimination by softening feces for easier removal and prevent constipation
IV. Perform/provide:	
A. Kegel exercises during the day 10 times, 4 times/day or 50 times, 2 times/day (tighten as if trying to hold urine and then relax)	A. Perineal strengthening exercises to treat stress incontinence
B. Information about pessary insertion and rationale	B. Pessary can be inserted to treat prolapse of uterus

NURSING DIAGNOSES

Risk for infection postoperatively related to inadequate primary defenses resulting from surgical wound within close proximity to contamination from urine or feces, stasis of body fluids resulting from urinary retention, invasive procedure of indwelling catheter to maintain decompression of bladder (vaginal hysterectomy), or inability to void resulting from tissue edema from surgical trauma

Altered urinary elimination postoperatively related to mechanical trauma of surgery (edema, pain, reduced muscle tone) resulting in urinary retention, bladder distention, and risk for infection

EXPECTED OUTCOMES
Absence of urinary tract infection and retention evidenced by return of normal urinary elimination pattern, surgical site intact and free of edema, foul-smelling drainage and healing, urine free of cloudiness and foul odor

INTERVENTION	RATIONALE
I. Assess for: A. Urine color, odor, amount with indwelling catheter in place, urinary frequency, urgency, cloudy, foul-smelling urine, bladder distention	A. Indwelling catheter usually in place postoperatively for several days until edema subsides, symptoms following catheter removal indicate retention or urinary tract infection
B. Pain, foul-smelling vaginal discharge	B. Indicates infection at surgical site
II. Monitor, describe, record: A. Temperature q4h (oral)	A. Elevation indicates infection
B. Urine or wound culture	B. Positive culture indicates infection
C. WBC	C. Increases indicate infection
III. Administer: A. Antimicrobial PO	A. Acts to destroy pathogens by inhibiting cell-wall synthesis

INTERVENTION	RATIONALE
B. Antipyretic PO	B. Acts to reduce temperature if needed
IV. Perform/provide:	
A. Place on bed rest in semi-Fowler's position	A. Prevents strain on suture line and increased intra-abdominal pressure
B. Catheter care TID	B. Prevents movement of pathogens up catheter into the bladder
C. Perineal care BID and following urination and defecation	C. Cleanses site and prevents possible wound contamination
D. Heat lamp to perineum for 20 minutes TID	D. Maintains dry wound area
E. Sitz bath BID	E. Promotes comfort of perineum and reduces edema
F. Refrain from invasive procedures such as enemas, rectal tube, thermometer, suppositories	F. Prevents trauma to wound area or introduction of contaminants
G. Douches as ordered using sterile technique	G. Prevents introduction of pathogens to surgical site
H. Techniques such as running warm water over perineum, running tap water, submerging of hands in a pan of water	H. Encourage urination after catheter removed
I. Catheterize for retention if symptoms appear (frequency)	I. Prevents stasis of urine leading to urinary infection

NURSING DIAGNOSIS
Knowledge deficit related to follow-up care, precautions to prevent infection or recurrence of cystocele or rectocele

EXPECTED OUTCOMES
Adequate knowledge of care and preventive measures evidenced by absence of complications or recurrence, verbalization of required daily care measures to maintain health status

INTERVENTION	RATIONALE
V. Teach patient/family:	
A. Pathophysiology of abnormal anatomical changes and surgical procedure	A. Provides baseline information and rationale for care
B. Precautions to take to prevent infection including: a. Wipe from front to back after urination and defecation	B. Prevents complications
b. Avoid douching, enemas, invasive procedures to rectal or vaginal area	b. Places pressure on and traumatizes suture line
c. Void q4h or when urge is felt	
C. Avoid straining at defecation, lifting or carrying heavy objects, coughing, bending at the waist, prolonged sitting, standing, or walking	C. Creates Valsalva response and places pressure on suture line by increasing intra-abdominal pressure
D. Low-residue diet, fluid intake of 2 to 3 L/day if allowed, offer sample diet menus with lists of foods to include and exclude	D. Prevents constipation causing pressure on posterior suture line

INTERVENTION	RATIONALE
E. Administer ordered douche slowly in small amounts and rotate nozzle	E. Prevents excessive pressure on suture line
F. Medication administration including name, action, dose, route, frequency, side effects to report	F. Ensures correct drug administration for optimal effect
G. Kegel exercises after healing is complete, sit on soft seat until healing is complete	G. Strengthens vaginal tone and perineal muscles to prevent recurrence
H. Resume intercourse in 4 to 6 weeks and inform of temporary loss of vaginal sensation that can last for several months	H. Prevents trauma prior to complete healing
I. Report incontinence, foul-smelling vaginal discharge or urine, persistent pain	I. Allows for early intervention for infection or recurrence of cystocele/rectocele

hysterectomy/salpingectomy/oophorectomy

DEFINITION

Hysterectomy is the surgical removal of the uterus through an abdominal incision. It can be a total hysterectomy (removal of the uterus and cervix) or panhysterectomy (removal of the uterus, cervix, fallopian tubes, and ovaries). It is performed to treat endometriosis, tumors (benign and malignant of the cervix, endometrium or muscle of the uterus), severe abnormal bleeding, and prolapse of the uterus. Hysterectomy done for prolapse can be done in conjunction with colporrhaphy through the vaginal route only if the uterus is to be removed. Salpingectomy is the surgical removal of one or both fallopian tubes and oophorectomy of one or both ovaries. Oophorectomy is done to treat ovarian cysts and malignant tumor of the ovary. This plan includes care for these procedures and can be used in association with COLPORRHAPHY/VAGINAL HYSTERECTOMY, PREOPERATIVE CARE, and POSTOPERATIVE CARE plans

NURSING DIAGNOSES

Anxiety preoperatively related to threat to self-concept resulting from possible sexual dysfunction, threat to health status if surgery advised (simple/radical hysterectomy, possible radiation therapy)

Body image disturbance postoperatively related to biophysical and psychosocial factors of hormonal imbalance and loss of body part resulting in loss of childbearing ability and/or feeling of femininity

Sexual dysfunction postoperatively related to altered body structure or function (surgery, radiation therapy) resulting in dyspareunia, change in achieving sexual satisfaction and positive relationship with partner

EXPECTED OUTCOMES

Anxiety within manageable levels and body image improved evidenced by verbalizations that anxiety and fear reduced and a more positive understanding of reproductive and sexuality losses, adaptation to hormonal changes with therapy, eventual participation in sexual intercourse and acceptance of improved libido and relationship with partner

INTERVENTION	RATIONALE
I. Assess for:	
A. Apprehension, anxiety level, fear of impotency, infertility, effect of loss on body image and sexuality	A. Provides data regarding perceptions about the effects of surgery and impact on personal life
B. Decreased libido, dyspareunia, vaginal bleeding	B. Hormone imbalance causes changes in body function
C. Feelings of sexual desirability, alterations in relationship with partner, self-worth as a whole person	C. Indicates degree of acceptance and adaptation to loss
III. Administer:	
A. Hormone PO	A. Acts to provide estrogen replacement if bilateral oophorectomy performed
IV. Perform/provide:	
A. Environment conducive to expression of feelings about sexuality changes, changes in life and acceptance by others	A. Provides opportunity to vent feelings and reduce fear and anxiety about sexuality inadequacy in private
B. Privacy and opportunity to interact with partner and others if requested	B. Improves and maintains relationship with partner
C. Encouragement and praise qualities and behaviors that have positive effect on self-image	C. Supports and reinforces adaptation to loss
D. Encourage participation in improving personal appearance, social activities	D. Enhances self-image and esteem

INTERVENTION	RATIONALE
E. Suggest methods of expressing sexual caring and activities	E. Assists to adjust to effect of surgery on feelings about sexual intercourse

NURSING DIAGNOSES

Altered urinary elimination postoperatively related to mechanical trauma of surgery (atony from edema) resulting in urinary retention and bladder distention, indwelling catheter resulting in risk for infection

Constipation related to surgical manipulation of bowel resulting in gas pain, reduced motility and inability to eliminate feces

EXPECTED OUTCOMES

Optimal voiding and bowel elimination pattern established evidenced by resumption of voiding without difficulty with absence of distention and residual urine, cloudy, foul-smelling urine, soft formed brown feces eliminated daily or q2days

INTERVENTION	RATIONALE
I. Assess for:	
A. Urine color, odor, amount with indwelling catheter in place, urinary frequency, urgency, cloudy, foul-smelling urine, bladder distention	A. Indwelling catheter usually in place postoperatively for several days until edema subsides, symptoms following catheter removal indicate retention or urinary tract infection
B. Pain, foul-smelling vaginal discharge	B. Indicates infection at surgical site
C. Bowel pattern preoperatively, gas pains, ability to eliminate gas and feces with amount and characteristics	C. Provides baseline data, postoperative gas and constipation are caused by the reduced motility of the gastrointestinal tract and lack of ambulation

INTERVENTION	RATIONALE
II. Monitor, describe, record:	
A. Temperature q4h (oral)	A. Elevation indicates infection
B. Urine or wound culture	B. Positive culture indicates infection
C. WBC	C. Increases indicate infection
III. Administer:	
A. Antimicrobial PO	A. Acts to destroy pathogens by inhibiting cell-wall synthesis
B. Antipyretic PO	B. Acts to reduce temperature if needed
C. Stool softener PO	C. Acts to soften feces for easier passage
IV. Perform/provide:	
A. Place on bed rest in semi-Fowler's position	A. Prevents strain on suture line and increased intra-abdominal pressure
B. Catheter care TID	B. Prevents movement of pathogens up catheter into the bladder
C. Perineal care BID and following urination and defecation	C. Cleanses site and prevents possible contamination from close proximity to anus
D. Fluid intake of 2 to 3 L/day	D. Promotes return to baseline urinary elimination and dilutes urine to prevent stasis leading to infection

INTERVENTION	RATIONALE
E. Techiques such as running warm water over perineum, running tap water, submerging of hands in a pan of water	E. Encourages urination after catheter removal
F. Catheterize for retention if symptoms appear (frequency) following voiding and reinsert indwelling catheter if residual continues or is more than 50 mL	F. Prevents stasis of urine leading to urinary infection
G. Enema for gas pains if ordered	G. Facilitates bowel motility to prevent constipation and provide relief for gas pains
H. Early ambulation with progressive increases	H. Promotes peristalsis and bowel elimination

NURSING DIAGNOSIS

Knowledge deficit related to follow-up care, precautions to prevent infection, resumption of varied activities, adaptation to and changes in self-image

EXPECTED OUTCOMES

Adequate knowledge of care and health measures evidenced by verbalization of progressive resolution of anxiety, sexuality, and self-concept concerns and compliance with resumption of physical activities without complications

INTERVENTION	RATIONALE
V. Teach patient/family:	
A. Pathophysiology of abnormal anatomical changes and reason for surgical procedure and effect on sexual function	A. Provides baseline information and rationale for care
B. Inform that feeling depressed and crying spells following surgery are not uncommon	B. Response to hormonal changes of vacillation in estrogen and progesterone levels
C. Inform that menstruation will cease, that hot flashes and other menopausal changes can occur	C. Effect of hysterectomy, symptoms of surgically induced menopause from bilateral oophorectomy
D. Inform that some spotting can occur for 2 weeks	D. Normal postoperative response until sutures absorbed

E. Precautions to take to prevent infection including:
  a. Wipe from front to back after urination and defecation
  b. Void q4h or when urge is felt
  c. Protect wound when bathing
	E. Prevents urinary or wound complications

F. Avoid straining at defecation, lifting of carrying heavy objects for 2 months, avoid prolonged standing, strenuous activities such as dancing	F. Allows for healing and prevents Valsalva response that places pressure on suture line by increasing intra-abdominal pressure

INTERVENTION	RATIONALE
G. Fluid intake of 2 to 3 L/day, include fiber in diet	G. Prevents constipation and promotes urinary elimination
H. Medication administration including name, action, dose, route, frequency, side effects to report	H. Ensures correct drug administration (hormone replacement) for optimal effect
I. Abdominal exercises daily	I. Strengthens muscles following surgery
J. Resume intercourse in 4 to 6 weeks or as physician instructs, avoid douching, tub baths until advised to resume	J. Prevents trauma prior to complete healing
K. Report incontinence, foul-smelling vaginal discharge or urine, persistent pain, vaginal bleeding	K. Allows for early intervention for infection or other complication
L. Suggest sex therapist, other counseling if appropriate	L. Provides support and assistance to overcome psychophysical problems

mastectomy/mammoplasty

DEFINITION

Mastectomy is the surgical removal of a breast performed to treat breast malignancy. Chemotherapy and radiation therapy can precede or follow the surgery. Approaches include a lumpectomy (removal of the tumor mass only), quadrantectomy (removal of a quarter of the breast that contains the tumor), total simple mastectomy (removal of the breast, pectoralis major fascia, and axillary tail of the breast), modified radical mastectomy (removal of the breast and axillary lymph nodes with preservation of the pectoralis major muscle), and radical and extended radical mastectomy (removal of the breast, pectoral and major muscles, axillary nodes plus the internal mammary lymph nodes with chest wall resection). Surgical reconstruction or mammoplasty procedures are available and can be performed during mastectomy surgery or at a later date depending on the women's preference, condition, and need to allay the emotional trauma associated with the mastectomy. Options include tissue expanders, implants, rotating the latissimus muscle, fashioning a flap from the abdominal muscle and skin, and can include nipples fashioned from grafts or tattooing procedures. This plan includes care of these procedures and can be used in association with the NEOPLASM (CHEMOTHERAPY/RADIATION THERAPY), PREOPERATIVE CARE, and POSTOPERATIVE CARE plans

NURSING DIAGNOSES

Anxiety related to change in health status causing inability to manage feelings of uncertainty, apprehension regarding prognosis (malignancy), change in self-concept resulting from loss of body part (mastectomy), situational crisis of decision to have reconstruction surgery (mammoplasty)

Ineffective individual coping related to inability to cope with change in life-style, personal vulnerability, possible chemotherapy or radiation therapy, loss of femininity resulting from mastectomy

Body image disturbance related to biophysical factor of missing body part, resulting in change in appearance (mutilation) and effect on sexuality

Dysfunctional grieving related to loss of physiopsychosocial well-being (actual loss of a body part) resulting in distress, sadness, denial, guilt, anger, depression

EXPECTED OUTCOMES

Anxiety and fear within manageable levels, development of coping and problem-solving skills, progressive adaptation to body image and lifestyle changes, initiation of grieving process evidenced by verbalizations that anxiety is decreasing, fear reduced, with willingness to participate in care and social activities, and receptivity to planning for postoperative care

INTERVENTION

I. Assess for:
   A. Apprehension, anxiety level, fear of mutilation and change in body appearance, effect on sexuality and femininity, feelings of inadequacy

   B. Use of coping mechanisms, stated fears of uncertainty of disease outcome, lifestyle changes

   C. Restlessness, diaphoresis, complaining, joking, withdrawal, talkativeness, increased P and R

   D. Personal resources to cope with stress, anxiety, and interest in learning to problem-solve, use of defense mechanisms

RATIONALE

   A. Provides data regarding perceptions about the loss and effects of surgery, anxiety can range from mild to severe and high level associated with loss of body part

   B. Assists in identifying inappropriate and appropriate use of coping skills, ineffective coping leads to depression and other psychosocial disorders

   C. Nonverbal expressions of anxiety when not able to communicate feelings

   D. Support systems and personal strengths assist in developing coping skills

INTERVENTION	RATIONALE
E. Feelings and response to change in role, ability to carry out role and participation in sexual/social activities, fear of stigmatization and rejection	E. Changes in body image and self-concept a common and serious problem with loss/changes in structure and function of a body part
III. Administer:	
A. Anti-anxiety agent PO	A. Acts to reduce anxiety level and provides calming effect and rest, depresses subcortical levels of CNS, limbic system
IV. Perform/provide:	
A. Environment conducive to expression of feelings about changes in body image, sexuality and rejection in private, avoid judgments and negative responses to feelings	A. Provides opportunity to vent feelings and reduce fear and anxiety about loss of body part and feelings of inadequacy in personal relationships
B. Allow time for expression of how loss of a breast affects lives of self and partner, encourage communication with partner in privacy	B. Identifies positive behaviors and time and willingness to adapt to change in appearance and life-style
C. Encourage participation in improving personal appearance, remain to assist with dressing and other personal activities, suggest resources for purchase of prosthesis, clothing, or other personal needs	C. Enhances self-image and esteem, provides alternatives to enhance body image

INTERVENTION	RATIONALE
D. Avoid verbal or nonverbal reactions to surgical site care or other procedures, display of distaste or alarm at surgical site	D. Promotes comfort with nurse–patient relationship
E. Privacy when dressings are changed, advise that feelings about loss of breast is normal, encourage to look at and care for wound at appropriate time	E. Reduces embarrassment caused by exposure of surgical site and use of a prosthesis
F. Inform of phantom pain sensation of missing breast that can be experienced, what activities to expect postoperatively, appearance of the breast reconstruction postoperatively	F. Reduces postoperative anxiety resulting from the unknown consequences of mastectomy/mammoplasty
G. Diversional activities such as relaxation exercises, TV, radio, music, reading, tapes, guided imagery, encourage to continue usual interests	G. Reduces anxiety and promotes comfort
H. Allow to participate in planning of care to maintain usual activities when possible, allow to participate in wound care as soon as possible	H. Allows for some control over situations, self-image can improve with involvement in self-care
I. Support grieving for loss of life-style and restrictions in activities, changes in physical appearance	I. Provides assistance in adaptation to changes imposed by loss of breast

INTERVENTION	RATIONALE
J. Suggest visit from one who has had a mastectomy and has made a successful recovery and rehabilitation, counseling if appropriate	J. Provides support and information from a reliable source

NURSING DIAGNOSES

Fluid volume excess related to compromised regulatory mechanism resulting from node resection causing lymphedema of the arm

Impaired physical mobility of arm on operative side related to pain and discomfort at incisional site, musculoskeletal impairment resulting from removal of pectoral fascia and muscles of more radical mastectomy procedures causing difficulty in performing ADL

Risk for infection related to inadequate primary defenses of node dissection associated with mastectomy or reaction to foreign body with mammoplasty resulting in edema and infection if arm or breast implant is traumatized or skin disrupted by abrasions or breaks

EXPECTED OUTCOMES

Optimal function of arm on operative side and absence of infection evidenced by normal size and shape of arm, full ROM of shoulder function with participation in ADL, and no redness, edema, purulent drainage from breast incisional or reconstructive site

INTERVENTION	RATIONALE
I. Assess for: A. Edema of arm on operative side, feeling of heaviness, loss of sensation, reluctance to attempt movement of arm, limited ROM of arm and shoulder	A. Reveals lymphedema of the arm following surgery caused by removal of axillary nodes and pressure or trauma to nerves from edema or during surgery; lymphedema can occur at a later time following surgery (secondary)

INTERVENTION	RATIONALE
B. Wound site for redness, swelling, warmth, purulent drainage, pain, changes at implant site or edematous arm	B. Indicates infectious process, usually occurs from cuts or trauma to edematous arm
C. Ability and interest in performing ADL especially personal grooming such as combing hair, bathing, brushing teeth, shampooing hair	C. Arm movement can be restricted temporarily for activities that require raising of the arm
II. Monitor, describe, record:	
A. Temperature q4h and PRN	A. Elevations indicate infection
B. WBC	B. Increases indicate infection
III. Administer:	
A. Antibiotic PO	A. Acts to destroy pathogens by inhibiting cell-wall synthesis
B. Analgesic PO, IM	B. Acts to control pain by interfering with CNS pathways, can be administered prior to arm exercises or activities
C. Diuretic PO	C. Acts on distal tubule to increase water excretion if edema becomes chronic
D. Antipyretic PO	D. Acts to reduce temperature if infection present

INTERVENTION	RATIONALE
IV. Perform/provide:	
A. Place in semi-Fowler's position with affected arm elevated on pillow, also place arm on pillow when sitting	A. Dependent arm position encourages fluid retention
B. Ambulate and flex and extend fingers postoperatively q1h and gradually increase to wrist and lower arm	B. Prevents muscle shortening and improves muscle tone, lymph and blood circulation
C. Increase exercises to include rope pulling, hair combing and brushing, turning rope in circle from door knob, finger crawl up wall, abduction and adduction of arm from 1 to 7 days postoperatively	C. Promotes full use of arm following mastectomy
D. ROM to upper arm to shoulder until axillary drain removed, then include abduction and external rotation of the upper arm and shoulder, pendulum swing, overhead pulley suspension, wall climbing exercises	D. Promotes mobility of arm and shoulder
E. Exclude arm from exercises if mammoplasty performed	E. Prevents complications associated with reconstruction to avoid disturbing the implant

INTERVENTION	RATIONALE
F. Assistance with ADL as needed with progressive performance of activities as condition improves	F. Promotes independence in self-care and control over own care
G. Place arm in sling when ambulating	G. Relieves tension on incision
H. Avoid injections, venipunctures, blood pressure taken in affected arm	H. Inhibits collateral lymph drainage and predisposes for infection
I. Physical therapy at 2 to 3 days postoperatively	I. Assists to regain full use of arm and shoulder

NURSING DIAGNOSIS

Risk for impaired skin integrity related to mechanical external factor of pressure of drainage tubes, possible ulceration at surgical site

Risk for injury related to physical internal factors of secretions or fluid accumulation, hematoma formation resulting from impaired wound drainage, deformed breast following mammoplasty resulting from trauma or necrosis at surgical site

EXPECTED OUTCOMES

Adequate wound healing with complications prevented evidenced by surgical drainage system patent with site clean, dry, and free of irritation and breakdown, skin intact at incisional site, absence of hematoma, seroma, or skin flap necrosis, successful results and healing of mammoplasty

INTERVENTION	RATIONALE
I. Assess for:	
A. Bleeding and drainage on dressing, redness, irritation of skin at site	A. Indicates status of wound healing or secretions that predispose to skin irritation and breakdown (dressings in place for 7 to 10 days in mammoplasty when nipple has been grafted to provide compression to the area)
B. Wound drainage, amount, color, consistency in drainage system q8h	B. Ensures drainage patency and progressive healing as drainage decreases or possible seroma or hematoma formation if drainage decreases (drains in place for 2 to 3 days following mammoplasty)
C. Edema, pain, change in color at incisional site, reduced drainage	C. Indicates hematoma formation resulting from trauma of surgery, bleeding from vessels
D. Skin flap that changes color to blue, red, or pallor or darkness, skin cool, foul odor, break in suture line	D. Indicates skin flap necrosis caused by impaired circulation to the wound, can predispose to extrusion of implant in mammoplasty
E. Change in shape of breast, reduced size, sensations or feeling of pressure from tissue expander	E. Indicates complication of tissue expander failure in mammoplasty

INTERVENTION	RATIONALE
IV. Perform/provide:	
A. Place in position of comfort that avoids lying on operative site	A. Prevents unnecessary pressure on wound and obstruction of drainage
B. Dressing changes using sterile technique and supplies, cleanse area around drains carefully and thoroughly, avoid disturbing graft during dressing change	B. Prevents contamination by pathogens
C. Empty drainage collection system noting all characteristics, especially amounts	C. Indicates characteristics of drainage to assess wound healing and absence of complications
D. Anchor drainage tubing at site with nonirritating tape, check for patency of drain, possible kinking of tubing, avoid pull on tube	D. Prevents leakage of secretions that irritate skin
E. Place articles within easy reach	E. Prevents need for reaching if shoulder movement restricted

NURSING DIAGNOSIS

Knowledge deficit related to follow-up care that includes wound, skin, prosthesis care, arm exercise regimen and resumption of activities, care of remaining breast, preparation for chemotherapy/radiation therapy, follow-up monitoring by physician

EXPECTED OUTCOMES

Knowledge and understanding of disease/surgical procedure, progressive grieving, and ongoing care with life-style modifications evidenced by compliance with planned postoperative therapy, proposed changes in activity/social routines and continued participation in arm exercises, verbalization of signs and symptoms to report

INTERVENTION	RATIONALE
I. Assess for:	
A. Readiness, willingness, and motivation to learn, discharge care and lifestyle changes	A. Learning can best take place if client is receptive and compliance is more likely to occur
B. Health practices, health beliefs, value orientations, family and partner interest and cooperation	B. Factors to incorporate into teaching plan to facilitate learning and compliance with care
IV. Perform/provide:	
A. Acknowledgment of perceptions in a nonjudgmental environment	A. Establishes nurse–patient relationship in an accepting environment
B. Explanations that are clear, accurate in understandable terms, small amount of information over time	B. Prevents misconceptions, erroneous attitudes and beliefs about disease
C. As much control over lifestyle change decisions as possible, include partner in discharge planning	C. Allows power to be given or retained by patient and significant others
D. Opportunities for demonstration and return demonstration/practice	D. Reinforces learning and ensures compliance of continued exercising
E. Teaching aids (pamphlets, video tapes, pictures, written instructions)	E. Reinforces learning

INTERVENTION	RATIONALE
F. Include partner in discussions and instructions for care after discharge	F. Allows for support and acceptance by significant other
G. Team of resource personnel/professionals	G. Psychological and sexual counselor, social worker, rehabilitation therapist, and others can assist in care and special needs and provide support for desired changes and adaptation to loss
V. Teach patient/family:	
A. Anatomy, pathophysiology, and progressive nature of the disease, options available for future reconstruction of breast	A. Promotes understanding of disease and options that facilitates compliance
B. Protection of arm from trauma, even if a minor cut or pin prick, and report any injury that causes redness, swelling, pain, purulent drainage, avoid burns from sun or cooking, wear gloves when cleaning or cooking, use an electric razor for legs and underarms	B. Affected arm prone to infection when circulation impaired
C. Inform that lymphedema can persist, elevate arm when sleeping, use elastic pressure gradient sleeve or intermittent pneumatic compression sleeve	C. Chronic condition can be present for lifetime, maintains maximum fluid volume reduction by mobilizing accumulation of fluid and assists in removal of the fluid

INTERVENTION	RATIONALE
D. Apply gentle manual massage around the implant moving it 4 to 6 times/day	D. Assists to maintain mobility of the implant and prevent fibrous capsule formation around implant as a response to the presence of a foreign substance
E. Administration and rationale of all prescribed medications (antibiotics, analgesics, diuretics) postoperatively, written schedule of times and dosages, side effects to expect and report	E. Promotes compliance of complete medication regimen
F. Continue arm and shoulder exercises and ROM daily following mastectomy, avoid exercises following mammoplasty for several weeks, and resume gradually as advised by physician	F. Maintains mobility of affected arm and prevents complications
G. Avoid wearing padded bra following mammoplasty, suggest padding bra following mastectomy and type of loose clothing to wear to obscure edematous arm or flat chest	G. Allows for implant to settle, enhances body image until prosthesis made following mastectomy
H. Handwash and wound care including dressing change, care of drainage system if applicable	H. Prevents transmission of pathogens to wound
I. Massage of healed incision with cocoa butter	I. Maintains softness of skin

INTERVENTION	RATIONALE
J. Inform of possible subsequent chemotherapy or radiation therapy	J. Customary treatments following surgery depending on staging or accepted protocol
K. Consider counseling or stress reduction program to assist in development of coping and problem-solving skills	K. Prevents depression associated with loss of body part
L. Remind of grieving process and time needed for each phase	L. Grieving can be delayed and should be completed for acceptance of loss
M. Resources for permanent prosthesis fitting and purchase	M. Provides information of when and where to obtain appropriate prosthesis
N. Monthly breast self-examination and mammography schedule, allow to practice	N. Ensures health of remaining breast by early detection of abnormality
O. Report temperature elevation, chills, changes in color or appearance of incision or implant, drainage, pain at site, change in ability to move shoulder, stiffness, insensitivity in affected arm to physician	O. Indicates possible complication of surgery for early intervention
P. Contact support groups such as Reach for Recovery of the American Cancer Association for information or educational materials	P. Provides assistance to reduce risk factors and maintain optimal health

orchiectomy

DEFINITION

Orchiectomy is the surgical removal of the testis and attached tunica, spermatic cord, and contents of the inguinal canal. A radical node dis-dection or retroperitonal lymphadenectomy can also be performed fol-lowing radiation for resistant tumor. It is done to diagnose or treat tes-ticular cancer or cryptorchidism. A testicular prosthesis can be inserted to replace the removed testicle. The risk factors associated with testicle malignancy is undescended testicles in children, especially if orchiopexy is not performed early and sons of mothers treated with medication to prevent pregnancy or miscarriage. This plan includes care following surgery and can be used in association with the PREOPERATIVE CARE and POSTOPERATIVE CARE plans

NURSING DIAGNOSES

Anxiety related to threat to self-concept resulting from sexual dysfunction (impotence, infertility, decreased ejaculation with lymphadenectomy), threat to health status if surgery advised (orchiectomy)

Body image disturbance related to biophysical and psychosocial fac-tors of change in body appearance resulting from loss of testis

EXPECTED OUTCOMES

Anxiety within manageable levels and body image improved evidenced by verbalizations that anxiety and fear reduced and a more positive under-standing of changes in sexual activity and sexuality needs

INTERVENTION	RATIONALE
I. Assess for: A. Apprehension, anxiety level, fear of impotency, infertility, effect of loss of ejaculation on sexual satisfaction, feelings about scrotal appearance	A. Provides data regarding perceptions about the effects of surgery
IV. Perform/provide: A. Environment conducive to expression of feelings about sexuality changes	A. Provides opportunity to vent feelings and reduce fear and anxiety about sexual inadequacy in private
B. Inform that erection and orgasm possible, reduced ejaculation only with lymphadenectomy (not always done)	B. Provides answers to concerns and misinformation, ejaculation changes caused by disruption of sympathetic nervous system pathways
C. Inform that a silicone prosthesis can be implanted in scrotum	C. Provides a normal appearance and enhances body image
D. Encourage participation in improving personal appearance, social activities	D. Enhances self-image and esteem

NURSING DIAGNOSIS
Knowledge deficit related to postoperative sexual function, ongoing treatments and preventive care

EXPECTED OUTCOMES
Adequate knowledge provided and understood evidenced by verbalizations and compliance with treatments and care

INTERVENTION	RATIONALE
V. Teach patient/partner:	
A. Inclusion of partner in discussions, encourage communication between patient and partner	A. Provides support and understanding between partners
B. Inform that remaining testis produces testosterone to maintain sexual drive and function	B. Provided by hyperplasia of remaining testis
C. Self-examination of the remaining testis monthly, allow to demonstrate and practice	C. Identifies abnormality of testis
D. Inform of possible need for radiation therapy, chemotherapy	D. Therapy prescribed depending on tumor staging
E. Availability of genetic counseling	E. Helpful in those desiring to have children
F. Report excessive anxiety, depression, sexual difficulties	F. Leads to an appropriate therapy or counseling referral

pelvic inflammatory disease

DEFINITION
Pelvic inflammatory disease (PID) is an infection of the pelvis involving the structure of one or all of the organs (pelvic peritoneum, veins, or connective tissue, uterus, fallopian tubes, and ovaries. It is caused by streptococcus, staphylococcus, gonococcus, chlamydia, or other infectious agents and can occur as the result of abortion, childbirth, sexual intercourse, and use of an intra-uterine device. Complications include abscess, adhesions, or infertility. This plan includes care of the acute infection and prevention of recurrences or transmission.

NURSING DIAGNOSES
Pain related to biologic injury agents of microbiologic invasion of pelvis resulting in infection/inflammation of structures or organs

Hyperthermia related to illness and increased metabolic rate resulting from infectious process

EXPECTED OUTCOMES
Pain and temperature reduced or controlled evidenced by decrease in request of analgesic, absence of restlessness, moaning, anxiety, and temperature within baseline parameters

INTERVENTION	RATIONALE
I. Assess for:	
A. Abdominal pain severity and characteristics, abdominal pressure or fullness, cramping in lower abdomen, spotting between menstrual periods, dyspareunia, purulent and foul-smelling vaginal discharge	A. Source of pain is abdominal and indicates acute PID
B. Dull, aching pain in lower abdomen, backache, menstrual abnormalities	B. Indicates chronic PID
C. Palpable mass in abdomen, pain and tenderness on vaginal examination	C. Indicates PID with fallopian tube or ovary enlargement
D. Nausea, vomiting, diaphoresis, restlessness, grimacing, moaning	D. Symptoms associated with severe pain, nonverbal expression of pain
E. Temperature elevation, chills, malaise, tachycardia	E. Associated with infectious process
II. Monitor, describe, record:	
A. Cultures of discharge	A. Identifies micro-organisms causing the infection and sensitivity to antibiotic therapy
B. VS and temperature q2–4h	B. Responses to severe pain and infection
C. WBC	C. Increased in acute infection

INTERVENTION	RATIONALE
III. Administer:	
A. Analgesic (narcotic) IM, PO	A. Acts to control pain before becoming severe and control gate closes
B. Antipyretic PO	B. Acts to reduce temperature
C. Antimicrobial IV, PO	C. Acts to destroy infectious agent by inhibiting cell-wall synthesis
D. Anti-inflammatory PO	D. Reduces inflammatory process and increases body defenses
IV. Perform/provide:	
A. Evaluation of effect of analgesic 30 minutes, $1\frac{1}{2}$, and 3 hours after administration	A. Determines response and need to repeat, increase, or change medication if pain is extremely severe
B. Dry heat to abdomen PRN, sitz bath if appropriate	B. Relieves pain by vasodilation to increase circulation to the site
C. Place in semi-Fowler's position or position of comfort	C. Promotes dependent drainage of pelvis
D. Encourage and assist in activities according to ability and pain episodes (10 minutes, q2h), and schedule activities 30 minutes following analgesic	D. Provides activity at optimal times to prevent or reduce pain
E. Cleanse perineal area after each elimination	E. Prevents spread of infection and promotes comfort

INTERVENTION	RATIONALE
F. Extra covers for chills, sponge bath if temperature is elevated	F. Provides warmth and reduces temperature
G. Quiet environment with opportunity for relaxation/ breathing techniques, guided imagery	G. Reduces stimuli and pain perception, provides distraction

NURSING DIAGNOSIS

Knowledge deficit related to information regarding prevention of recurrence, transmission of infection

EXPECTED OUTCOMES

Adequate information and increased level of knowledge of disease and care evidenced by verbalizations of measures to take to control or prevent infection and the absence of recurring pelvic infection

INTERVENTION	RATIONALE
V. Teach patient/family:	
A. Pathophysiology of PID, factors that contribute to infection	A. Promotes knowledge and understanding of disease
B. Handwashing technique and proper disposal of pads	B. Prevents transmission of infection
C. Inform sexual partner of infection and need for examination, how organisms are introduced into reproductive tract, use of condoms	C. Prevents transmission to or from partner

INTERVENTION	RATIONALE
D. Hygienic care such as cleansing genitalia with soap and water, wipe from front to back, change pads and tampons frequently	D. Provides measures to prevent infection
E. Importance of periodic examination and physician visits, resumption or restriction of sexual intercourse	E. Provides opportunity for prevention or early treatment of infection
F. Inform of risk for infertility with repeated infections	F. Provides information that appropriate precautions can prevent complications
G. Report vaginal bleeding, discharge characteristics, pain in lower abdomen	G. Provides for early treatment of recurrence

penile implantation

DEFINITION
A penile implantation is the surgical insertion of a penile prosthesis performed to treat erectile dysfunction. It allows for a sustained erect penis for sexual function. The prosthesis can be semi-rigid, consisting of a pair of silicone rods resulting in a permanent semi-erection firm enough to allow for penetration. Another is the self-contained prosthesis consisting of a pump, cylinder, and a bag filled with fluid. The penis can assume a relaxed position until inflated by pumping the fluid from the bag to the shaft creating an erection and then returning the fluid to the bag, again relaxing the penis, by pressing a valve. Impotency can be psychogenic or physical in origin caused by diabetes mellitus, spinal cord trauma, atherosclerosis, radiation therapy, or surgery. This plan includes the surgical care of these procedures and can be used in association with the SPINAL CORD TRAUMA, DIABETES MELLITUS, PREOPERATIVE CARE, and POSTOPERATIVE CARE plans

NURSING DIAGNOSES
Sexual dysfunction related to altered body function (disease process, trauma, surgery, radiation, or psychogenic) preoperatively resulting in impotence

Altered sexuality patterns related to altered structure and function (surgical implantation of penile prosthesis) postoperatively resulting in changes in sexual behaviors and activity

Body image disturbance related to biophysical factor of change in sexual activity, appearance and embarrassment of a permanent semi-erection with semi-rigid prosthesis insertion

EXPECTED OUTCOMES
Resolution of impotence following surgery and progressive adaptation to change in sexual activity and pattern evidenced by verbalizations of feeling of improved sexual performance and relationship with partner with correct use of the implant device, ability to conceal semi-erection

INTERVENTION	RATIONALE
I. Assess for:	
A. Psychological functioning, impotence, feelings about sexual inadequacy, underlying medical conditions	A. Provides data regarding sexual dysfunction and possible cause
B. Feelings associated with implant and change in functioning of penis, sexual expression and satisfaction	B. Reveals effect of implant on body image, self-worth, and sexuality
IV. Perform/provide:	
A. Attentive, nonjudgmental environment to express feelings about the implant	A. Provides opportunity to vent feelings without embarrassment
B. Encourage expression of how implant affects lives of self and partner	B. Identifies positive behaviors and willingness to adapt to change in function
C. Privacy during self-care, offer pajama bottoms to wear	C. Prevents embarrassment of exposure of penile semi-erection
D. Referral to sex therapist or psychologist if appropriate	D. Provides support and counseling to treat psychogenic impotence

NURSING DIAGNOSIS
Knowledge deficit related to follow-up surgical care, operation of prosthesis and resumption of sexual activity

EXPECTED OUTCOMES
Adequate information and understanding of sexual practices with a penile implant evidenced by successful progression to satisfactory sexual experiences

INTERVENTION	RATIONALE
V. Teach patient/partner:	
A. Include partner in instruction and demonstrations	A. Maintains relationship with sexual partner
B. Operation of pump using a model to inflate and deflate the device, allow to practice inflation and deflation of penile device for 4 to 6 weeks	B. Promotes acceptance and satisfactory use of prosthesis, will maintain pump position and promote fibrous tissue growth around implant
C. Amount of pressure to use for inflation	C. Excessive pressure will obstruct fluid flow
D. Inform that adaptation to implant takes time	D. Promotes patience and acceptance of change in function
E. Suggest wearing snug-fitting underwear with penis placed in an upward position on abdomen, loose trousers	E. Assists to conceal semi-rigid prosthesis
F. Advise to begin sexual activity 6 to 8 weeks after surgery with physician's permission, use adequate lubrication	F. Allows for healing and prevents undue trauma to penis after surgery

prostatectomy
(perineal/retropubic/suprapubic/transurethral)

DEFINITION

Prostectomy is the partial or total removal of the prostate gland. Its approach is determined by age, signs and symptoms, size, and location of the enlarged gland or mass. It is done to correct urinary obstruction associated with benign prostatic hypertrophy, chronic urinary retention, chronic urinary tract infections, impaired renal function resulting from chronic urinary obstruction, and prostate malignancy. The perineal procedure is performed to remove the gland mass low in the pelvis via an incision between the anus and scrotum to treat prostatic cancer. Retropubic resection is done to remove the gland via a low abdominal incision without involvement of the bladder to remove a large mass and treat a urethral stricture. Superpubic resection is done to remove a large mass and correct bladder pathology. Transurethral resection (most common approach) is done via a cystoscope inserted through the urethra for partial removal of a moderately hypertrophic gland to treat benign hypertrophic prostate or a small malignant mass that causes compression of the urethra, urethral stricture, or scarring of the bladder neck resulting in chronic urinary problems. A radical prostatectomy includes removal of the gland, seminal vesicles, vas deferens, bladder neck cuff, and lymph nodes via the perineal or retropubic approach to treat prostatic malignancy. Those at risk include men over 50 years of age. This plan includes the surgical care of these procedures and can be used in association with the PREOPERATIVE CARE, POSTOPERATIVE CARE plans, PROSTATIC HYPERTROPHY plan for medical care, and NEOPLASM (INTERNAL/EXTERNAL CHEMOTHERAPY/RADIATION THERAPY) plan

NURSING DIAGNOSES

Anxiety related to threat to or change in health status causing inability to manage feelings of uncertainty and apprehension regarding uncertain prognosis (malignancy), ability to manage urinary/bowel problems (incontinence)

Ineffective individual coping related to inability to cope with change in urinary elimination pattern, change in sexuality pattern/function, and future life-style changes

Body image disturbance related to biophysical factor of change in structure and function of body part (prostatectomy, urinary catheter), embarrassment of effect on sexual performance (sterility, retrograde ejaculation, impotence) resulting from a specific surgical procedure

EXPECTED OUTCOMES

Anxiety and fear within manageable levels, development of coping and problem-solving skills, body image improved evidenced by verbalizations that anxiety is decreasing, fear reduced, participation in care activities and receptive to planning for postoperative care, changes in urinary/bowel elimination and sexual function, and management of chronic anxiety

INTERVENTION	RATIONALE
I. Assess for:	
A. Level of anxiety, use of coping mechanisms, stated fears of uncertainty of disease outcome, life-style changes	A. Anxiety can range from mild to severe and high level associated with diagnosis of malignancy; assists in identifying inappropriate use of coping skills
B. Restlessness, diaphoresis, complaining, joking, withdrawal, talkativeness, increased P and R	B. Nonverbal expressions of anxiety when not able to communicate feelings
C. Personal resources to cope with stress, anxiety, and interest in learning to problem-solve, use of defense mechanisms	C. Support systems and personal strengths assist to develop coping skills

INTERVENTION	RATIONALE
D. Feelings and response to change in role and ability to carry out role, participate in care/activities, fears expressed of sexual inadequacy (impotence, sterility)	D. Changes in body image and self-concept a common and serious problem with changes in structure and function of a body organ
E. Negative expressions about the changes in lifestyle, feelings, or preoccupation with the change	E. Responses to anticipated changes (negative or positive)

III. Administer:

A. Anti-anxiety agent PO	A. Acts to reduce anxiety level and provides calming effect and rest, depresses subcortical levels of CNS, limbic system

IV. Perform/provide:

A. Environment conducive to rest, time to express fears and anxiety, avoid anxiety-producing situations	A. Decreases stimuli that cause stress/anxiety, venting of feelings decreases anxiety
B. Suggest new methods to enhance coping skills and problem solving, allow to externalize and identify those that help	B. Offers alternative coping strategies that allow for release of anxiety and fear
C. Positive feedback regarding progress made, focus on abilities rather than inabilities	C. Provides support for adaptive behavior, promotes self-worth and responsibility

INTERVENTION	RATIONALE
D. Avoid verbal or nonverbal reactions to expressions of concerns	D. Promotes comfort with nurse–patient relationship
E. Privacy when dressings or catheter care is provided, advise that feelings are normal	E. Reduces embarrassment caused by exposure of surgical/catheter site
F. Diversional activities such as relaxation exercises, TV, radio, music, reading, tapes, guided imagery, encourage to continue usual interests	F. Reduces anxiety and promotes comfort
G. Allow to participate in planning of care to maintain usual activities when possible	G. Allows for some control over situations
H. Inform of what to expect following surgery regarding catheters, incontinence, sexual changes, and when improvements can be expected, include significant other in discussion of concerns	H. Reduces self-doubts and concerns about functional status and relationship with partner

NURSING DIAGNOSIS

Pain related to biologic injury agents of trauma of surgery resulting in bladder spasms, irritation of bladder distention by catheter and bladder irrigation; stress on incision caused by pressure or straining

EXPECTED OUTCOMES

Pain reduced or controlled evidenced by decrease in request for analgesic, absence of restlessness, moaning, anxiety, and catheter obstruction

INTERVENTION	RATIONALE
I. Assess for:	
A. Sharp, intermittent suprapubic pain, leakage of urine around catheter, bladder distention palpated, rate of bladder irrigation	A. Indicates bladder spasms or urinary retention causing pain, rapid infusion of continuous irrigation causes spasms
B. Catheter patency, tension on catheter	B. Indicates possible obstruction from blood clots, pulling or traction on the catheter causes pain from pressure on the bladder neck
C. Pain and characteristics at incisional site	C. Indicates pain caused by surgical trauma to tissue, can be increased by movement, exertion during bowel elimination, pressure from sitting on perineal incision
D. Restlessness, grimacing, moaning, withdrawal	D. Symptoms associated with pain, nonverbal expression of pain
III. Administer:	
A. Analgesic IM, PO	A. Acts to control pain before becoming severe and control gate closing
B. Antispasmodic PO, SUP	B. Acts to increase bladder capacity in presence of spasms by action on detrusor muscle, relieves suprapubic pain

INTERVENTION	RATIONALE
IV. Perform/provide:	
A. Place in semi-Fowler's position or position of comfort, pillow to sit on	A. Promotes comfort to incisional site by reducing pressure at area
B. Evaluation of effect of analgesic 30 minutes, $1\frac{1}{2}$, and 3 hours after administration	B. Determines response and need to repeat, increase, or change medication if pain not managed
C. Sitz bath following removal of catheter and/or drains	C. Relieves pain by vasodilation to increase circulation to the site
D. Encourage and assist in activities according to ability and pain acuity and schedule activities 30 minutes following analgesic	D. Provides activity at optimal times to prevent or reduce pain
E. Irrigate to remove clots, maintain continuous irrigation rate, or reduce if return is not red	E. Irrigations irritate bladder and rapid infusion causes spasms, obstructed irrigation system causes distention and pain
F. Reduce catheter traction when appropriate	F. Reduces pressure on neck of bladder
G. Avoid kinking, twisting, or pulling on catheter, tape to leg or abdomen	G. Prevents irritation to bladder mucosa and tension or pull on catheter causing pain
H. Quiet environment with opportunity for relaxation/breathing techniques, guided imagery	H. Reduces stimuli and pain perception, provides distraction

NURSING DIAGNOSES

Sexual dysfunction related to altered body function (disease process, trauma of surgery) resulting in impotence (perineal resection), sterility, temporary retrograde ejaculation

Altered sexuality patterns related to altered structure and function resulting in changes in sexual behaviors and activity (reduced libido), difficulty in adapting to changes in sexuality

EXPECTED OUTCOMES

Resolution of and progressive adaptation to change in sexual activity and pattern evidenced by verbalizations of feeling of improved sexual performance and relationship with partner, correction of dysfunction and sexual satisfaction achieved

INTERVENTION	RATIONALE
I. Assess for: A. Surgical procedure, impotence, erectile dysfunction or absence of erection, sterility, decreased libido, feelings about sexual inadequacy	A. Provides data regarding sexual dysfunction and possible cause, transurethral approach does not usually result in sexual dysfunction; dysfunction is result of damaged parasympathetic nerves or removal of parts in more radical surgical procedures
B. Feelings associated with change in relationship with partner, sexual expression and satisfaction	B. Reveals effect of surgery on body image, self-worth, and sexuality
IV. Perform/provide: A. Attentive, nonjudgmental environment to express feelings about the sexuality concerns	A. Provides opportunity to vent feelings without embarrassment

INTERVENTION	RATIONALE
B. Encourage expression of how sexuality changes affects lives of self and partner	B. Identifies positive behaviors and willingness to adapt to change in function
C. Privacy during self-care, offer pajama bottoms to wear	C. Prevents embarrassment of exposure of catheter and drainage system
D. Alternate expression of sexuality such as massage, use of assistive aids, possible penile implant	D. Allows for sexual relations if impotence exists
E. Alternate positions to use when intercourse allowed and inform that comfort increases as healing progresses (usually 6–8 weeks)	E. Prevents pressure on surgical site
F. Retrograde ejaculation occurs during orgasm with semen discharged into the bladder, urine will be cloudy after intercourse temporarily	F. Results from trauma to the internal sphincter and semen passes into the bladder rather than the urethra
G. Referral to sex therapist or psychologist if appropriate	G. Provides support and counseling to treat psychogenic impotence

NURSING DIAGNOSES

Altered urinary elimination related to mechanical trauma of surgery resulting in edema, indwelling catheter to ensure bladder emptying resulting in irritation of surrounding tissues, possible obstruction causing retention, distention and discomfort; removal of catheter resulting in urinary retention, incontinence, dribbling

  Risk for infection related to inadequate primary defenses (stasis of urine) resulting from retention and inability to completely empty bladder, invasive procedure of superpubic drains placement, indwelling catheter placement and irrigations

Hyperthermia related to illness and increased metabolic rate resulting from infectious process (urinary bladder)

EXPECTED OUTCOMES
Optimal voiding elimination pattern with continence established and absence of infection following catheter removal evidenced by resumption of voiding of adequate amounts without difficulty and absence of retention and residual urine, cloudy, foul-smelling urine, temperature elevation

INTERVENTION	RATIONALE
I. Assess for:	
A. Urine color, odor, amount with indwelling catheter in place, catheter patency with absence of urine in tubing, low output, bladder fullness or distention, cloudy, foul-smelling urine	A. Indwelling catheter usually in place postoperatively for about 3 days until edema subsides
B. Redness, edema, pain, purulent drainage from wound, breaks or irritation around suprapubic catheter	B. Indicates infection at incision and catheter insertion site
C. Retention, bladder distention, frequency, incontinence, inability to control dribbling, cloudy, foul-smelling urine following catheter removal	C. Indicates need for urinary rehabilitation following removal of catheter caused by effect of surgery on sphincter muscle tone; symptoms following catheter removal indicate retention or urinary tract infection
D. Temperature elevation, chills, malaise, tachycardia	D. Associated with infectious process

INTERVENTION	RATIONALE
II. Monitor, describe, record: A. Temperature q4h (oral)	A. Elevation indicates infection
B. Urine or wound culture	B. Positive culture indicates infection
C. WBC	C. Increases indicate infection
III. Administer: A. Antimicrobial PO	A. Acts to destroy pathogens by inhibiting cell-wall synthesis
B. Antipyretic PO	B. Acts to reduce temperature if needed
IV. Perform/provide: A. Place on bed rest in semi-Fowler's position	A. Promotes comfort and return of continuous irrigation fluid by gravity
B. Catheter care TID	B. Prevents movement of pathogens up catheter into the bladder
C. Maintain patent catheter drainage system, with NS if blocked, place collection bag below bladder level, avoid kinking of tubing, maintain closed system, tape securely to prevent movement	C. Prevents urinary retention and backflow of urine leading to discomfort and urinary bladder infection
D. Perineal care BID and following urination and defecation	D. Cleanses site and prevents possible contamination from close proximity to anus

INTERVENTION	RATIONALE
E. Dressing change and wound care using sterile technique and supplies	E. Prevents transmission of pathogens to wound
F. Fluid intake of 2 to 3 L/day	F. Promotes return to baseline urinary elimination and dilutes urine to prevent stasis leading to infection
G. Extra covers for chills, sponge bath if temperature elevated	G. Provides warmth and reduces temperature
H. Place urinal within easy reach or offer to assist to bathroom q2h	H. Promotes return to baseline pattern following catheter removal
I. Techniques such as running warm water over perineum, running tap water, submerging of hands in a pan of water, allowing to stand to void	I. Encourages urination after catheter removal
J. Catheterize for retention if symptoms appear (frequency) following voiding and reinsert indwelling catheter if residual continues or is more than 50 mL	J. Prevents stasis of urine leading to urinary infection
K. External catheter device with closed drainage system	K. Provides method to use instead of indwelling catheter for incontinence

NURSING DIAGNOSIS

Knowledge deficit related to follow-up care that includes resumption of activities, urinary catheter and drainage system care or management of incontinence

EXPECTED OUTCOMES

Knowledge and understanding of disease/surgical procedure, and ongoing care with life-style modifications evidenced by verbalizations of understanding and compliance with proposed daily activities and participation in bladder control rehabilitation

INTERVENTION	RATIONALE
I. Assess for: A. Readiness, willingness, and motivation to learn, discharge care and life-style changes	A. Learning can best take place if client is receptive and compliance is more likely to occur
B. Health practices, health beliefs, value orientations, age	B. Factors to incorporate into teaching plan to facilitate learning and compliance with care
IV. Perform/provide: A. Acknowledgment of perceptions in a nonjudgmental environment	A. Establishes nurse–patient relationship in an accepting environment
B. Explanations that are clear, accurate in understandable terms, small amount of information over time	B. Prevents misconceptions, erroneous attitudes and beliefs about disease
C. As much control over life-style change decisions as possible, include partner in discussions and discharge planning	C. Allows power to be given or retained by patient and reinforces relationship with significant other
D. Teaching aids (pamphlets, video tapes, pictures, written instructions)	D. Reinforces learning

INTERVENTION	RATIONALE
E. Team of resource personnel/professionals	E. Social worker, sexual counselor, urinary rehabilitation therapist, and others can assist in teaching specific care and providing support for desired changes

V. Teach patient/family:

INTERVENTION	RATIONALE
A. Anatomy, function of the prostate, pathophysiology, and nature of the disease, age-related factors causing signs and symptoms	A. Promotes understanding of disease that facilitates compliance
B. Accurate information about effect of procedure on sexual function and suggested temporary remedies	B. Prevents misinformation causing unnecessary fear and anxiety
C. Handwash and care of wound and catheter/closed drainage system if in place	C. Prevents transmission of pathogens that cause infection
D. Administration and rationale of all prescribed medications (antimicrobials, antispasmotics, urinary antiseptics), written schedule of times and dosages, side effects to expect and to report	D. Promotes compliance of complete medication regimen
E. Fluid intake of 10 to 12 glasses/day, but avoid drinking prior to bedtime and going out, high-fiber diet if constipated	E. Maintains daily fluid needs and return to urinary elimination pattern and prevents straining caused by constipation

INTERVENTION	RATIONALE
F. Use protective pads, waterproof undergarment, external device when leaving home	F. Prevents embarrassment of dribbling or incontinence during socialization
G. Perineal exercises 10 to 20 times q2h, practice starting and stopping during voiding	G. Strengthens sphincter muscle tone and improves urinary control
H. Limit strenuous activity for 4 to 6 weeks such as lifting heavy objects, prolonged walking or sitting, sexual intercourse	H. Prevents postoperative complication (formation of clot)
I. Take steps to arrange for urinary retraining program if ordered or provide written instructions to prevent incontinence (urinate q2–3h, void when urge is felt, distribute fluid intake to accommodate daily routine, stand to void until bladder completely empty, avoid alcohol and caffeine-containing beverages)	I. Supports attempts to maintain continence
J. Report temperature elevation, chills, continued loss of bladder control or distention, blood in urine, other complaints to physician	J. Indicates possible complication of urinary elimination
K. Maintain schedule for physician appointments, screening tests for prostate disease	K. Allows for ongoing monitoring of surgery and general health

prostatic hypertrophy

DEFINITION

Benign prostatic hypertrophy (BPH) is the enlargement of the prostate gland common in men over 50 years of age. The greatest risk factor is age with possible causes believed to include diet, heredity, hormone changes (androgen). The gland gradually enlarges by the growth of normal cells causing hyperplasia that compresses the urethra at the neck of the bladder resulting in the obstruction of urinary flow. Although other complications can develop, this is the most common one. This plan includes care of this condition and can be used in association with PROSTATECTOMY care plan

NURSING DIAGNOSES

Anxiety related to threat to self-concept resulting from urgency and dribbling causing inability to prevent incontinence, threat to health status if surgery advised (prostatectomy)

Body image disturbance related to biophysical and psychosocial factors of embarrassment of possible incontinence at inopportune times resulting from change in urinary function and pattern

EXPECTED OUTCOMES

Anxiety within manageable levels and body image improved evidenced by verbalizations the voiding pattern established with minimal urgency and absence of dribbing or incontinence

INTERVENTION	RATIONALE
I. Assess for: A. Concerns of inability to control voiding pattern, fear of socializing outside of home, sexual change	A. Promotes expression of feelings about urine loss causing embarrassment

INTERVENTION	RATIONALE
B. Anxiety level and effect on daily life and control of urination	B. Anxiety can range from mild to severe and can occur if not near a bathroom when needed
IV. Perform/provide:	
A. Explanations of cause of urgency and dribbing	A. Reduces anxiety level
B. Wear protective garment if leaving home	B. Prevents soiling clothing if unable to hold urine or not sure of opportunity to reach bathroom
C. Advise fluid schedule of 100 mL q2–3h if concerned about urgency	C. Prevents excessive filling of bladder
D. Void before leaving home	D. Prevents need to void while enroute
E. Allow time to void and continue until bladder empty even if stream is slow and dribbling	E. Prevents residual and bladder filling in short time

NURSING DIAGNOSES

Urinary retention related to blockage resulting from pressure of enlarged prostate gland on urethra, development of bladder diverticula causing incomplete emptying of the bladder

Altered urinary elimination related to mechanical trauma of obstructive process resulting in retention, frequency, urgency, incontinence

Urge incontinence related to overdistention of bladder resulting from decreased bladder capacity as prostate enlarges

Risk for infection related to inadequate primary defenses (stasis of urine) resulting from retention and inability to completely empty bladder

EXPECTED OUTCOMES

Optimal urinary elimination and absence of urinary bladder infection evidenced by absence of symptoms of urinary obstruction and signs and symptoms of infection

INTERVENTION	RATIONALE
I. Assess for:	
A. Urinary frequency, urgency, hesitancy in starting urination, dribbling, voiding in small amounts (less than 100 mL), nocturia, incontinence or inability to reach toilet in time with an accidental loss of urine	A. Symptoms of urinary obstruction and retention associated with prostatic hypertrophy
B. Bladder distention, residual urine, absence of voiding, feeling of bladder fullness and discomfort	B. Indicates urinary retention
C. Frequency, urgency, burning on urination, hematuria, cloudy, foul-smelling urine, presence of catheter	C. Indicates urinary bladder infection resulting from urinary stasis (residual)
II. Monitor, describe, record:	
A. Urinalysis and culture	A. Culture results of bacterial count of >100,000/mL indicates infection, an increase in RBC and WBC in urinalysis indicates abnormality
B. CBC, BUN, electrolytes, creatinine	B. Reveals compromised renal function or excessive bleeding
C. Cystoscopy, intravenous pyelography (IVP)	C. Reveals renal function, structure and function of ureters and bladder

INTERVENTION	RATIONALE
D. Urethral pressue profile	D. Reveals obstruction
III. Administer: A. Antimicrobial PO	A. Destroys pathogens by inhibiting cell-wall synthesis or interfering with biosynthesis of proteins
IV. Perform/provide: A. Restrict large amounts of fluid at bedtime or rapid intake of fluids	A. Prevents nocturia, possible overdistention, incontinence, or urinary retention
B. Encourage 2 to 3 L/day fluid intake if allowed, spread over the 24 hours in small amounts	B. Dilutes urine and prevents infection
C. Privacy, access to toilet	C. Prevents embarrassment and possible urge incontinence
D. Hot sitz bath	D. Relieves symptoms
E. Catheterize as appropriate if unable to determine residual urine following voiding or if patient is unable to void	E. Relieves overdistention and restores urinary flow
F. Prepare for surgical procedure for partial or total removal of prostate gland	F. Relieves obstruction of urinary flow

NURSING DIAGNOSIS

Knowledge deficit related to measures for prevention of physical and psychological discomfort and promotion of optimal urinary elimination

EXPECTED OUTCOMES
Optimal urinary elimination without complications evidenced by times and amounts of elimination pattern within baseline determinations, absence of incontinence and urinary bladder infection

INTERVENTION	RATIONALE
V. Teach patient/family:	
A. Advise to void as soon as urge is felt	A. Prevents loss of bladder tone if bladder is distended
B. Carefully avoid drinking large amounts of water at one time	B. Results in rapid distention of bladder causing retention
C. Avoid alcoholic drinks	C. Results in acute urinary retention as it has a diuretic effect
D. Follow instructions given for access to bathroom, wearing protective garments or pads	D. Prevents accidental loss of urine and embarrassment
E. Avoid over-the-counter cold medications (sympathomimetics)	E. Tends to affect hypertrophic prostate
F. Report hematuria, anuria, dysuria, cloudy, foul-smelling urine	F. Indicates infection, rupture of blood vessels stretched by bladder overdistension

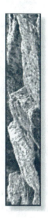

Ophthalmologic/Otologic Systems Standards

ophthalmologic/otologic systems data base

HISTORICAL DATA REVIEW
Past events:
1. Acute and/or chronic ophthalmologic/otologic disease or disorders, presence of other diseases that affect these systems (diabetes, thyroid disorders, infectious process, hypertension)
2. Chronic signs and symptoms related to eye or ear disorders (pain, headache, multiple colds, drainage, swelling, redness, changes in visual or auditory perception or refractive disorders)
3. Diabetes, retinoblastoma, retinitis pigmentosa of family members
4. Childhood disorders (strabismus, eye trauma, chronic otitis media or sinusitis), immunizations for measles, mumps, influenza
5. Allergies that affect eyes or ears (chemicals, dust, pollens, cosmetics)
6. Occupational/environmental, leisure activities and hobbies with hazardous exposure to eyes or ears and use of safety goggles, sunglasses, protective eargear
7. Medications (prescription and over-the-counter) for eye or ear conditions, medications taken with ototoxic effects
8. Hospitalization and feelings about care, surgery associated with eye(s) or ear(s) structure or function

Present events:
1. Medical diagnoses associated with or affecting ophthalmologic/otologic function
2. Known or suspected eye disorders (cataracts, glaucoma, color visual deficits, retinal detachment, macular degeneration, congenital disorders, infection, visual deficits/presbyopia and corrective lenses [eyeglasses or contact lenses])
3. Eye changes (floaters, double vision, flashing lights, redness, pain, photophobia, burning, scratchy feeling, dryness, tearing, drainage)
4. Known or suspected ear disorders (infection, vestibular disorder, con-

ductive or sensorineural hearing loss/presbycusis and corrective device [in the ear or canal, post-auricular, on eyeglasses, or implanted])
5. Ear changes (pain, drainage, tinnitus, vertigo, balance, equilibrium)
6. Activities of daily living (self-care) affected by visual or auditory deficits, effect on self-esteem, ongoing treatment regimens

PHYSICAL ASSESSMENT DATA REVIEW

1. Symmetry, alignment, and movement of eyes, eyelids, eyebrows, eyelashes; symmetry, alignment, size of external ears and pinna
2. Eye conjunctiva, sclera, cornea color, texture, surface irregularities, edema, lesions, dryness or moistness, lacrimal gland color, and edema; ear skin color, smoothness, deformity, masses, lesions
3. Iris and pupil color, roundness, equal reaction to light and accommodation (PERRLA), ocular movements, ocular muscle movements, visual acuity (Snellen), peripheral vision, intra-ocular fluid pressure
4. Ophthalmoscopic examination of eyes for red reflex, optic disc, retinal veins and arteries
5. Ear canals for color, edema, drainage, cerumen, foreign objects, auditory acuity, conductive hearing loss, vestibular acuity
6. Otoscopic examination for eardrum color, bulging, retraction, perforation

NURSING DIAGNOSES CONSIDERATIONS

1. Anxiety
2. Diversional activity deficit
3. Risk for infection
4. Risk for trauma
5. Knowledge deficit
6. Self-care deficits
7. Self-esteem disturbance
8. Sensory/perceptual alterations (visual, auditory)
9. Social isolation

GERIATRIC CONSIDERATIONS

Visual and auditory changes in geriatric patients depend on the effects of the aging process and disorders of other systems on sensory structure and function that result in perceptual abnormalities. Ophthalmologic and otologic changes associated with aging that should be considered when assessing the geriatric patient include:

1. Reduced fat around eye resulting in the globe sinking deeper into socket and thinning and wrinkling of lids
2. Tympanic membrane sclerosis or atrophy, increased rigidity of middle ear bones resulting in difficulty in hearing high-frequency sounds, hearing if noise is present, sound distortion, and phonetic regression; cerumen contains more keratin and becomes harder and more easily impacted
3. Decreased size and responsiveness to light intensities of the pupils resulting in difficulty in seeing at night or slower adaptation to the dark, constriction response becomes slightly delayed
4. Decreased sensitivity of cones in retina resulting in difficulty in color discrimination and a blending of colors at opposite ends of the color spectrum
5. Decreased lacrimal gland secretion resulting in conjunctiva becoming dry and lacking luster with tiny vessels visible
6. Sclera yellowish with pigmented deposits, cornea becomes less translucent and more spherical, can develop white-yellow deposits at periphery
7. Decreased elasticity of lens and more opacity resulting in cataract formation, reduced focus and accommodation, loss of peripheral vision, decreased tolerance to glare and night vision, decreased ability to differentiate visual detail and colors
8. Anterior chamber becomes shallower, yellowish plaques appear near inner canthus

DIAGNOSTIC LABORATORY TESTS AND PROCEDURES

1. Skull x ray, magnetic resonance imaging (MRI), computerized tomography (CT), ultrasonography, visual evoked response, electroretinography, exophthalmometry, fluorescein angiography, visual and auditory acuity tests, visual field tests, tonometry, slit lamp examination, refraction, vestibular tests, electronystagmography, otoscopy, ophthalmoscopy
2. Culture of fluids from eye or ear, smears and laboratory examination, tissue biopsy

MEDICATIONS

1. Anticarbonic anhydrases: acetazolamide
2. Anticholinesterase agents: isofluophate, demecarium bromide
3. Antihistamines: diphenhydramine
4. Antimicrobials: penicillins, cephalosporins, optic or ophthalmic topical antibiotics
5. Antivertigo agents: diazepam, antivert
6. Beta-blockers/alpha-adrenergics: timolol maleate, epinephrine
7. Corticosteroids: ophthalmic prednisolone
8. Miotics: pilocarpine hydrochloride, carbachol
9. Mydriatics: phenylephrine hydrochloride, cyclopentolate hydrochloride

cataract/intra-ocular lens insertion

DEFINITION
Cataract formation is the development of opacity of the lens. It is most commonly caused by aging but can also result from disorders such as diabetes mellitus, neurodermatitis, galactosemia, Down syndrome, or in association with ocular disorders such as retinitis, retinal detachment, iridocyclitis. Other causes include corticosteroid therapy, trauma, infrared light, radiation, and infectious conditions such as measles, mumps, chickenpox, or hepatitis. The formation of cataracts occurs over time beginning with opacity that allows for some light to enter (immature) and ending with complete opacity (mature) that reduces vision to a blur or complete obliteration of objects. The surgical procedure includes the extraction of the lens and a portion of the lens capsule by emulsification and then suctioning to remove the lens material. This is followed by the insertion of a new lens into the posterior chamber. This plan includes care for the visually impaired and, if surgery is performed, can also be used in association with the PREOPERATIVE CARE and POSTOPERATIVE CARE plans

NURSING DIAGNOSES
Sensory/perceptual alterations (visual) related to altered status of sense organs (cataracts) causing anxiety, progressively reduced visual reception

Sensory/perceptual alterations (visual) related to altered status of sense organ (eye) postoperatively resulting from eye dressing or use of protective cover over operative eye

EXPECTED OUTCOMES
Optimal visual acuity maintained with eyeglasses preoperatively and improved visual acuity postoperatively evidenced by adaptation to correction resulting in normal or near normal vision

INTERVENTION	RATIONALE
I. Assess for:	
A. Visual acuity testing, blurred vision, photophobia, aversion to glare, diplopia, distortion of red reflex by ophthalmoscopy	A. Signs and symptoms of cataracts determined primarily by ongoing periodic visual acuity testing
B. Ability to perform ADL based on visual perception, reading, driving, and other visual limitations	B. Visual changes cause difficulty in performing daily routine activities
C. Perception of quality of vision and effect on life-style	C. Determining factor for consideration of cataract surgery
D. Dressing dry, secure, and in place	D. Protects eye postoperatively from trauma or contamination
II. Administer:	
A. Mydriatic TOP eye drops	A. Acts to dilate pupils by contracting eye muscles or iris preoperatively to facilitate surgery
B. Cycloplegic TOP eye drops	B. Acts to paralyze ciliary muscles preoperatively
C. Antibiotic TOP eye drops or ointment	C. Acts to prevent infection of the eye postoperatively
D. Anti-inflammatory TOP eye drops	D. Acts to reduce inflammation postoperatively
E. Analgesic PO, TOP eye drops	E. Acts to control postoperative eye pain

INTERVENTION	RATIONALE
IV. Perform/provide:	
A. Safe environment with orientation to furniture placement, articles in convenient places, no bright lights or glare	A. Prevents bumping into objects or falling causing injury
B. Glasses with periodic changes based on physician testing of visual acuity and slit lamp examination	B. Facilitates vision during cataract formation and postoperatively
C. Eye dressing usually removed the next day by physician	C. Provides immediate protection to the operative eye with temporary obstruction of vision
D. Use of metal shield during sleep and prevents activities such as rubbing eye	D. Protects operative eye from accidental trauma

NURSING DIAGNOSIS
Knowledge deficit related to discharge care including, eye care, eye medications, activities, and follow-up appointments with physician for monitoring of healing, visual acuity, and change in corrective glasses

EXPECTED OUTCOMES
Compliance with postoperative follow-up care evidenced by compliance with prescribed regimen and adaptation to corrections in vision

INTERVENTION	RATIONALE
V. Teach patient/family:	
A. Administration of eye medications orally or by eye drops or ointment instillation procedure using sterile technique and allow to return demonstration, frequency and amount, length of time to apply medications	A. Enhances healing and prevents complications of infection, edema, and increased intraocular pressure
B. Inform to use protective covering and how to tape it in place, when to use it	B. Prevents accidental trauma to eye
C. Avoid bumping the eye, lifting heavy objects and straining, and sleeping on the operative side	C. Measures to prevent trauma to eye
D. Report itching, unrelieved pain to physician	D. Pain can indicate increased intraocular pressure
E. Keep appointments with physician, usually 2 consecutive days following surgery, 1 week and then 1 month, and 6 to 12 months thereafter	E. Monitors healing process, changes of dressing, acuity testing and changes in visual correction that varies with each patient

corneal disorders/keratoplasty

DEFINITION

Corneal disorders include dystrophies affecting all layers, keratitis affecting the epithelium that can develop into infections and ulcerations, and keratonconus affecting the shape. All can be successfully treated with corneal transplantation or keratoplasty. The procedure involves the surgical removal of the cornea and transplantation of a donor cornea. Type of corneal grafts include penetrating, lamellar, and keyhole lamellar. This plan includes care for disorders affecting the cornea and, if surgery is performed, can also be used in association with the PREOPERATIVE CARE and POSTOPERATIVE CARE plans

NURSING DIAGNOSES

Anxiety related to threat to health status resulting from changes in visual acuity preoperatively and possible loss of vision or transplant rejection postoperatively

Sensory/perceptual alterations (visual) related to altered status of sense organs resulting from corneal dysfunction preoperatively and trauma and treatment of surgery postoperatively causing altered visual reception and transmission, anxiety, and possible falls (covering over operative eye)

EXPECTED OUTCOMES

Optimal visual acuity maintained preoperatively and improved visual acuity postoperatively evidenced by adaptation to corneal transplant and absence of failure of the graft, injury or trauma to the operative eye

INTERVENTION	RATIONALE
I. Assess for:	
A. Level of anxiety, feelings about expectations of transplant	A. Moderate levels of anxiety expected preoperatively, can reach high levels as vision fails and patient waits for weeks or months for donor tissue to become available for transplant
B. Visual acuity, blurred vision, photophobia, tearing, dry eyes, cloudy appearance and edema of eye	B. Signs and symptoms of corneal disorders resulting in varying degrees of visual failure and monitored by ongoing periodic visual acuity testing and eye examinations
C. Ability to perform ADL based on visual perception, reading, driving, and other visual limitations	C. Visual changes cause difficulty in performing daily routine activities
D. Perception of quality of vision and effect on life-style	D. Determining factor for consideration of corneal surgery
E. Dressing dry, secure, and in place, presence of drainage	E. Protects eye postoperatively from trauma or contamination
II. Monitor, describe, record:	
A. Slit lamp examination	A. Performed by physician to view corneal damage
B. Fluorescein stain	B. Reveals corneal surface defects

IV. Perform/provide:

INTERVENTION	RATIONALE
A. Quiet, supportive environment and answer any questions honestly and clearly, clarify information as needed	A. Reduces anxiety and fear of unknown, promotes relaxation
B. Orient to surroundings and place articles within reach, assist with care or other needs	B. Provides support when vision impaired
C. Safe environment with strategic furniture placement in convenient places, absence of clutter, throw rugs, daylight or additional lighting in areas as needed, clear pathways, rails and other assists to ambulate and use stairs	C. Prevents bumping into objects or falling
D. Aids such as large-numbered telephones, large-lettered books and newspapers	D. Enhances reading and provides diversional activity and contact with the community
E. Eye dressing usually removed the next day by the physician	E. Immediate protection to operative eye
F. Use of metal shield during sleep or prevent activities such as rubbing eye	F. Protects operative eye from accidental trauma

NURSING DIAGNOSES

Pain related to physical injuring agent of surgical procedure (keratoplasty), biological injuring agent of infectious process (keratitis)

Risk for infection related to inadequate primary defenses resulting from cornea surgery, compromised cornea barrier resulting from disease or trauma

EXPECTED OUTCOMES
Pain reduced or controlled evidenced by verbalizations that discomfort relieved by analgesics, absence of infectious process evidenced by a clean wound free from edema, irritation, and drainage

INTERVENTION	RATIONALE
I. Assess for: A. Pain severity, duration, with eye movement, dry eyes, inability to close eyelids, scratchiness in eye, purulent drainage	A. Associated with eye infection or a predisposition to infection
B. Pain severity, if unrelieved by analgesics, redness, edema, changes in vision postoperatively	B. Associated with corneal transplant that can indicate infection, increasing intraocular pressure, or graft rejection
III. Administer: A. Antibiotic TOP eye drops or ointment	A. Acts to prevent or treat infection of the eye pre- or postoperatively by preventing cell wall synthesis causing destruction of micro-organisms
B. Anti-inflammatory TOP eye drops	B. Acts to reduce inflammation postoperatively
C. Analgesic PO, TOP eye drops	C. Acts to control postoperative eye pain or pain resulting from keratitis
D. Mydriatic TOP eye drops	D. Acts to decrease spasms of ciliary body to reduce pain

INTERVENTION	RATIONALE
IV. Perform/provide:	
A. Warm or cool compress to eye	A. Reduces lid and conjunctival edema and removes secretions
B. Cleanse around eye with warm water and soft gauze pad	B. Removes excessive tearing that can dry and result in lids sticking together
C. Eye shield over operative eye	C. Prevents accidental rubbing or bumping of eye causing injury and pain
D. Sterile technique for all dressing changes, administration of eye medications	D. Prevents transmission of pathogens to eye
E. Schedule eye drop administration to allow for rest periods	E. Promotes uninterrupted rest and sleep when medications administered frequently

NURSING DIAGNOSES

Knowledge deficit related to discharge care including, eye care, eye medications, activities, signs and symptoms to report, and follow-up appointments with physician for monitoring of healing and visual acuity

EXPECTED OUTCOMES

Compliance with postoperative follow-up care evidenced by compliance with prescribed regimen and verbalization of visual or other changes to assess and report indicating complications

INTERVENTION	RATIONALE
V. Teach patient/family:	
A. Administration of eye medications by eye drops or ointment instillation procedure using sterile technique, allow to return demonstration, frequency and amount, length of time to apply medications	A. Enhances healing and prevents complications of infection, edema
B. Inform to use protective covering and how to tape it in place, when to use it, wear glasses or sunglasses for eye protection	B. Prevents accidental trauma to eye, usually used for 1 month following surgery
C. Avoid bumping the eye, lifting heavy objects and straining, and sleeping on the operative side, rubbing eye or squeezing eyelids	C. Measures to prevent trauma to eye
D. Cleanse eye area with warm water and wash cloth	D. Promotes cleanliness and removes any dried secretions
E. Report unrelieved pain, redness, edema, decrease in visual acuity	E. Indicates increased intraocular pressure, graft rejection
F. Assess vision daily using a familiar object to view and report any decrease in visual perception of object	F. Allows for evaluation of changes in vision following corneal transplant

INTERVENTION	RATIONALE
G. Inform that sutures remain in place for 6 months or longer, that improved vision can be experienced immediately with gradual improvement as healing continues, and that glasses or contact lenses can be prescribed to enhance vision	G. Time it takes for healing and to monitor graft rejection can be up to one year
H. Keep appointments with physician, usually 2 consecutive days following surgery, 1 week and then 1 month, or scheduled thereafter depending on individual	H. Monitors healing process, changes of dressing, acuity testing, and changes in visual correction that vary with each patient
I. Modification of home environment with safety precautions such as lighting, removal of rugs, clutter, clear pathways, use of ambulatory aids	I. Prevents injury if vision impaired

glaucoma/trabeculectomy

DEFINITION

Glaucoma is a disorder characterized by increased intraocular pressure, atrophy of the optic nerve, eventually leading to loss of vision. The pressure increase is caused by the amount and rate of production (hyper-production) of aqueous fluid and the maintenance of outflow of the fluid from the eye (obstruction). It is classified as open- or closed-angle glaucoma. Most are treated medically by improving outflow. Surgery, a filtering procedure, such as trabeculectomy can be performed when medical regimens have not been successful in preventing progression of the disease. Surgical procedures allow for relief of pressure by creating an outflow process (new opening or implantation device). This plan includes care for the prevention of visual impairment in those with glaucoma and, if surgery is performed, can also be used in association with the PREOPERATIVE CARE and POSTOPERATIVE CARE plans

NURSING DIAGNOSES

Sensory/perceptual alterations (visual) related to altered status of sense organs (glaucoma) causing anxiety, progressively reduced visual reception

Sensory/perceptual alterations (visual) related to altered status of sense organ (eye) postoperatively resulting from eye dressing or use of protective cover over operative eye, complication of infection

EXPECTED OUTCOMES

Optimal visual acuity maintained with ophthalmic medication regimen and adaptation to visual loss preoperatively and maintenance of visual acuity postoperatively evidenced by absence of further loss of vision, performance of special eye care and resumption of usual activities and daily routines

INTERVENTION	RATIONALE
I. Assess for:	
A. Visual acuity, changes in vision, peripheral vision or blind spots at the periphery, medications taken currently that can affect angle closure (antihistamines), intra-ocular pressure testing by tonometry	A. Signs and symptoms of glaucoma determined primarily by ongoing periodic eye pressure and visual acuity testing
B. Ability to perform ADL based on visual perception, reading, driving, and other visual limitations	B. Visual changes cause difficulty in performing daily routine activities
C. Ability to administer own eye medication on a routine daily basis	C. Medical regimen includes facilitating aqueous outflow with medications
D. Perception of quality of vision and effect on life-style	D. Determining factor for consideration of trabeculectomy surgery
E. Dressing dry, secure, and in place	E. Protects eye postoperatively from trauma or contamination
II. Monitor, describe, record:	
A. Slit lamp examination with tonometry, gonioscopy by physician	A. Views eye for corneal cloudiness, turbidity of aqueous, measures intra-ocular pressure, determines the depth and circumference of the chamber angle
III. Administer:	
A. Sympathomimetic TOP eye drops	A. Acts to increase aqueous outflow

INTERVENTION	RATIONALE
B. Miotic TOP eye drops	B. Acts to increase outflow by constricting the pupil
C. Beta blocker TOP eye drops	C. Acts to decrease aqueous secretion
D. Carbonic anhydrase inhibitor PO	D. Acts to decrease production of aqueous fluid
E. Antibiotic TOP eye drops or ointment	E. Acts to prevent infection of the eye postoperatively
F. Anti-inflammatory TOP eye drops	F. Acts to reduce inflammation postoperatively
G. Analgesic PO, TOP eye drops	G. Acts to control postoperative eye pain

IV. Perform/provide:

A. Safe environment with orientation to furniture placement, articles in convenient places or changed for convenience of patient	A. Prevents bumping into objects or falling
B. Supervision of eye drops or ointment administration with correct frequency and amounts as planned and reviewed with patient input	B. Ensures that medication regimen is followed as this is the most important aspect of eye care
C. Eye dressing in place with use of metal shield during sleep	C. Protects operative eye from accidental trauma
D. Sterile technique for all procedures performed for eye care, cleanse eye with saline if needed	D. Prevents transmission of pathogens that cause infection

INTERVENTION	RATIONALE
E. Assist in performing ADL as needed while encouraging self-care as appropriate	E. Promotes independence and control over situations

NURSING DIAGNOSIS
Knowledge deficit related to discharge care including, eye care, eye medications, activities, and follow-up appointments with physician for monitoring of healing, visual acuity, and change in intra-ocular pressure

EXPECTED OUTCOMES
Compliance with postoperative follow-up care evidenced by correct administration of medication regimen and adaptation to change or correction in vision

INTERVENTION	RATIONALE
V. Teach patient/family:	
A. Coping skills to adapt to vision changes, improvement or declines	A. Manages grief and anxiety associated with any further visual loss
B. Administration of eye medications by eye drops or ointment instillaton procedure using sterile technique, allow to return demonstration, frequency and amount, length of time to apply medications	B. Enhances healing and prevents complications of infection, edema, increased intraocular pressure
B. Inform to use protective covering and how to tape it in place, when to use it and rationale for its use	B. Prevents accidental trauma to eye postoperatively
C. Clease around eye with warm water and soft cloth	C. Promotes cleanliness and removes secretions

INTERVENTION	RATIONALE
D. Avoid bumping the eye, lifting heavy objects and straining, and sleeping on the operative side	D. Measures to prevent trauma to eye
E. Report unrelieved pain, nausea, reduced visual acuity, redness, edema, drainage, blurring of vision	E. Indicates increased intraocular pressure or infection
F. Keep appointments with physician as scheduled pre- and postoperatively	F. Monitors healing process, changes of dressing, and changes in vision and pressure that varies with each patient

ocular enucleation

DEFINITION

Ocular enucleation is the complete removal of the eyeball. The removal of the entire eyeball and surrounding soft supporting tissues is known as ocular exenteration. The procedure is usually done to treat malignancy, glaucoma, sympathetic ophthalmia, eye infections, or eye trauma/injury. A plastic shell is placed in the socket following removal to serve as a support until a prosthesis or implant can be fitted and inserted. The surgery can be combined with postoperative radiation therapy. This plan can be used in association with the PREOPERATIVE CARE, POSTOPERATIVE CARE, and NEOPLASM (CHEMOTHERAPY/EXTERNAL or INTERNAL RADIATION) plans

NURSING DIAGNOSES

Ineffective individual coping related to situational crises of visual deficit (loss of eye) and psychophysiological changes, inability to manage stress, cope with change in appearance, and effect on life-style

Body image disturbance related to biophysical and psychosocial perceptual factors causing changes in physical appearance/sensory functions (eye prosthesis, visual deficit)

EXPECTED OUTCOMES

Progressive acknowledgment and adaptation to changes in visual function and ability to cope evidenced by verbalizing positive statements about changes and expressed feeling of adapting to loss and use of eye prosthesis, development and utilization of coping skills, return of personal interest in appearance and social participation

INTERVENTION	RATIONALE
I. Assess for:	
A. Use of coping mechanisms, stated fears of uncertainty of disease outcome, lifestyle changes, reactions to loss of vision in one eye	A. Assists in identifying inappropriate use of coping skills, feelings of grief over losses associated with eye removal and visual changes
B. Negative expressions about loss, feelings of helplessness, withdrawal from social activities	B. Indicates difficulty in coping and decrease in self-esteem and body image
C. Personal resources to cope with stress of change and interest in learning to problem-solve	C. Support systems and personal strengths assist to develop coping skills
D. Feelings about possible role change, participation in activities, and need to modify life-style	D. Decline in self-esteem common in those with visual deficits
IV. Perform/provide:	
A. Environment conducive to rest, expression of fears and concerns, avoid anxiety-producing situations	A. Decreases stimuli that cause stress, venting of feelings assists to cope with changes
B. Listen and clarify perceptions and information given, correct misconceptions and assist to understand condition and surgery	B. Promotes successful resolution of crisis and establishes positive coping mechanisms

INTERVENTION	RATIONALE
C. Allow time to verbalize feelings of denial, anger, fear, or resentment, comments about appearance and possible loss of abilities in a nonjudgmental environment	C. Promotes temporary use of defense mechanisms to assist in reducing negative feelings
D. Discuss strengths and abilities with sincerity and honesty, allow to participate in planning care routines	D. Promotes self-esteem without undermining trust and allows for control over situations
E. Suggest new methods to enhance coping skills and problem solving, allow to externalize and identify those that help	E. Offers alternative coping strategies that allow for release of anxiety and promote hope
F. Encouragement and positive feedback regarding progress made, focus on abilities rather than disabilities	F. Provides support for adaptive behavior, promotes self-worth and responsibility
G. Support grieving for loss of life-style and changes in appearance and sensory perception	G. Provides assistance in adaptation to changes imposed by condition

NURSING DIAGNOSES
Pain related to physical injuring agent of surgical procedure (ocular enucleation), biologic injuring agent of infectious process

Risk for infection related to inadequate primary defenses resulting from eye surgery, compromised body protective resources resulting from eye disease or trauma

EXPECTED OUTCOMES
Pain reduced or controlled evidenced by verbalizations that discomfort relieved by analgesics, absence of infectious process evidenced by a clean wound free from edema, irritation, and drainage

INTERVENTION	RATIONALE
I. Assess for:	
A. Pain severity, duration, with eye movement, redness, edema, visual changes preoperatively	A. Associated with eye infection or a predisposition to infection
B. Pain severity, if unrelieved by analgesics, redness, edema, purulent drainage, changes in vision postoperatively	B. Associated with post-operative site that can indicate infection, pain caused by trauma of surgery
C. Visual acuity of remaining eye, alterations in depth perception postoperatively	C. Provides information about need for safety measures to prevent falls or restrictions caused by visual deficit
III. Administer:	
A. Antibiotic TOP eye drops or ointment in socket, IM postoperatively	A. Acts to prevent or treat infection of the eye pre- or postoperatively by preventing cell wall synthesis causing destruction of micro-organisms
B. Anti-inflammatory IM, PO	B. Acts to reduce inflammation postoperatively
C. Analgesic PO, IM	C. Acts to control postoperative eye pain or pain caused by infection
IV. Perform/provide:	
A. Observation of pressure dressing for bleeding, inform the client that the dressing is removed the next day	A. Applied following surgery to protect operative eye from immediate injury or hemorrhage

INTERVENTION	RATIONALE
B. Warm or cool compress to eye q4h after dressing removed	B. Reduces lid and conjunctival edema and removes secretions
C. Cleanse eye with warm water and soft gauze pad, avoid allowing water to touch socket	C. Removes drainage that can dry and cause discomfort
D. Eye shield over operative eye until prosthesis is fitted	D. Prevents accidental rubbing or bumping of eye causing injury and pain, concern over appearance of the site
E. Sterile technique for all dressing changes and administration of eye medications	E. Prevents transmission of pathogens to eye

NURSING DIAGNOSIS

Knowledge deficit related to discharge care, including eye prothesis use and care, eye medications, activities, signs and symptoms to report, and follow-up appointments with physician for monitoring of healing and visual acuity of remaining eye, prosthetist for making and fitting of prosthesis

EXPECTED OUTCOMES

Compliance with postoperative follow-up care evidenced by compliance with prescribed regimen and verbalization of visual or other changes to assess and report, adaptation to care and use of eye prosthesis

INTERVENTION	RATIONALE
V. Teach patient/family:	
A. Type of surgery and procedure performed, if prosthesis will be needed and type	A. Promotes knowledge and decreases anxiety and possible misinformation

INTERVENTION	RATIONALE
B. Administration of eye medications by eye drops or ointment instillaton procedure using sterile technique, allow to return demonstration, frequency and amount, length of time to apply medications	B. Enhances healing and prevents complications of infection
C. Inform to use protective covering and how to tape it in place, when to use it, to wear impact-resistant glasses	C. Prevents accidental trauma to eye, can be used for 6 weeks following surgery or until prosthesis is fitted to cover site and prevent aversion to it
D. Avoid bumping the eye, lifting heavy objects and straining, and sleeping on the operative side, rubbing eye	D. Measures to prevent trauma to eye and accidental injury
E. Cleanse eye area with warm water and wash cloth	E. Promotes cleanliness and removes any dried secretions
F. Report pain, redness, edema, changes in depth perception	F. Indicates infection and visual acuity changes in remaining eye
G. Inform that depth perception is affected and care should be taken when driving, walking, and participating in activities	G. Assists to adjust to monocular vision

INTERVENTION	RATIONALE
H. Procedure to remove, cleanse, insert, and store prosthesis, allow to return demonstration and practice prosthesis care procedures as follows:	H. Provides proper care of prosthesis for most effective use
a. Remove by pulling down on lower lid and applying slight pressure to allow prostesis to fall into a cupped hand held against the cheek under eye, or use a suction cup to remove the prosthesis	
b. Cleanse with mild soap under running water using fingers	
c. Reinsert by applying slight pressure to upper bony orbit to raise upper lid and placing top of prosthesis under upper lid, pulling down on lower lid and applying slight pressure on lower prosthesis, which slips into the lower lid	
I. Keep appointments with physician or prosthetist as scheduled	I. Monitors healing process, changes or adjustments needed in prosthesis
J. Modification of home environment with safety precautions such as lighting, removal of rugs, clutter, clear pathways, use of ambulatory aids if needed and depending on visual acuity of remaining eye	J. Prevents injury if vision impaired

rhegmatogenous retinal detachment/scleral buckling

DEFINITION

A hole or tear in the retina causing separation or detachment of the retina allowing fluid accumulation that separates it from a blood supply. The detachment can increase over time and result in loss of function and necrosis of the retinal tissues. It can be caused by vitreous traction, atrophy of the vitreous, aphakia and myopia, cataract extraction, diabetic retinopathy, tumor, degenerative disease (lattice), or eye trauma. It is treated by cryopexy or laser treatment to seal an existing hole prior to detachment or surgical scleral buckling that returns the retina's contact with the choroid. This plan includes care to prevent further loss of vision and following surgical intervention to prevent complications and promote adaptation to the return of vision. It can be used in association with the PRE-OPERATIVE CARE and POSTOPERATIVE CARE plans

NURSING DIAGNOSES

Sensory/perceptual alterations (visual) related to altered status of sense organs (retinal detachment) causing anxiety, sudden change in visual acuity

Sensory/perceptual alterations (visual) related to altered status of sense organ (eye) postoperatively resulting from eye dressing or use of protective cover over operative eye, inflammation and swelling, slowness in improvement or return of vision

Anxiety related to threat to health status resulting from changes in visual acuity and extension of the tear preoperatively, and fear associated with possible redetachment and loss of vision postoperatively

EXPECTED OUTCOMES

Optimal visual acuity maintained preoperatively and return of visual acuity postoperatively evidenced by adaptation to change in vision or loss of vision and ability to resume activities following surgical correction

INTERVENTION	RATIONALE
I. Assess for:	
A. Visual acuity testing, sudden floaters or dark spots, flashes of light or an obliteration of the field of vision	A. Indicates degree of detachment of the retina, blood and retinal cells are freed when a tear occurs and cause shadows on the retina resulting in floating spots; visual loss depends on location of the tear
B. Level of anxiety, expressed apprehension, fear about loss of vision	B. Anxiety can range from mild to severe and affect ability to cope with vision losses and to adapt to visual changes
C. Ability to perform ADL based on visual perception, reading, driving, and other visual limitations	C. Visual changes cause difficulty in performing daily routine activities
D. Perception of quality of vision and effect on life-style	D. Determining factor for consideration of surgery to correct retinal detachment
E. Dressing dry, secure, and in place	E. Protects eye postoperatively from trauma or contamination
III. Administer:	
A. Mydriatic TOP eye drops	A. Acts to dilate pupils by contracting eye muscles or iris preoperatively to facilitate surgery
B. Anti-inflammatory TOP eye drops	B. Acts to reduce inflammation postoperatively
C. Diuretic IV	C. Acts to reduce intraocular pressure postoperatively

INTERVENTION	RATIONALE
IV. Perform/provide:	
A. Accepting environment for expression of concerns and for questions about tear or repair procedure	A. Provides venting of fears and feelings that decrease anxiety level
B. Bed rest, place head down in sidelying position	B. Prevents further detachment and allows retinal opening to be in lowest part of the eye
C. Safe environment with assistance when needed, place articles within reach, introduce to the environment with furniture placement, bathroom, rails, or aids for ambulation	C. Provides support when eyes are covered
D. Cover both eyes with pads, if uncovered, avoid reading	D. Prevents increased detachment from movement of eyes
E. Eye dressing usually removed the next day by the physician	E. Immediate protection to operative eye
F. Use of metal shield during sleep or activities	F. Continues protection of operative eye from accidental trauma

NURSING DIAGNOSES

Pain related to physical injuring agent of surgical procedure (scleral buckling), biologic injuring agent of inflammation/infectious process

Risk for infection related to inadequate primary defenses resulting from eye surgery, compromised internal protective systems against infection resulting from disease or trauma

EXPECTED OUTCOMES

Pain reduced or controlled evidenced by verbalizations that discomfort relieved by analgesics, absence of infectious process evidenced by eye free from edema, irritation, and drainage

INTERVENTION	RATIONALE
I. Assess for:	
A. Pain severity, redness, swelling of the lids and conjunctiva, ecchymosis of lids	A. Associated with eye inflammation or predisposition to infection during postoperative period
B. Pain, redness, purulent drainage	B. Associated with infection postoperatively
III. Administer:	
A. Antibiotic TOP eye drops or ointment	A. Acts to prevent or treat infection of the eye pre- or postoperatively by preventing cell wall synthesis causing destruction of microorganisms
B. Anti-inflammatory TOP eye drops	B. Acts to reduce inflammation postoperatively
C. Analgesic PO, TOP eye drops	C. Acts to control postoperative eye pain or pain resulting from keratitis
D. Cycloplegic TOP eye drops	D. Acts to decrease spasms of ciliary body to reduce pain and prevents formation of iris adhesions
IV. Perform/provide	
A. Warm or cool compress to eye QID	A. Reduces lid and conjunctival edema and pain

INTERVENTION	RATIONALE
B. Cleanse around eye with warm water and soft gauze pad	B. Removes excessive tearing that can dry and result in lids sticking together
C. Eye shield over operative eye	C. Prevents accidental rubbing or bumping of eye causing injury and pain
D. Sterile technique for all dressing changes and administration of eye medications	D. Prevents transmission of pathogens to eye

NURSING DIAGNOSIS

Risk for trauma related to internal factor of poor vision causing possible falls

  Impaired physical mobility related to visual perceptual impairment preoperatively and imposed restricted activity postoperatively resulting in inability to perform ADL and participate in occupation/social activities

EXPECTED OUTCOMES

Adequate sensory input and safe movement within restrictions and visual deficit evidenced by absence of injury and physical exertion during progressive restoration of visual loss following surgery

INTERVENTION	RATIONALE
I. Assess for:	
A. Ability to perform ADL, activity restrictions and duration expected, activities that are allowed	A. Activity restrictions needed if an air or gas bubble has been injected during surgery to apply pressure on the retina from the inner aspect of the eye
B. Hazards in the environment that can predispose to falls and trauma	B. Prevents possible trauma or injury

INTERVENTION	RATIONALE
IV. Perform/provide:	
A. Bed rest, side rails up	A. Prevents falls from bed
B. Avoid movements such as shaving, combing hair, coughing	B. Prevents damage or extension to repaired tear
C. Position to allow for maximal pressure on the retina by gravitational force during the day and sleep postoperatively for a few days	C. Positioning if air or gas bubble has been injected to allow for absorption
D. Assist with ADL and allow for progressive self-care	D. Promotes independence in self-care and control of situation
E. Read to patient, use touch for comfort, radio for diversion	E. Provides stimulation and prevents boredom
F. Assist with ambulation, clear pathways, rearrange furniture or aquaint with placement of items that can be used for support when walking	F. Prevents falls or injury from bumping into furniture

NURSING DIAGNOSIS
Knowledge deficit related to discharge care, including eye care, eye medications, activities, and follow-up appointments with physician for monitoring of healing, visual acuity, and complications

EXPECTED OUTCOMES
Adequate knowledge of postoperative follow-up care evidenced by compliance with prescribed regimen and adaptation to corrections in vision or loss in vision

INTERVENTION	RATIONALE
V. Teach patient/family:	
A. Optimal vision can take up to 3 months to achieve and activities can usually be resumed in 3 to 6 weeks	A. Surgery is successful with proper care dependent on extent and duration of detachment prior to surgery
B. That warm or cold compresses continue and eye be washed with warm water and soft cloth to cleanse	B. Assists to resolve swelling and redness that can take a few weeks to resolve
C. Administration of eye medications by eye drops or ointment instillaton procedure using sterile technique, allow to return demonstration, frequency, and amount, length of time to apply medications	C. Enhances healing and prevents complications of infection, edema, increased intraocular pressure
D. Inform to use protective covering or eyeglasses, how to tape them in place, and when to use this protection	D. Prevents accidental trauma to eye after dressing removed
E. Avoid bumping the eye, lifting heavy objects and straining, sleeping on the operative side, and air travel	E. Measures to prevent trauma to eye or change pressure in the eye
F. Modify home environment by removing rugs, poor lights, cords, or items in pathways, rails or aids for ambulation	F. Prevents falls and trauma by removing safety hazards

INTERVENTION	RATIONALE
G. Report any visual changes or changes in the appearance of the eye to the physician	G. Provides for early intervention if redetachment occurs
H. Keep appointments with physician as scheduled	H. Monitors healing process, changes in visual acuity

tympanoplasty/ossiculoplasty

DEFINITION

Tympanoplasty is the surgical restoration of a conductive hearing loss by reconstruction of the middle ear using a graft to repair and close a perforation in the tympanic membrane to produce an intact tympanum. It is done to treat tympanosclerosis caused by deposits in the membrane resulting from persistent middle ear infections (otitis media) or damage to the membrane caused by trauma. It can also be done in association with the ossiculoplasty procedure. Ossiculoplasty is the surgical reconstruction of necrotic ossicles by the use of prostheses to reconnect the ossicles or rebuild the ossicles in order to carry sound. Stapedectomy is a procedure of the middle ear rarely done today to correct otosclerosis or sclerosis of the stapes. This plan includes care for the hearing impaired and surgery performed to correct conductive hearing loss and can be used in association with the PREOPERATIVE CARE and POSTOPERATIVE CARE plans

NURSING DIAGNOSES

Anxiety related to threat to health status resulting from chronic middle ear disorders and changes in auditory acuity preoperatively

Sensory/perceptual alterations (auditory) related to altered status of sense organs resulting from preoperative disease and trauma, and surgery postoperatively resulting from edema, packing in the operative ear

EXPECTED OUTCOMES

Optimal auditory acuity maintained preoperatively and improved acuity postoperatively evidenced by return of hearing, comprehension, correct responses to communications, and verbalizations of decreased anxiety and understanding of speech interactions with others

INTERVENTION	RATIONALE
I. Assess for:	
A. Level of anxiety, feelings about hearing loss and expectations of surgery	A. Moderate levels of anxiety expected preoperatively
B. Auditory acuity testing, complaints of inability to hear, improper responses, feelings of frustration, improvement in responses when moving closer, use of hearing aid, lipreading	B. Signs and symptoms of hearing loss and possible techniques to use for communication
C. Ability to perform activities with auditory perception deficit such as driving, working, socializing	C. Auditory changes cause difficulty in performing daily routine activities
D. Perception of quality of hearing and effect on lifestyle	D. Determining factor for consideration of ear surgery
E. Dressing dry, secure, and in place, presence of drainage	E. Protects ear postoperatively from trauma or contamination
II. Monitor, describe, record:	
A. Culture of ear drainage	A. Identifies infectious agent in chronic middle ear problems
B. Audiometric hearing tests	B. Measures hearing loss
IV. Perform/provide:	
A. Quiet, supportive environment, answer any questions honestly and clearly, clarify information as needed	A. Reduces anxiety and fear of unknown, promotes relaxation

INTERVENTION	RATIONALE
B. Offer paper and pencil, cards, magic slate	B. Alternate methods of communication if hearing deficit severe
C. Safe environment that is noise free, well-lighted	C. Enhances hearing and/or lipreading
D. Face patient when talking, speaking into the best ear, speaking slowly and slightly louder, using simple, short sentences	D. Enhances hearing and facilitates communication
E. Encourage lipreading, use of hearing aid if appropriate	E. Promotes auditory perception
F. Inform that dressing will be in place and that diminished hearing will last several weeks postoperatively	F. Protects operative ear, edema and blood accumulation in ear causes diminished hearing

NURSING DIAGNOSES

Risk for infection related to inadequate primary defenses resulting from ear surgical incision, frequent middle ear exposure to upper respiratory infections leading to infection

Risk for injury related to internal factor of regulatory function resulting in dislodgment of prosthesis and leakage of perilymph around the prosthesis causing vertigo and potential falls

EXPECTED OUTCOMES

Absence of infectious process and injury evidenced by operative ear free from edema, pain, pressure, and purulent drainage, no tinnitus or trauma resulting from vertigo or falls

INTERVENTION	RATIONALE
I. Assess for:	
A. Pain severity, duration in ear, edema, drainage, auditory changes preoperatively	A. Associated with ear infection or a predisposition to infection
B. Pain severity, if unrelieved by analgesics, feeling of pressure, vertigo, tinnitus, changes in hearing and foul-smelling purulent drainage from ear postoperatively	B. Associated with ear postoperatively that can indicate infection or dislodgment of prosthesis
C. Auditory acuity of remaining ear	C. Provides information about need for safety measures to prevent falls postoperatively or restrictions caused by auditory deficit
II. Monitor, describe, record:	
A. Temperature q4h	A. Elevations indicate infection
B. WBC	B. Increases indicate infection
III. Administer:	
A. Antibiotic PO, IM	A. Acts to prevent or treat infection of the eye pre- or postoperatively by preventing cell wall synthesis causing destruction of micro-organisms
B. Anti-inflammatory PO, IM	B. Acts to reduce inflammation postoperatively

INTERVENTION	RATIONALE
C. Analgesic PO, IM	C. Acts to control postoperative eye pain or pain caused by ear infection
D. Antipyretic PO	D. Acts to reduce temperature during middle ear infection

IV. Perform/provide:

INTERVENTION	RATIONALE
A. Bed rest for 24 hours with restricted movements and lying on unoperative ear postoperatively	A. Prevents prosthesis dislodgment
B. Slow position changes, move head and upper body at the same time, avoid looking down when walking, and watching quick-moving objects	B. Reduces vertigo and possible fall
C. Observation of ear dressing, usually a cotton ball, for serosanguineous drainage, but can be a dressing that completely covers the ear	C. Applied following surgery to protect and support ear
D. Inform that noises such as cracking or popping or some pain in the ear or side of the face can be experienced immediately following the surgery	D. Common postoperatively and are considered normal responses
E. Inform to cough or sneeze with the mouth open, and blow the nose one side at a time	E. Prevents increased pressure within the ears

INTERVENTION	RATIONALE
F. Sterile technique for all dressing changes, administration of ear medications, or irrigations	F. Prevents transmission of pathogens to ear
G. Suggest holding to rails or furniture and sit down immediately if vertigo present	G. Prevents falls if dizzy or feeling faint

NURSING DIAGNOSIS

Knowledge deficit related to discharge care, including ear care, medications, activities, measures to prevent complications, and follow-up appointments with physician for monitoring of healing and auditory acuity, signs and symptoms to report

EXPECTED OUTCOMES

Adequate information about postoperative follow-up care evidenced by compliance with ear care procedures and preventive measures resulting in absence of complications during healing period and progressive return of auditory acuity

INTERVENTION	RATIONALE
V. Teach patient/family:	
A. Administration of medications orally and by ear drops or ointment instillation procedure using sterile technique, allow to return demonstration, frequency and amount, length of time to apply medications	A. Enhances healing and prevents complications of infection
B. Changing of cotton ball daily, noting drainage or bleeding and report to physician	B. Prevents accidental insertion of anything that can injure ear and allows for early treatment of a complication

INTERVENTION	RATIONALE
C. Cover ear or wear aids to eliminate noise	C. Protects ear from noisy or cold environments or introduction of infectious agents
D. Avoid touching dressing or allowing ear or dressing to get wet for 2 weeks, use two cotton balls with petroleum jelly on one to repel water when bathing or shampooing	D. Prevents contamination of wound and could retard healing process
E. Avoid water in the ear from swimming or diving, avoid flying for at least 1 week	E. Prevents introduction of infectious agents or change in pressure in the ears
F. Avoid physical activities for 1 week and more strenuous exercises for at least 3 to 4 weeks	F. Prevents possible trauma to ear
G. Blow nose gently, one side at a time, and sneeze or cough with mouth open, avoid straining at defecation for at least 1 to 2 weeks	G. Prevents increased pressure in ears
H. Report any decreased hearing, pain or drainage from ear	H. Allows for early intervention to care for possible complications
I. Avoid exposure to upper respiratory diseases	I. Predisposes to contamination via eustachian tube
J. Keep appointments with physician as scheduled	J. Monitors healing process, changes of dressing, and changes in auditory acuity or correction that varies with each patient

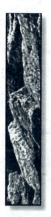

Integumentary System Standards

integumentary system data base

HISTORICAL DATA REVIEW
Past events:
1. Acute and/or chronic integumentary disease or disorders, presence of other diseases that affect the system (diabetes, vascular, collagen or renal disorders, blood dyscrasia)
2. Chronic signs and symptoms related to integumentary disorders (pain, color changes, swelling, drainage, dryness, rash, pruritis, lesions, bruising, urticaria, masses, nail changes, alopecia)
3. Eczema, skin reactions, or other integumentary disorders of family members
4. Allergies and effect on skin (erythema, urticaria, blisters, pruritis)
5. Recent exposure to infectious diseases, immunization status
6. Occupational/environmental exposure to skin irritants (sun, cold, plants), skin, hair, nail cleansing and care routine (soap, shaving cream, lotions, perfumes, bath oils, powders, cosmetics, shampoo, hair rinse, hair tint, sprays, nail polish)
7. Nutritional status, travel and activity, life-style factors that predispose to skin disorders
8. Medications including popular topical preparations (prescriptions and over-the-counter) for integumentary conditions
9. Hospitalizations and feelings about care, surgery associated with integumentary system and incisional skin scars

Present events:
1. Medical diagnoses associated with or affecting integumentary structure or function, proposed reconstructive or cosmetic surgery
2. Skin, hair, scalp, nail abnormalities and changes in existing condition
3. Appearance of skin, hair, nails for color, lesions, rashes, masses, infectious process, eruptions, itching, ecchymoses, breakdown
4. Activities of daily living and effect on skin, hair, nail cleanliness and integrity, effect on body image and self-esteem

PHYSICAL ASSESSMENT DATA REVIEW

1. Skin cleanliness, odor, color, texture, dryness, oiliness, temperature, turgor, tenderness, scaling, crusting, exudate, edema, lesions and type, breaks, excoriation, nevi, warts, lipomas, keloids, cellulitis
2. Hair cleanliness, texture, infestation, dandruff
3. Nail cleanliness, angle, thickness, brittleness, infection
4. Type, degree or severity, and extent of burn injury (size, depth, location)

NURSING DIAGNOSES CONSIDERATIONS

1. Altered nutrition: less than body requirements
2. Altered tissue perfusion (peripheral)
3. Body image disturbance
4. Bowel incontinence
5. Functional incontinence
6. Risk for impaired skin integrity
7. Risk for infection
8. Risk for injury
9. Impaired skin integrity
10. Knowledge deficit

GERIATRIC CONSIDERATIONS

Integumentary changes in geriatric patients depend on body build and nutritional/fluid status all of which determine the amount of fat in the subcutaneous tissue layer. Common skin problems in the elderly include breakdown or decubiti, easy bruising, and skin discolorations that are disturbing to self-esteem and body image because they are so visible. Integumentary changes associated with aging that should be considered when assessing the geriatric patient include:

1. Decreased subcutaneous fat especially over the arms and legs resulting in loss of body insulation and support for vessels
2. Decreased skin elasticity resulting in sagging, wrinkles, facial and neck lines, elongated ear lobes, ptosis of eyelids, reduced skin turgor resulting in stiffness and loss of pliability
3. Increased skin dryness, thinning, vascular fragility resulting in risk for itching, bruising, and trauma
4. Epidermal tissue overgrowth resulting in senile telangiectasia and

hyperkeratotic warts, increased skin pigmentation (aging spots) on exposed areas
5. Increased nail ridging, thickening of toenails with lifting of nail plate, increased thickening, brittleness, and splitting of finger nails resulting in risk for fungal infections, decreased nail growth and strength
6. Decreased hair follicle density resulting in loss of head, axillary and pubic hair, increased hair growth in ears, nares, and eyebrows
7. Decreased circulation to the skin resulting in reduced blood supply of oxygen and nutrients, decreased cell replacement resulting in delayed wound healing and risk for decubiti
8. Skin atrophy with decreased vascularity and elasticity resulting in loss of water content and storage in skin layers, decreased water content resulting in dryness causing rough, scaly texture and pruritis
9. Decreased tactile perception of pain and decreased sebaceous and sweat gland activity resulting in dry skin and reduced ability of body to cool itself
10. Decreased melanin production and estrogen after menopause resulting in graying of hair or hair growth on face respectively

DIAGNOSTIC LABORATORY TESTS AND PROCEDURES

1. Skin tissue biopsy and laboratory examination, patch test, skin surface light examination
2. Skin culture, smears, complete blood count (CBC), electrolyte panel

MEDICATIONS

1. Anti-acne agents: benzoyl peroxide, tretinoin, isotretinoin
2. Antimicrobials: erythromycin, polymyxin/bacitracin, nystatin, permethrin, tetracycline, penicillin, acyclovir
3. Antipruritics: phenol, camphor, calamine, boric acid, aluminum acetate, potassium permanganate
4. Antiseptics: acetic acid, hydrogen peroxide, chlorhexidine gluconate
5. Corticosteroids: betamethasone, hydrocortisone, triamcinolone acetonide, diflorasone
6. Emollients: vaseline, neutrogena, aquaphor
7. Keratolytics: lactic acid, salicylic acid
8. Skin protectorants: PABA, benzophenone (sun), zinc oxide, opsite, duoderm (physical)

decubitus ulcer

DEFINITION

Decubitus ulcer, also known as pressure sore, is a state of risk for or actual skin breakdown caused by sustained pressure, friction, or shearing forces that damage the skin. Other factors involved in skin damage include inadequate nutrition, reduced circulation and sensation, aging skin, exposure to excretions/secretions, and effects of medications. The most common sites are the sacrum, iliac crests, heels, elbows, scapulae, ears, and head. Ulcer formation varies in degrees and progresses in stages beginning with redness of the skin surfaces to breaks or disruptions leading to destruction of the skin layers (epidermis and dermis)

NURSING DIAGNOSIS

Risk for impaired skin integrity related to external factors of shearing forces and pressure, immobilization (enforced bed rest), excretions and secretions (urinary and fecal incontinence), and internal factors of altered circulation, nutritional state (obesity, emaciation), sensation (tactile), and lack of protective tissue at skeletal prominences

EXPECTED OUTCOMES

Skin integrity preserved with preventive measures implemented evidenced by intactness, and no redness, irritation, or excoriation

INTERVENTION	RATIONALE

I. Assess for:

A. Skin areas exposed to pressure (bony prominences), moisture resulting from incontinence, edema or changes in tactile sensation, presence of redness, blanching, excoriation, rash, or breaks

A. Data base inclusions of early signs and symptoms leading to skin breakdown

IV. Perform/provide:

A. Turn or change position q2h or more often, shift weight while sitting q1h, and limit sitting time to 1 hour

A. Prevents prolonged pressure on areas causing ischemia as blood supply is reduced leading to high risk for tissue breakdown

B. Head of bed elevation to no more than 30 degrees, limit this position based on extent of immobility

B. Prevents shearing caused by sliding down in bed resulting in the skin remaining in one position while underlying tissues alter their position

C. Sheepskin between skin and linens, apply a light layer of cornstarch to sheet, use a lift sheet to assist in moving or changing positions in bed

C. Prevents friction to skin caused by contact with sheets or pulling along the linens when changing positions that can tear fragile skin

D. Position and support areas with foam, eggcrate, water or air mattress, gel or air seat cushions

D. Protects areas by reducing or controlling pressure to skin when lying in bed or sitting in a chair

E. Change linens when wet or soiled, apply sheets smoothly and snugly

E. Ensures dry smooth bed by eliminating wrinkles to prevent pressure to skin

INTERVENTION	RATIONALE
F. Wash and rinse perineal area with warm water and mild soap, pat dry, following incontinence, apply protective ointment to perineum, collecting device if possible and practical	F. Maintains dryness of skin prone to irritation from body excretions
G. Change damp dressings and empty drainage devices as needed	G. Protects skin from excessive moisture that causes breakdown and provides medium for infectious agents
H. Apply a moisturizer or lotion to skin following bathing with a mild oil base soap or add to bath water	H. Reduces drying of skin when moisture on the skin is reduced from evaporation
I. Assist with or perform ROM, encourage activities and mobility as tolerated, and use of overhead trapeze to facilitate movement in bed	I. Promotes circulation and prevents joint contractures and muscle mass loss
J. Spray benzoin or apply other ointments or pastes to areas at risk	J. Provides barrier to protect skin from exposure to irritants
K. Nutritional and fluid intake based on height, weight, frame, and general health status	K. Provides for well-nourished, hydrated skin state that is more likely to resist breakdown
L. Avoid massage of pressure areas, use of donuts or heat lamps	L. Known to cause more damage to skin than prevent skin breakdown

INTERVENTION	RATIONALE
V. Teach patient/family:	
A. Report any changes in skin color, texture, irritation, lesions, rashes, or breaks, weakness and increasing immobility	A. Indicates risk for skin breakdown and allows for early preventive measures

NURSING DIAGNOSIS

Impaired skin integrity related to external mechanical factors of shearing forces and pressure, immobilization, and internal factors of altered nutritional state, circulation, presence of excretions/secretions causing disruption of skin surface or destruction of skin layers

EXPECTED OUTCOMES

Decubitus treated without complication evidenced by progressive healing of tissues and decrease in the size, absence of infection at decubitus site, effective application of a combination of dressings to cover and protect area, maintain moisture, and/or absorb excess exudate

INTERVENTION	RATIONALE
I. Assess for:	
A. Type, area, and extent of breakdown, type of treatment and frequency ordered, measured size of ulcer, and drainage characteristics	A. Provides information of stage of decubitus formation necessary prior to determining and performing care
B. General health status and potential for healing	B. Healing depends on adequate fluid and nutrition, circulatory status
II. Monitor, describe, record:	
A. Measurement of ulcer size as appropriate, at least weekly	A. Provides information of progress of wound healing or extension of ulcer

INTERVENTION	RATIONALE
IV. Perform/provide:	
A. Handwashing prior to any skin care procedures	A. Prevents transmission of pathogens to the decubitus site
B. Place in positions that avoid allowing contact of skin irritation, breaks or tissue destruction with bed linens	B. Prevents pressure on areas that already reveal some stage of decubitus ulcer
C. Shave area at site of skin irritation or breaks prior to treatment if needed	C. Prevents contamination and use of tape to secure dressings without pulling the hair
D. Use disposable gloves to carefully remove dressing and discard in proper receptacle	D. Proper removal and disposal of soiled dressings by universal precautions
E. Wash and rinse the skin around breakdown with warm water and pH neutral or commercial cleanser, pat dry, gently massage area, and again discard gloves in hazardous disposal bag	E. Cleanses and removes debris at treatment site
F. Put on sterile gloves and use sterile technique and sterile supplies for all care of open wounds	F. Prevents contamination of area by micro-organisms that can cause infection
G. Apply ointments, sprays, or pastes to skin around break in skin	G. Protects skin around ulcer from moisture and further breakdown

INTERVENTION	RATIONALE
H. Apply a dry Telfa dressing and secure with tape, or use transparent permeable adhesive dressing to the ulcer	H. Dressing treatment for stages I & II
I. Cleanse and irrigate with saline from cleanest to least clean area	I. Treatment for later stages of ulcer
J. Apply medication, debriding agent or gelatin sponge; hydrocolloid, hydrogel, or polyurethane foam	J. Treatment for breakdown involving destruction of deeper layers of tissue to prevent infection or absorb secretions to enhance healing
K. Dispose of gloves and all used supplies and articles in a properly labeled container for hazardous waste	K. Complies with universal precautions to prevent transmission on pathogens
L. Include vitamin C and additional protein and calories in daily dietary intake	L. Promotes wound healing

erysipelas/cellulitis

DEFINITION
Erysipelas is an acute inflammation of the skin and lymphatics. It is usually caused by beta-hemolytic streptococcus (group A). Cellulitis is also an inflammation of the skin that involves deeper tissue layers. It is usually caused by a different strain of streptococcus. Those at greatest risk are the older adult and those with disorders such as diabetes, open wounds, or malnutrition

NURSING DIAGNOSES
Pain related to biologic injuring agent (infectious process)

Hyperthermia related to infection of superficial and/or deeper skin layers/tissue causing stimulation to the regulating center in the hypothalamus

Impaired tissue integrity related to factor of microbial invasion and spread causing pain, destruction of skin layers

EXPECTED OUTCOMES
Relief or control of pain and temperature reduced and within baseline parameters evidenced by verbalizations that pain absent and comfort increased following analgesic, temperature in range of 98.6°F (37°C) maintained; progressive healing of lesions evidenced by skin intact with reduced edema, redness, blistering and control of spread of infection

INTERVENTION	RATIONALE
I. Assess for:	
A. Pain, type (superficial or deep), severity, site(s)	A. Reveals pain descriptors associated with inflammation/ infection

INTERVENTION	RATIONALE
B. Elevated temperature, chills, malaise, diaphoresis	B. Indicates signs and symptoms of infectious process
C. Skin redness that spreads and appears as a plaque with sharp borders	C. Indicates superficial eruptions usually on the face or extremities associated with erysipelas
D. Skin redness, edematous area that spreads and has no borders, blistering, nodular area	D. Indicates inflammation associated with cellulitis

II. Monitor, describe, record:

A. VS and temperature q4h	A. Decreased BP, increased P, associated with high temperature elevation can occur with the rapid spread of infection facilitated by enzyme activity
B. WBC, differential	B. Elevation of WBC indicates presence of infectious process
C. Wound culture and sensitivities	C. Identifies causative agent to determine antibiotic regimen

III. Administer:

A. Antipyretic PO	A. Acts to reduce temperature and promote comfort
B. Analgesic PO	B. Acts to reduce pain according to severity
C. Antimicrobial PO, IV	C. Acts to interfere with cell wall synthesis and cause death of pathogens

INTERVENTION	RATIONALE
IV. Perform/provide:	
A. Calm, restful environment with optimal warm temperature and ventilation, warm blankets and change of damp linens or clothing	A. Prevents stimuli that increase pain and chilling associated with fever
B. Bed rest if pain present or rest periods before and after activity	B. Exertion and fatigue increase pain perception
C. Position of comfort with support of extremity	C. Decreases pain and discomfort
D. Application of warm soaks to affected area	D. Promotes comfort and reduces edema and inflammation by vasodilation
E. Backrub, sponge bath, relaxation techniques	E. Cooling measures to decrease temperature and promote comfort
F. Fluid intake of 2 to 3 L/day as permitted, warm fluids if chilled	F. Replaces fluid lost from diaphoresis as temperature increases or persists

NURSING DIAGNOSIS
Knowledge deficit related to lack of information about follow-up care and prevention of transmission of infectious agents or recurrence of infection in the same area

EXPECTED OUTCOMES
Adequate knowledge and skills acquired and performed evidenced by compliance with treatment regimen and progressive return to wellness

INTERVENTION	RATIONALE
V. Teach patient/family:	
A. Take temperature and allow for return demonstration and report any elevation, administration of anti-pyretic based on elevations	A. Monitors for elevation that can indicate recurrence of infection
B. Antibiotic administration as ordered for full course of medication, with dosage, frequency, route, side ef-fects	B. Destroys micro-organisms by interfering with cell wall synthesis
C. Handwash technique with antiseptic soap prior to and following care procedures	C. Prevents transmission of pathogens
D. Disposal of used articles, dressings, proper care of clothing and linens utilizing universal precautions	D. Prevents cross-contamina-tion as a result of care pro-cedures
E. Report recurrence of le-sions, edema, redness in areas	E. Allows for early interven-tion to treat possible recur-rence caused by lymphatic obstruction since lymphat-ics are involved in the in-fections

rhytidectomy/blepharectomy

DEFINITION

Rhytidectomy, also known as "face lift," is the surgical redistribution of facial and neck tissue and includes the excision of excess soft tissue. It is done for cosmetic reasons to remove wrinkles, treat scarring, remove redundant tissue caused by palsy or trauma, any of which can create body image disturbances. Blepharectomy is the surgical redistribution and excision of eyelid tissue done for cosmetic reasons to enhance body image or treat ptosis of the lid(s) to enhance visual perception. Both can be done at the same time as well as separately under local or general anesthesia depending on the anticipated extent of surgery. This plan includes care specific to these procedures and can be used in association with the PREOPERATIVE CARE and POSTOPERATIVE CARE plans

NURSING DIAGNOSES

Anxiety related to threat to or change in health status, self-concept, preoperatively causing inability to manage feelings of uncertainty and apprehension regarding uncertain outcome, and postoperatively causing stress from unsatisfactory outcome and possible disfigurement

Body image disturbance related to biophysical factor of dissatisfaction with appearance preoperatively and change in facial appearance and acceptance of outcome of surgery postoperatively

EXPECTED OUTCOMES

Anxiety controlled or within manageable levels and improved body image evidenced by verbalizations that feeling more relaxed and satisfied with results of surgery following wound healing

INTERVENTION	RATIONALE
I. Assess for: A. Level of anxiety, use of coping mechanisms, stated fears of uncertainty of disease outcome, inappropriate use of coping skills	A. Anxiety can range from mild to severe, assists in identifying level of anxiety associated with surgery and change in appearance
B. Restlessness, complaining, joking, withdrawal, talkativeness, increased P and R	B. Nonverbal expressions of anxiety when not able to communicate feelings
C. Personal resources to cope with stress, anxiety	C. Support systems and personal strengths assist to manage anxiety
D. Feelings and response to change in appearance, satisfaction with results of plastic surgery	D. Changes in body image and self-concept a common and serious problem with facial surgery and possible disfigurement
III. Administer: A. Anti-anxiety agent PO	A. Acts to reduce anxiety level and provides calming effect and rest, depresses subcortical levels of CNS, limbic system
IV. Perform/provide: A. Environment conducive to rest, expression of fears and anxiety, avoid anxiety-producing situations	A. Decreases stimuli that cause stress/anxiety, venting of feelings decreases anxiety
B. Suggest new methods to enhance coping skills and problem solving, allow to externalize and identify those that help	B. Offers alternative coping strategies that allow for release of anxiety and fear

INTERVENTION	RATIONALE
C. Privacy when dressings removed or changed, remain during the procedure	C. Reduces anxiety caused by first glimpse of surgical incisions
D. Allow to participate in planning of care to maintain usual activities when possible	D. Allows for some control over situations

NURSING DIAGNOSES

Risk for infection related to inadequate primary defenses (surgical incision)

Pain related to physical injury agent of surgery resulting from pressure of edema, possible hematoma

Sensory/perceptual alterations (visual) related to altered visual perception preoperatively by ptosis causing obstruction of vision and postoperatively by edema causing temporary obstruction of vision

EXPECTED OUTCOMES

Adequate defenses and wound healing with complications prevented evidenced by temperature, WBC within normal range, absence of redness, swelling, purulent drainage at wound site(s), pain controlled with analgesic and progressive return of baseline visual perception as edema subsides

INTERVENTION	RATIONALE
I. Assess for:	
A. Wound site(s) for edema, hematoma formation, color, drainage	A. Indicates possible infectious process or complication
B. Pain severity, type and frequency, itching around eyes, pain or tightness on side of face	B. Moderate pain usually experienced and itching can be caused by some corneal swelling, facial pain indicates hematoma formation

INTERVENTION	RATIONALE
C. Facial and eyelid edema, visual acuity affected by edema	C. Results from surgical trauma
II. Monitor, describe, record: A. Temperature q4h and PRN	A. Elevations indicate infection
B. WBC	B. Increases indicate infection
III. Administer: A. Antibiotic PO	A. Acts to prevent cell wall synthesis to destroy microorganisms in the prevention or treatment of infection
B. Antipyretic PO	B. Acts to reduce temperature
C. Analgesic PO	C. Acts to control pain associated with the surgical procedure
IV. Perform/provide: A. Hair shampoo and thorough washing of the face preoperatively	A. Cleanses areas involved in the surgical procedure
B. Elevate head of bed to position of comfort	B. Reduces edema and promotes rest
C. Ice or cold compress to face or eyes for 24 to 48 hours postoperatively	C. Reduces edema by vasoconstriction
D. Soft foods for 24 to 48 hours, avoid unnecessary interactions	D. Minimizes talking and chewing to achieve better result by finer scars

INTERVENTION	RATIONALE
E. Use sterile technique for wound care including equipment and supplies, facial dressing is usually removed within 24 to 48 hours and the face gently washed	E. Prevents contamination by pathogens
F. Assistance with care if vision is obstructed by edema if needed	F. Promotes independence and control over care

NURSING DIAGNOSIS
Knowledge deficit related to follow-up care and promotion of wound healing and successful outcome

EXPECTED OUTCOME
Adequate knowledge acquired for postoperative care evidenced by compliance with restrictions and allowed activities with progressive return to wellness

INTERVENTION	RATIONALE
V. Teach patient/family:	
A. Maintain elevated head of bed for at least 1 week	A. Minimizes edema and promotes comfort
B. Gently wash face with mild soap and warm water, pat dry, apply lotion as needed, avoid touching the surgical site(s)	B. Prevents contamination of suture line during healing process
C. Shampoo hair gently with mild soap and warm water 48 hours postoperatively	C. Promotes cleanliness and comfort

INTERVENTION	RATIONALE
D. Continue application of ice or cold wash cloth to eyes for 48 hours postoperatively	D. Continues to reduce edema and discomfort
E. Avoid bending over from the waist down, restrict activity for 1 month	E. Reduces risk for increasing edema
F. Suggest wearing sunglasses, scarf on head, or other measures to cover discoloration or edema, instruct to avoid bumping eyes when using sunglasses	F. Conceals swelling and bruising that occur around the eyes
G. Inform to keep appointment to remove sutures in 5 to 10 days	G. Allows time for healing and reduced edema

skin graft

DEFINITION
Skin graft is the surgical removal of skin from part of the body and transplantation to another part of the body (autograft), or from another person (homograft). Types of skin grafts commonly used are sheet or meshed grafts. Grafts are used in the management of burns, plastic surgery to correct scarring and provide cover for large areas of a defect. This plan includes care specific to skin graft procedures and can be used in association with the PREOPERATIVE CARE and POSTOPERATIVE CARE plans

NURSING DIAGNOSES
Anxiety related to threat to or change in health status, self-concept preoperatively causing inability to manage feelings of uncertainty and apprehension regarding uncertain outcome, and postoperatively causing stress from unsatisfactory outcome (graft rejection or death of graft)

Body image disturbance related to biophysical factor of burn wound or scarring preoperatively, and change in appearance resulting from skin graft(s) and acceptance of outcome postoperatively

EXPECTED OUTCOMES
Anxiety controlled or within manageable levels and improved body image evidenced by verbalizations that feeling more relaxed, new skin adhering to underlying tissue evidenced by progressive wound healing with graft in contact with adjacent skin and minimal scarring or disfigurement, verbalization of satisfaction with results of surgery

INTERVENTION	RATIONALE
I. Assess for:	
A. Level of anxiety, use of coping mechanisms, stated fears of uncertainty of disease outcome, inappropriate use of coping skills	A. Anxiety can range from mild to severe, assists in identifying level of anxiety associated with surgery and change in appearance
B. Restlessness, complaining, joking, withdrawal, talkativeness, increased P and R	B. Nonverbal expressions of anxiety when not able to communicate feelings
C. Personal resources to cope with stress, anxiety	C. Support systems and personal strengths assist to manage anxiety
D. Feelings and response to change in appearance, satisfaction with results of surgery	D. Changes in body image and self-concept a common and serious problem with burns, wound coverings, and the possible scarring and disfigurement
III. Administer:	
A. Anti-anxiety agent PO	A. Acts to reduce anxiety level and provides calming effect and rest, depresses subcortical levels of CNS, limbic system
IV. Perform/provide:	
A. Environment conducive to rest, expression of fears and anxiety, avoid anxiety-producing situations	A. Decreases stimuli that cause stress/anxiety, venting of feelings decreases anxiety

INTERVENTION	RATIONALE
B. Suggest new methods to enhance coping skills and problem solving, allow to externalize and identify those that help	B. Offers alternative coping strategies that allow for release of anxiety and fear
C. Privacy when dressings removed or changed, remain during the procedure	C. Reduces anxiety caused by first glimpse of surgical incisions
D. Allow to participate in planning of care to maintain usual activities when possible	D. Allows for some control over situations
E. Assist to be realistic about expectations of graft results	E. Reduces disappointment and depression if graft fails

NURSING DIAGNOSES

Risk for infection related to inadequate primary defenses (burn or surgical incision sites)

Pain related to physical injury agent of burn wound (extent and depth of injury) or graft sites, especially donor site

Impaired skin integrity related to external factor of injury and plastic surgery (skin graft), internal factors of altered circulation, blood or serum accumulation under graft causing a floating graft

EXPECTED OUTCOMES

Adequate defenses and wound healing with complications prevented evidenced by temperature, WBC within normal range, absence of redness, swelling, purulent drainage at wound site(s), and adherence of graft to wound, verbalization that pain controlled with analgesic

INTERVENTION	RATIONALE
I. Assess for: A. Wound site(s) for edema, color, purulent drainage	A. Indicates possible infectious process or complication

INTERVENTION	RATIONALE
B. Bleeding or serum beneath the graft	B. Prevents adherence of graft to the wound site that can cause death or partial loss of graft
C. Pain severity, type and frequency, stage of healing of graft, pain during wound care procedures	C. Pain experience depends on the depth and extent of injury and wound healing with severe pain at new donor sites because of exposed nerve endings
II. Monitor, describe, record:	
A. Temperature q4h and PRN	A. Elevations indicate infection
B. WBC	B. Increases indicate infection
C. Graft culture	C. Identifies pathogens responsible for infection
III. Administer:	
A. Antibiotic PO, TOP	A. Acts to prevent cell-wall synthesis to destroy microorganisms in the prevention or treatment of infection
B. Antipyretic PO	B. Acts to reduce temperature
C. Analgesic PO, IM	C. Acts to control pain associated with the surgery
IV. Perform/provide:	
A. Use sterile technique for all care, equipment and supplies for wound, handwash prior to any contact or care	A. Prevents contamination by pathogens

INTERVENTION	RATIONALE
B. Ensure that dressings are secure, avoid loosening the dressings or allowing the patient to lie on them	B. Provides proper amount of pressure to wound if compression dressing is applied following surgery
C. Elevate position of graft site(s), immobilize to avoid movement and pressure for 3 to 7 days following skin graft surgery	C. Prevents disturbance of graft and possible damage to allow time for the graft to adhere to wound
D. Gently roll a sterile cotton swab from the center to outer part of graft, or assist with aspiration of fluid from under the graft with a syringe and needle	D. Removes small amount or large accumulation of blood or serum under the autograft
E. Heat lamp, bed cradle to site	E. Dries and protects site if fine-mesh gauze dressing is applied
F. Administer analgesic prior to painful procedures such as dressing change, exercises	F. Allows for optimal pain relief when needed
G. Relaxation techniques, music, guided imagery	G. Provides nonpharmacological methods to reduce pain
H. Adequate nutritional intake based on age, sex, weight, extent of injury and surgery	H. Increased energy requirements for wound healing
I. Assist with activities, avoid ROM until graft healing achieved	I. ROM postponed as this can disturb graft, but limited activities allowed

NURSING DIAGNOSIS
Knowledge deficit related to follow-up care and promotion of wound/graft healing and successful outcome

EXPECTED OUTCOMES
Adequate knowledge acquired for postoperative care evidenced by compliance with recommended activities and positioning requirements with progressive return to function with minimal deformity and scarring

INTERVENTION	RATIONALE
V. Teach patient/family:	
A. Avoid touching the surgical site(s), perform handwash prior to contact with surgical area, instruct in sterile technique for wound care if appropriate	A. Prevents contamination of suture line during healing process
B. Reinforce exercise and positioning routines, provide written instructions to follow	B. Provides correct information to ensure return to functional level
C. Application and removal of splints if used (static or dynamic)	C. Provides immobilization and proper positioning, prevent contractures
D. Participate in formal rehabilitation program if advised, ordered	D. Promotes return to optimal functional level
E. Suggest or reinforce suggestion for a couseling referral	E. Enhances psychosocial recovery and movement through the grieving process
F. Inform to keep appointments with physician as scheduled	F. Permits monitoring of healing and modification of treatment regimen if needed

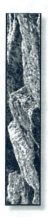

Bibliography

Black JM and Matassarin-Jacobs E. *Luckmann and Sorensen's Medical–Surgical Nursing: A Psychophysiologic Approach,* ed 4. Philadelphia, WB Saunders, 1993

Bryant R. *Acute and Chronic Wounds: Nursing Management,* St. Louis, Mosby-Year Book, 1992

Deglin JH and Vallerand AH. *Davis's Drug Guide for Nurses,* ed 4. Philadelphia, FA Davis, 1995

Doenges ME and Moorhouse MF. *Nurse's Pocket Guide: Nursing Diagnoses with Interventions,* ed 3. Philadelphia, FA Davis, 1991

Fischbach F. *A Manual of Laboratory and Diagnostic Tests,* ed 4. Philadelphia, JB Lippincott, 1992

Kim MJ, McFarland GK, and McLane AM. *Pocket Guide to Nursing Diagnoses,* ed 5. St. Louis, Mosby-Year Book, 1992

Lewis S et al. *Manual of Psychosocial Nursing Interventions: Promoting Mental Health in Medical-Surgical Settings.* Philadelphia, WB Saunders, 1990

Lewis SM and Collier IC. *Medical–Surgical Nursing: Assessment and Management of Clinical Problems,* ed 3. St. Louis, Mosby-Year Book, 1992

McCloskey JC and Bulechek GM. *Nursing Interventions and Classification (NIC).* St. Louis, Mosby-Year Book, 1992

McFarland GK and McFarlane EA. *Nusing Diagnosis and Intervention: Planning for Patient Care,* ed 2. St. Louis, Mosby-Year Book, 1993

Moore MC. *Pocket Guide to Nutrition and Diet Therapy,* ed 2. St. Louis, Mosby-Year Book, 1992

Phippen ML and Wells P. *Perioperative Nursing Practice.* Philadelphia, WB Saunders, 1994

Rorden JW and Taft E. *Discharge Planning Guide for Nurses,* Philadelphia, WB Saunders, 1990

Rudy EB and Gray VR. *Handbook of Health Assessment,* ed 3. Norwalk, CT, Appleton & Lange, 1991

Skidmore-Roth Linda. *Mosby's Nursing Drug Reference,* St. Louis, Mosby-Year Book, 1995

Swearingen PL. *Manual of Nursing Therapeutics: Applying Nursing Diagnoses to Medical Disorders,* ed 2. St. Louis, Mosby-Year Book, 1990

Thomas CJ (ed). *Taber's Cyclopedic Medical Dictionary,* ed 17. Philadelphia, FA Davis, 1989

Ulrich SP, Canale SW, and Wendell SA. *Medical–Surgical Nursing Care Planning Guides,* ed 3. Philadelphia, WB Saunders, 1994

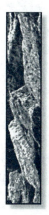

Appendix A
Abbreviations

ABG	Arterial Blood Gases	COPD	Chronic Obstructive Pulmonary Disease
ADL	Activities of Daily Living	CSF	Cerebrospinal Fluid
A.M.	Morning		
AP	Anteroposterior	cu	Cubic
BID	2 Times a Day	CVA	Cerebrovascular Accident
BP	Blood Pressure		
bpm	Beats per Minute	ECG	Electrocardiogram
C	Centigrade/ Celsius	EEG	Electroencephalogram
Ca	Calcium		
CAD	Coronary Artery Disease	F	Fahrenheit
		g	Gram
CBC	Complete Blood Dount	GFR	Glomerulofiltration Rate
CDC	Centers for Disease Control	GI	Gastrointestinal
		HCl	Hydrochloric Acid
CHF	Congestive Heart Failure	Hb	Hemoglobin
Cl	Chloride	Hct	Hematocrit
cm	Centimeter	Hg	Mercury
CNS	Central Nervous System	HIV	Human Immunodeficiency Virus
CO	Cardiac Output	ICP	Intracranial Pressure
CO_2	Carbon Dioxide		

IM	Intramuscular	PO	By Mouth, Orally
INH	Inhalation	PRN	when needed
I&O	Intake and Output	QD	Every Day, Daily
IPPB	Intermittent Positive Pressure Breathing	q2h, q3h	Every 2, 3, or 4 Hours
IV	Intravenous	q4h	
K	Potassium	QID	4 Times a Day
kg	Kilogram	R	Respiration
L	Liter	RLQ	Right Lower Quadrant
lb	Pound	ROM	Range of Motion
LLQ	Lower Left Quadrant	RUQ	Right Upper Quadrant
LOC	Level of Consciousness	SC	Subcutaneous
LUQ	Left Upper Quadrant	sec	Second
mcg/μg	Microgram	SLG	Sublingual
mEq	Milliequivalent	Sp. gr.	Specific Gravity
MI	Myocardial Infarction	S&S	Signs and Symptoms
min	Minute	T	Temperature
mg	Milligram	TID	3 Times a Day
mL	Milliliter	TOP	Topical
mm	Millimeter	TPN	Total Parenteral Nutrition
Na	Sodium		
NANDA	North American Nursing Diagnosis Association	TPR	Temperature, Pulse, Respiration
N/G	Nasogastric	URI	Upper Respiratory Infection
NPO	Nothing By Mouth		
O_2	Oxygen	UTI	Urinary Tract Infection
OTC	Over the Counter	VS	Vital Signs
P	Pulse, Phosphorus	WBC	White Blood Count
PERL	Pupils Equal, React to Light	WNL	Within Normal Limits
		<	Less Than
PID	Pelvic Inflammatory Disease	>	More Than
P.M.	Afternoon	/	Per

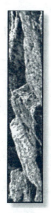

Appendix B
Index of Nursing Diagnoses, Eleventh NANDA Conference (1994)

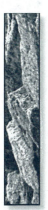

Index

coronary artery disease-related,
119–121
diabetes mellitus-related, 508–511
gastrectomy/gastroplasty-related,
626–629
heart failure-related, 138–140
hepatitis-related, 636–638
hypertension-related, 157–160
hysterectomy-related, 768–770
inflammatory bowel disease-
related, 655–657
inflammatory heart disease-related,
170–172
intracranial/spinal infections-
related, 387–388
intracranial trauma-related,
391–394
laryngectomy-related, 221–224
liver cirrhosis-related, 597–599
mastectomy/mammoplasty-related,
775–779
myocardial infarction, 173–176
neoplasm-related, 60–63
orchiectomy-related, 789–790
outpatient perioperative care-
related, 2–5
pancreatitis-related, 668–670
peptic ulcer-related, 678–680
pneumothorax-related, 255–258
preoperative care-related,
11–14
prostatectomy-related, 800–803
prostatic hypertrophy-related,
814–815
rhegmatogenous retinal detach-
ment/scleral buckling-related,
847–849
rhytidectomy/blepharectomy-
related, 877–879
seizure disorder-related,
411–413
skin graft-related, 883–885
spinal cord trauma-related,
419–422

tympanoplasty-related, 855–857
urinary diversion-related, 340–343
Aphasia, 369
Appendectomy, 563
Appendicitis/ruptured appendix/
appendectomy, 563–570
definition of, 563
fluid volume deficit, 565–567
knowledge deficit, 569–570
infection risk, 567–568
nutritional alterations, 565–567
pain, 563–565
skin integrity impairment, 567–568
Arterial bypass, 130–137
activity intolerance, 130–133
definition of, 130
knowledge deficit, 136–137
pain, 130–133
peripheral tissue perfusion alteration, 133–135
skin integrity impairment, 133–135
Arterial circulation to extremities, diminished, 130–137, 692
activity intolerance, 130–133
definition of, 130
knowledge deficit, 136–137
pain, 130–133
peripheral tissue perfusion alteration, 133–135
skin integrity impairment, 133–135
Arteriosclerosis obliterans, 130
Arthritis, 704–716, 747
activity intolerance, 710–713
anxiety, 704–706
body image disturbances, 704–706
chronic pain, 706–709
coping styles, 704–706
definition of, 704
knowledge deficit, 713–716
physical mobility impairment,
710–713
self-care deficit, 710–713
Ascites
liver cirrhosis-related, 597, 603

Aspiration risk
  cerebrovascular accident-related,
    362–365
  laryngectomy-related, 218–221
  postoperative-related, 18–21
  spinal cord trauma-related,
    422–424
Asthma, 200–217
Atherosclerosis, 692
  pain-related, 121

Benign prostatic hypertrophy (BPH),
    814
Bile, 588, 591
Blepharectomy, 877–882
Body image disturbance
  amputation-related, 692–696
  arthritis-related, 704–706
  bowel resection/diversion-related,
    571–574
  cancer-related, 83–86
  cerebrovascular accident-related,
    356–359
  gastrectomy/gastroplasty-related,
    626–629
  hepatitis-related, 636–638
  hyperthyroidism/hypothyroidism-
    related, 539–541
  hysterectomy-related, 768–770
  laryngectomy-related, 221–224
  liver cirrhosis-related, 597–599
  mastectomy-related, 775–779
  ocular enucleation-related,
    840–842
  orchiectomy-related, 789–790
  osteoporosis-related, 743–745
  penile implantation-related,
    797–798
  prostatectomy-related, 801–803
  prostatic hypertrophy-related,
    814–815
  rhinoplasty/septoplasty, 285–286

rhytidectomy/blepharectomy-
    related, 877–879
  skin graft-related, 883–885
  urinary diversion-related, 341–343
Bowel diversion, 571–585
Bowel incontinence
  cerebrovascular accident-related,
    372–375
  spinal cord trauma-related,
    429–433
Bowel resection/diversion, 571–585,
    615, 655
  anxiety, 571–574
  body image disturbance, 571–574
  coping styles, 571–574
  definition of, 571
  fluid volume deficit, 579–581
  infection risk, 574–578
  knowledge deficit, 582–585
  nutritional alterations, 579–581
  skin integrity impairment, 574–578
Brain abscess, 380
Breathing pattern alterations
  anemia-related, 479–481
  chronic obstructive pulmonary
    disease-related, 200–203
  heart failure-related, 145–147
  liver cirrhosis-related, 603–606
  pleuritis-related, 238–240
  pneumonia-related, 242–245
  pneumothorax-related, 255–258
  postoperative-related, 18–21
  pulmonary embolis-related,
    261–246
  pulmonary resection-related,
    269–272
  rhinoplasty/septoplasty, 283–285
  spinal cord trauma-related,
    422–424
  thyroidectomy-related, 544–546
  transient ischemic attacks-related,
    447–449
Bronchitis, chronic, 200–217

short

Fatigue
  cancer-related, 81–83
  heart failure-related, 147–149
Fear
  chronic obstructive pulmonary dis-
      ease-related, 204–206
  neoplasm-related, 60–62
  preoperative care-related,
      11–14
Feeding self-care deficit
  cerebrovascular accident-related,
      362–365
Fissure, 557
Fistulectomy, 557
Fluid volume deficit
  acquired immunodeficiency syn-
      drome-related, 465–468
  anemia-related, 483–485
  appendicitis/ruptured appendix/
      appendectomy-related,
      565–567
  bowel resection/diversion-related,
      579–581
  cancer-related, 68–72
  cerebrovascular accident-related,
      362–365
  cholecystitis/cholelithiasis/ chole-
      cystectomy-related, 588–591
  chronic renal failure-related,
      302–307
  hepatitis-related, 638–642
  inflammatory bowel disease-
      related, 659–662
  intracranial/spinal infections-
      related, 382–383
  intracranial trauma-related,
      403–405
  liver cirrhosis-related, 600–603
  pancreatitis-related, 672–675
  postoperative-related, 32–34
  renal/urinary tract
      calculi/litholapaxy-related,
          327–330
      infections-related, 335–337

Fluid volume excess
  chronic renal failure-related,
      302–307
  heart failure-related, 140–145
  hyperthyroidism/hypothyroidism-
      related, 538–539
  liver cirrhosis-related, 603–606
  mastectomy-related, 775–779
  renal/urinary tract infections-
      related, 335–337
Folic acid deficiency, 479
Fractures, cast/traction, 717–727
  definition of, 717
  diversional activity deficit, 724–726
  infection risk, 719–722
  knowledge deficit, 726–727
  pain, 717–719
  peripheral neurovascular dysfunc-
      tion risk, 719–722
  physical mobility impairment,
      722–724
  self-care deficit, 722–724
  skin integrity impairment, 719–722
  trauma/injury risk, 724–726

Gallbladder
  disease, 668
  inflammation, 586
  stones, 586
  See also Cholecystitis; Cholelithi-
      asis; Cholecystectomy
Gas exchange impairment
  anemia-related, 479–481
  chronic obstructive pulmonary dis-
      ease-related, 200–203
  heart failure-related, 145–147
  pneumothorax-related, 255–258
  pulmonary embolis-related,
      261–246
  pulmonary resection-related,
      269–272
Gastrectomy/gastroplasty, 626–635,
      678